Current Neurology
VOLUME 4

Current Neurology

VOLUME 4

Edited by

Stanley H. Appel, M.D.

Professor and Chairman
Department of Neurology
Baylor College of Medicine
Houston, Texas

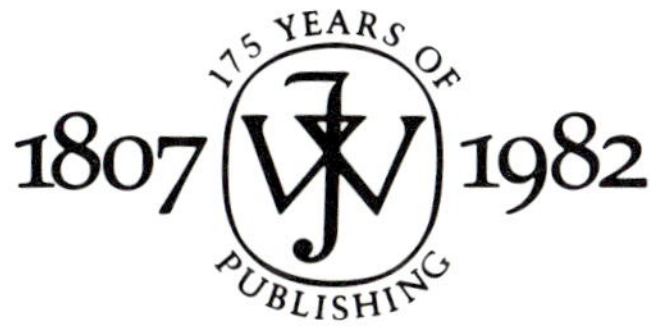

A WILEY MEDICAL PUBLICATION

JOHN WILEY & SONS / New York • Chichester • Brisbane • Toronto • Singapore

ISBN 0-471-09556-7

ISSN 0161-780X

Printed in the United States of America

10 9 8 7 6 5 4 3 2 1

Produced by Cale—Prince Communications, Inc.,
an affiliate of Harwal Publishing Co.

Contributors

Stanley H. Appel, M.D.
Professor and Chariman,
   Department of Neurology
Baylor College of Medicine
Houston, Texas

Richard M. Armstrong, M.D.
Assistant Professor of Neurology
Baylor College of Medicine
Houston, Texas

John P. Blass, M.D., Ph.D.
Professor of Neurology and Medicine
Division of Chronic and Degenerative
   Diseases
Cornell University Medical College
New York, New York

Nikolai Bogduk, B.Sc (Med), M.B.
Lecturer in Anatomy
University of Queensland
St. Lucia, Queensland, Australia

Robert E. Burke, M.D.
Fellow in Neurology
Columbia University College of Physicians
   and Surgeons
New York, New York

Ivan Diamond, M.D., Ph.D.
Professor of Neurology, Pediatrics
   and Pharmacology
University of California School of Medicine
San Francisco, California

Stanley Fahn, M.D.
H. Houston Merritt Professor of Neurology
Columbia University College of Physicians
   and Surgeons
New York, New York

Marvin A. Fishman, M.D.
Professor of Pediatrics and Neurology
Director, Section of Pediatric Neurology
Baylor College of Medicine
Chief, Neurology Service
Texas Children's Hospital
Houston, Texas

Candace J. Gibson, Ph.D.
Research Associate, Department
   of Nutrition and Food Sciences
Massachusetts Institute of Technology
Cambridge, Massachusetts

Daniel G. Glaze, M.D.
Assistant Professor of Pediatrics
Instructor in Neurology
Baylor College of Medicine
Houston, Texas

Janette Goddard, M.D.
Assistant Professor of Pediatrics
Baylor College of Medicine
Houston, Texas

Eli S. Goldensohn, M.D.
Professor of Neurology
Columbia University College of Physicians
  and Surgeons
New York, New York

John H. Growdon, M.D.
Associate Professor of Neurology
Tufts New England Medical Center
Boston, Massachusetts

Thomas K. Koch, M.D.
Department of Neurology
University of California School of Medicine
San Francisco, California

James W. Lance, M.D., F.R.C.P., F.R.A.C.P.
Professor of Neurology
University of New South Wales
Kensington, New South Wales, Australia

Gajanan Nilaver, M.D.
Assistant Professor of Neurology
Columbia University College of Physicians
  and Surgeons
New York, New York

Timothy A. Pedley, M.D.
Associate Professor of Neurology
Columbia University College of Physicians
  and Surgeons
New York, New York

Stanley B. Prusiner, M.D.
Associate Professor of Neurology
University of California School of Medicine
San Francisco, California

Donald H. Silberberg, M.D.
Professor and Chairman,
  Department of Neurology
University of Pennsylvania
  School of Medicine
Philadelphia, Pennsylvania

Sandro Sorbi, M.D.
Research Associate, Department of
  Neurology
Division of Chronic and Degenerative
  Diseases
Cornell University Medical College
New York, New York

Earl A. Zimmerman, M.D.
Professor of Neurology
Columbia University College of Physicians
  and Surgeons
New York, New York

Preface

In recent decades a growing interest in neurology and the neurosciences has been evidenced in many ways. There has been a rapid expansion in research and in publications and journals devoted to this subject. This increase in knowledge is so striking that even the most skillfully prepared clinician has difficulty in keeping abreast of the current aspects of neurophysiology, biochemistry, neuropharmacology, and their application to clinical neurology.

Our continuing effort in this series is to review advances in neurology. Our approach continues to be selective rather than all-encompassing. This year we emphasize neuroendocrinology and neuropeptides, pain and pain syndromes, and dietary management by the use of neurotransmitter precursors as an approach to therapy. We also have reviewed the latest advances in seven other areas.

Rather than include all subjects each year, we will review most subjects on a two- to three-year cycle. In this way we can continue to focus on major research areas which have implications for specific clinical problems. This present volume should help to maintain and to enhance our increasingly sophisticated approach to neurological disease.

Stanley H. Appel, M.D.

Contents

Current Neurology
VOLUME 4

1
Neuromuscular Disorders

Richard M. Armstrong and Stanley H. Appel

Three topics are reviewed in this chapter: lipid myopathies, polymyositis, and malignant hyperthermia.

The role of lipids in the metabolism of muscle has been examined in the past 10 years, and disorders of lipid metabolism, which result in myopathy, have been identified. Deficiencies of carnitine and carnitine palmityl transferase (CPT) are examples of these. The metabolism of lipids is complex, and undoubtedly additional causes of lipid myopathy will be defined as additional cases are identified.

Polymyositis remains a controversial area in terms of diagnostic criteria and management. While it appears to be an autoimmune condition, its pathogenesis is not understood, and the approach to treatment is highly variable. Corticosteroids are frequently used, sometimes in conjunction with immunosuppressive chemotherapy, and more recently, plasmapheresis has been employed in some cases.

Malignant hyperthermia is recognized with increasing frequency. Although it is primarily a problem for the anesthetist, the neurologist may be consulted for assistance with diagnosis and counseling of affected family members. The acute episode can be managed effectively, and family members who are at risk can be identified.

LIPID STORAGE MYOPATHIES

That an abnormality of lipid metabolism could cause myopathy was suggested in 1969 (1). Subsequently, the role of lipids in muscle metabolism has been recognized, and some clinical correlates of disordered lipid metabolism have been defined.

Lipids are a major source of energy for muscle at rest and during prolonged activity. Free fatty acids derived from triglycerides and very low-density lipoproteins of blood or triglycerides, which are stored within the muscle cell undergo acylation with carnitine. They are then transported across the mitochondrial membrane where they undergo β-oxidation and subsequently enter the Krebs cycle. Carnitine is essential as the carrier for transport of medium and long-chain fatty acids across the inner mitochondrial membrane. Carnitine is derived from diet and from endogenous synthesis. The synthesis requires lysine and methionine and occurs in liver, testes, and kidney. Deficiencies of carnitine (2) and of CPT (3) have been identified and are discussed below.

The muscle cell can esterify free fatty acids into triglycerides, which are stored as intracellular lipid droplets within the muscle fiber. These can subsequently be broken down and utilized by muscle. The lipid droplets are more frequent in type 1 fibers and can be stained with a number of stains for neutral fat (Oil Red O, Sudan Black, and Nile blue sulfate). In addition to endogenous stores, free fatty acids may be derived from the blood. The blood triglycerides are broken down to free fatty acids by lipoprotein lipase, which is located in the endothelial cells of capillaries. Lipoprotein lipase activity has been demonstrated in human muscle (4). An intracellular triglyceride lipase has been characterized in adipose tissue but has not been studied in detail in skeletal muscle (5).

Free fatty acids within the muscle cell are activated to fatty acyl-coenzyme A (CoA). Fatty acyl-CoA synthetase, which is located in the outer mitochondrial membrane, catalyzes the reaction and acts mainly on long-chain fatty acids (6, 7). Activated fatty acids are then transferred to carnitine by acylcarnitine transferase which is bound to the outer surface of the inner mitochondrial membrane. This allows transfer across the inner mitochondrial membrane. A second acylcarnitine transferase converts the fatty acyl carnitine to fatty acyl CoA which then undergoes β-oxidation resulting in acetyl CoA which enters the Krebs cycle (8). The β-oxidation is catalyzed by a series of four enzymes located in the mitochondrial matrix. At least two of these are present in multiple forms with specificity for acyl CoA's of different chain lengths (9, 10).

Acylcarnitine transferases also have multiple forms with maximal affinity for short-, medium-, or long-chain fatty acids (11). The last, CPT, exists in two forms. One, CPT-I is bound to the outer surface and the other, CPT-II, is bound to the inner surface of the inner mitochondrial membrane (12, 13). Functional differences can be demonstrated between these two forms. It is not known if they are identical enzymes whose activity is modified by their location within the membrane or if they are different enzymes under separate genetic control. Fig. 1 presents a schematic representation of lipid metabolism in muscle [see also Table 1] (14).

Carnitine Deficiency

Although carnitine is present in many foods including beef, the daily human requirements are met chiefly by biosynthesis, mainly in liver and kidney. Two essential amino acids, lysine and methionine, are required for biosynthesis. The newly synthesized carnitine is actively transported into skeletal and cardiac muscle allowing for higher concentration of carnitine in these tissues than in serum. Impaired biosynthesis, transport or excessive catabolism,

and release from cell and body fluids could theoretically account for carnitine deficiency.

At present two types of carnitine deficiency are recognized: myopathic carnitine deficiency (type I lipid storage myopathy) and systemic carnitine deficiency.

Myopathic Carnitine Deficiency

This is characterized clinically by a progressive generalized weakness which is usually evident during childhood. While affecting mainly the proximal limb and truncal muscles, there may be involvement of the facial and pharyngeal muscles as well. The weakness is slowly progressive, but there may be episodic worsening from which there is some recovery. An elevated serum creatine kinase (CK) and myopathic electromyogram (EMG) confirm the diagnosis of a myopathy but are not diagnostic (15–18).

Diagnosis is based upon pathological and biochemical studies. Morphologically there is an increased number of lipid droplets within the muscle fibers. This can be estimated on light microscopy by staining for neutral fats. The amount of lipid can be quantitated morphometrically from electron micrographs (19). Biochemically, the carnitine content of the muscle is reduced to a third or less of the normal values, but plasma carnitine levels are normal or only slightly decreased (14). The triglyceride content of the muscle is increased, but the pattern is normal. In muscle extracts the oxidation of fatty acids is impaired but can be corrected by the addition of carnitine (20). In myopathic carnitine deficiency, it is postulated that the defect may be one of faulty transport of carnitine into muscle (12). In 1 case when carnitine transport was measured it was normal, but in this instance the faulty oxidation of fatty acids was not corrected with the addition of carnitine (17). In other cases the addition of carnitine has corrected the faulty oxidation of fatty acids.

Two forms of treatment have been used with some success. Corticosteroids were effective in at least 3 cases (16, 17, 20) but were not effective in 2 others (1, 21–23). Corticosteroids increase the uptake of carnitine in tissue culture which may explain the beneficial effect observed in vivo (23). Similarly, orally administered carnitine has been bene-

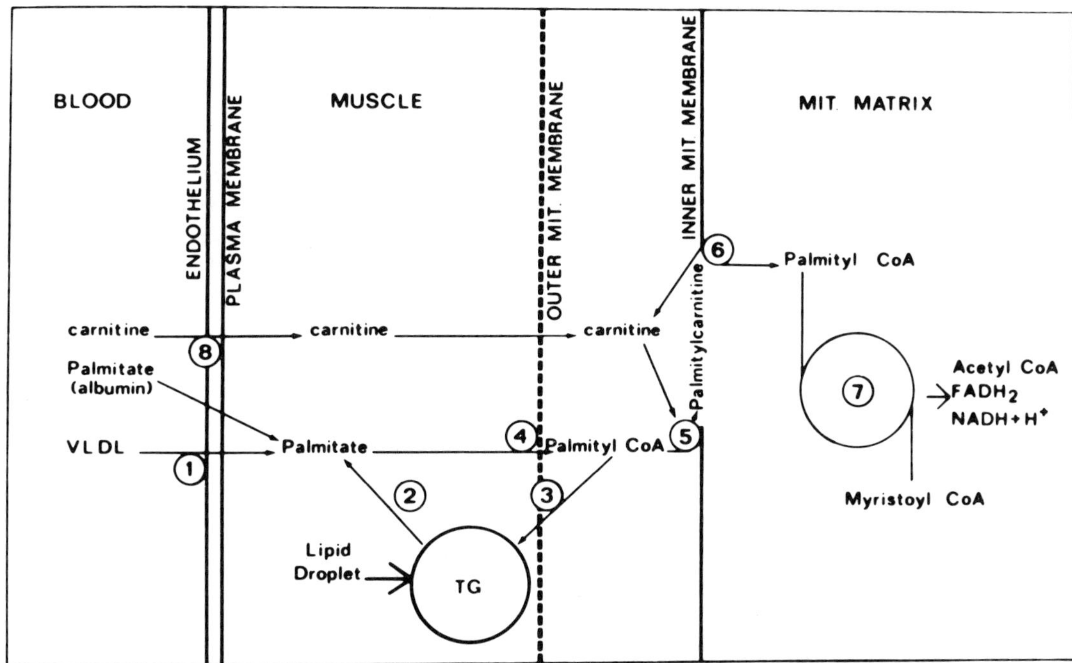

Figure 1. This is a schematic representation of the principal pathways of lipid metabolism in muscle. Palmitate is used as a typical long-chain fatty acid. Exogenous, blood-borne substrates are represented by fatty acids bound to albumin and by triglycerides in the form of very low-density lipoproteins (VLDL). Endogenous lipid stores are tryglycerides (TG) in lipid droplets. Enzymes or enzyme complexes are indicated by circled numbers adjacent to the membranes to which they are bound. MIT = mitochondrial. 1 = lipoprotein lipase. 2 = tri-, di-, and monoglyceride lipase. 3 = synthesis of triglycerides from long-chain acyl-CoA requiring glycerol 1 phosphate, and three enzymes, glycerol-phosphate acyltransferase, phosphatidate phosphatase, and diglyceride acyltransferase. 4 = palmityl CoA synthetase. 5 = carnitine palmityltransferase (CPT)-I. 6 = CPT-II. 7 = β-oxidation pathway, including acyl-CoA dehydrogenase enoyl-CoA hydratase, β-hydroxyacyl-CoA dehydrogenase, and β-keto-acyl-CoA thiolase. 8 = the active transport system of carnitine into muscle. (Reprinted with permission from Dimauro S, et al: Disorders of lipid metabolism in muscle. *Muscle Nerve* 3:369-388, 1980.)

Table 1.

No.	Tests Compared	Correlation Coefficient	t Value	P Value
33	Halothane against caffeine	0.38	2.28	<0.05
34	Halothane against halothane/ caffeine	0.70	5.58	<0.001
32	Halothane against caffeine suxamethonium	0.47	2.88	<0.01
31	Caffeine against halothane/ caffeine	0.55	3.58	<0.01
29	Caffeine against halothane/ suxamethonium	0.26	1.41	NS
30	Halothane/caffeine against caffeine/suxamethonium	0.36	2.18	<0.05

ficial in some cases (24, 25). In 1 case with normal muscle carnitine, but all other features of lipid storage, treatment with carnitine resulted in clinical improvement (26).

Systemic Carnitine Deficiency

This was first described in 1975. It manifests as a progressive myopathy similar to that of myopathic carnitine deficiency, but there are superimposed episodes of acute hepatic encephalopathy (27). In these cases, the carnitine levels are decreased in muscle, plasma, and liver.

Out of 8 patients with this disease, 6 have died of cardiorespiratory failure; 5 before 20 years old. In 2 cases the condition was aggravated in late pregnancy or postpartum. In addition to the accumulation of lipid in the muscle fibers, some, but not all, cases have increased lipid in the liver tissue obtained by biopsy. In three autopsied cases lipid accumulation was found in muscle, liver, heart, and tubular epithelial cells of the kidney. In all cases, the plasma carnitine levels have been low and hepatic concentrations have also been low when measured (14). In this condition, a defect in hepatic synthesis has been suggested but is not proven.

Oral administration of carnitine was effective in the case reported by Karpati, and after 3½ years it was discontinued without detriment (14). While serum levels of carnitine increased during treatment, the muscle and liver concentrations were unaltered. In another case the same dose of carnitine was ineffective (28).

Mixed Forms of Carnitine Deficiency

These have also been reported. Cases typical of systemic carnitine deficiency with normal plasma carnitine levels, and cases with low plasma carnitine without liver disease have been observed. These observations and the variable response to therapy with carnitine indicate that within this group of lipid storage myopathies there may be a great deal of biochemical heterogeneity and that defects at different sites in the lipid metabolism may produce similar clinical pictures for which appropriate therapy may be quite different.

Carnitine deficiency may occur as a result of malnutrition and liver disease (29) or as a consequence of renal failure and dialysis (30). Administration of carnitine to these patients has not been uniformly successful in correcting the deficiency and the high plasma triglycerides. In some cases such therapy has aggravated the weakness, possibly by impairing neuromuscular transmission (31). It has also been described in association with mitochondrial dysfunction (32–35). Lipid accumulation has been noted in association with mitochondrial abnormalities when carnitine levels were not measured or were normal. Three cases of congenital ichthyosis, myopathy, and lipid storage have been described (36–39). In these cases, muscle and plasma carnitine levels were normal as was CPT.

Although myopathic and systemic carnitine deficiencies are partially characterized, there is considerable biochemical variability within these two groups. The diverse features of the mixed and secondary cases and of cases with lipid storage within muscle, which are without abnormalities of carnitine or CPT, suggest that each case must be evaluated in as much detail as possible. Such analysis may define further specific defects and facilitate the development of rational therapies for these disorders.

Carnitine Palmityl Transferase Deficiency

DiMauro has reviewed 21 cases in which deficiency of the acylcarnitine transferase, CPT, has been documented (14). Clinically these cases are characterized by recurrent myoglobinuria which is usually precipitated by prolonged exercise, fasting, or exposure to cold. There is a striking male preponderance (20 of 21 cases). During the acute episode there is swelling, tenderness, and weakness of affected muscles. Any muscle group may be involved, and respiratory failure may occur. Interictally there is no weakness or EMG abnormality. In contrast to myophosphorylase and phosphofructokinase deficiencies these patients tolerate brief, vigorous exercise and do not develop contracture with the ischemic exercise test. Between attacks CK levels are normal, but plasma lipids and triglycerides may be elevated. Lipid accumulation, when present, in the muscle fibers is less pronounced than in carnitine deficiency, and most often the muscle appears to be normal (37).

CPT levels in muscle were reduced in all cases, but using radioactive assays, residual activity of 5% to 24% was present (14). The defect is expressed in leukocytes, (40, 41) platelets, (41) and cultured fibroblasts (41, 42). It is not established whether CPT-I and -II are selectively involved or if both are involved. To date various reports have supported each of these possibilities (3, 41, 43, 44).

Impaired utilization of long-chain fatty acids would result from a defect of CPT. It is consistent, then, that fasting or prolonged exercise, circumstances in which lipid metabolism predominates in muscle, would provoke an attack. Fasting may be used as a provocative test. Fasting for 36–72 hours is associated with a delayed rise of serum ketone bodies, increased serum CK, increased triglycerides, and cholesterol in some, but not all, patients. High carbohydrate, low fat diet, and restriction of activity may offer some protection from attacks.

There is a report of twin girls who presented clinically as typical cases of CPT deficiency, but they had normal CPT levels and normal palmityl CoA synthetase (14, 45). This again highlights the need for careful documentation of each case of these relatively uncommon conditions in an attempt to define the precise abnormality in each case.

The genetic basis for these conditions is not known. In the carnitine deficiencies and other lipid storage conditions there are some instances of consanguinity, but the data to date allow no meaningful analysis. In the 21 cases of CPT deficiency, 20 occurred in males, and in this group there were 3 pairs of brothers. Further studies of parents and sibs may allow determination of whether this disease is transmitted as an autosomal or sex-linked recessive trait.

POLYMYOSITIS/DERMATOMYOSITIS

The inflammatory myopathies, designated as polymyositis or dermatomyositis, (P/DM) form a significant group in any neuromuscular clinic and may present a challenge to diagnosis and management. The estimated incidence is 5 per million per year (46). Approximately one-fifth of these will present before 15 years of age, and two-thirds will present after 45 years of age.

Diagnostic Criteria and Classification

The criteria used for diagnosis vary from time to time and from clinic to clinic, and this has caused confusion and complicated attempts at evaluation of therapies and analysis of the clinical course. Bohan and coworkers (47) have proposed a set of diagnostic criteria and a classification which are useful in that they allow definition of relatively homogeneous groups. This should facilitate analysis of individual clinical studies and allow meaningful comparisons between different centers. It is recognized that certain cases are at best "probable," and treatments must be highly individualized, but adherence to such a classification for purposes of analysis and reporting of data should be encouraged.

The diagnostic criteria suggested by Bohan are:

1. There is an onset of symmetrical weakness of limb-girdle and anterior neck flexor muscles, which is progressive over weeks to months.

2. There is muscle biopsy evidence of necrosis of fibers of both fiber types.

3. There is an elevation in serum of skeletal muscle enzymes (CK, lactate dehydrogenase [LDH]).

4. There are EMG abnormalities of motor unit potentials (short, small, and polyphasic), spontaneous activity (fibrillation potentials), and increased insertional activity with bizarre high frequency repetitive discharges.

5. There are dermatological changes: an edematous, violaceous to erythematous rash of eyelids and malar areas (heliotrope rash); erythema, scaling, dermal atrophy, and dusky red streaking of the knuckles, elbows, knees, forehead, neck, and chest (Gottron's sign); and periungual telangiectasias.

On the basis of these criteria, the individual case may be classified under polymyositis as *definite* with four criteria without rash; *probable*, three criteria without rash; and *possible*, two criteria without rash. Dermatomyositis would be *definite* with three or four criteria with rash; *probable*, two criteria with rash; and *possible*, one criteria with rash.

Dermatomyositis is the more easily defined and recognized condition. The presence of one type of the described skin lesions is a diagnostic requirement in association with the sporadic onset of progressive, symmetrical weakness of the proximal limb muscles. The skin lesions are well described and may consist of an edematous, violaceous to erythematous rash of eyelids and malar areas "heliotrope rash"; erythema, scaling dermal atrophy, and dusky red streaking of the knuckles, elbows, knees, forehead, neck, and chest (Gottron's sign); periungual telangiectasias; or a photosensitive eruption similar to that seen in lupus erythematosus (48, 49).

In addition to the positive criteria set out above, there are conditions which should be excluded as diagnostic possibilities before making the diagnosis of polymyositis:

1. The presence of central or peripheral neurological disease such as postinfectious polyneuropathy or motor neuron disease (amyotrophic lateral sclerosis) should be considered in the differential but can generally be excluded on the basis of clinical picture, electrodiagnostic studies, and examination of the spinal fluid.

2. Patients should be excluded if they present with a slowly progressive unrelenting muscle disease in which there is a positive family history, and if the clinical picture is similar to one of the recognized types of muscular dystrophy. The history, clinical course, and muscle biopsy should allow differentiation.

An inflammatory component in the muscle biopsy of a patient with muscular dystrophy may give rise to confusion (50–52). An inflammatory response to degenerating muscle is expected, and at times it may be a prominent feature in a dystrophic biopsy. In polymyositis, muscle fiber hypertrophy is usually absent but may be a prominent feature in dystrophic muscle. The type of inflammatory cell may also be helpful. In polymyositis, the cells may be predominantly mononuclear lymphocytes. The factors that determine whether or not an autoimmune response will be initiated and propagated in response to muscle damage and degeneration are not known. It is to be expected that on occasion an autoimmune response might be initiated in a patient with underlying dystrophy. This may be the explanation for the occasional case of dystrophy which appears to be steroid responsive, but the eventual course of the disease is not significantly altered. The presence of a vasculitis is helpful in differentiating between P/DM and muscular dystrophy in children (53, 54). Some investigators have used a trial of steroids to differentiate between an inflammatory myopathy and a dystrophy.

3. The muscle biopsy may demonstrate pathology such as sarcoid granulomas, eosinophilic fasciitis or myositis, specific infectious agents, or specific myopathies.

It is essential that each biopsy be evaluated with care for any of these possibilities. Sarcoidosis may manifest clinically as a polymyositis or dermatomyositis (55–57). The diagnosis of sarcoid may be made when granulomas are found in the muscle biopsy or when other manifestations of sarcoid become evident. Granulomas in muscle are found in a number of cases of sarcoidosis in which there is no clinical symptomatology to suggest myositis. Eosinophilic fasciitis or polymyositis may be evident on biopsy and should be considered separately from P/DM (58, 59).

There have been several reports in the recent literature which reaffirm that toxoplasmosis may manifest itself as a picture very similar to that of polymyositis or dermatomyositis (60–62). Response of the muscle symptoms to therapy specific for toxoplasmosis is clear in some cases and suggests a casual relationship. Some cases do not respond. A survey of 69 patients with P/DM suggests that there is an increased incidence of complement fixing toxoplasma antibodies which correlates with high IgM levels, but the significance of this to the pathogenesis of P/DM is not known (63).

4. Metabolical or endocrinological abnormalities must also be excluded, including the abnormalities of glycogen storage which occur in muscle and lipid myopathies, and endocrine function, including thyroid, adrenal, and parathyroid glands, must be carefully evaluated. In addition, myopathies secondary to exogenous corticosteroids must be excluded.

Another iatrogenic cause for P/DM type of myopathy is penicillamine (64, 65). This may be an immunologically mediated effect. It is reversed after withdrawal of the penicillamine. In 1 case subsequent challenge with ampicillin exacerbated the condition (64). It has also been suggested that bacille Calmette Guérin (BCG) vaccination may result in dermatomyositis (66). The latter is not established as a causal factor, but each case of P/DM merits careful analysis of the history for possible etiologic factors.

Having excluded the above-mentioned conditions, the physician may diagnose patients as having definite, probable, or possible P/DM. Patients may be further subdivided on the basis of associated conditions and age. Bohan suggests the following division: group 1, primary idiopathic polymyositis; group 2, primary idiopathic dermatomyositis; group 3, P/DM associated with neoplasia; group 4, childhood P/DM associated with vasculitis; and group 5, P/DM associated with collagen vascular disease.

The separation of groups 1 and 2 may be considered arbitrary, but the presence or absence of skin lesions allows easy separation of these two. It is useful to maintain this division in an attempt to make the populations as homogeneous as possible.

Identification of group 3 continues to stimulate discussion in regard to the possibility of a malignancy generating a P/DM syndrome as a secondary or remote effect. The reported incidence of malignancy in patients with P/DM ranges from 15%–26% (47, 67, 68). There is no compelling evidence for a significant relationship, and in recent years there has been a de-emphasis of exhaustive searches for malignancy in patients presenting with P/DM. Routine evaluation with a careful history, physical, examination, chest x-ray, blood studies, and those special studies appropriate to specific symptoms or signs are probably sufficient.

Banker's classic review of childhood P/DM identified vasculitis as a significant component in many childhood cases (50, 69). The vasculitis also involves systems other than muscle. Vasculitis is rarely a prominent feature in adult cases. It is thus appropriate to retain this as a separate diagnostic category.

It is recognized that a number of patients with P/DM may also manifest abnormalities consistent with one of the collagen vascular disorders. If it is accepted that these conditions are the result of an autoimmune process, it is not surprising that on occasion both occur together. P/DM may be the presenting complex of a collagen vascular disorder or may complicate the course of a previously diagnosed disorder such as systemic lupus or rheumatoid arthritis.

Therapy

There is a significant morbidity and mortality associated with P/DM. Mortality has been reported to range from 14%–28% or more (47, 70, 71). The weakness may be severe enough to prevent ambulation or result in respiratory failure and impaired swallowing. Polymyositis may also be associated with diffuse interstitial lung disease (72, 73). Cardiac involvement occurs in P/DM, but it is relatively uncommon as a significant complication in the course of the disease. Complete heart block and infarction have been reported recently, and cardiomyopathy may occur (74–76). The course is highly variable, and the natural history of the disease cannot be predicted accurately in an individual case.

Most patients who are diagnosed as definite or probable P/DM will be treated with corticosteroids. Although there has not been a randomized and controlled study to demonstrate the efficacy of corticosteroids, many patients appear to respond. Few clinicians would not treat with corticosteroids in cases which have significant clinical weakness and functional impairment (70, 77). Exceptionally, one might consider treating a minimally involved patient with nonsteroidal anti-inflammatory drugs, rest, and careful clinical monitoring. Delay in the initiation of treatment may contribute to a bad prognosis.

The therapeutic regimen for corticosteroid therapy varies widely, but an initial daily dose of 60–100 mg of prednisone is a reasonable starting point. If this dosage results in significant clinical improvement within a few (4–8 weeks) then with careful monitoring of the clinical condition the dose may be gradually tapered over a period of months until a much lower dose is reached and a satisfactory response is sustained (77, 78). Some suggest that maintenance at 10–20 mg per day for 2 or more years is desirable (79). As an alternative to reducing the daily dose, consideration may be given to moving the dosage to an alternate day program. Alternate day administration of steroids may be used in treating the childhood cases as an attempt to ameliorate or offset the complications of corticosteroids in the growing child.

Measurement of myoglobin and muscle enzymes (creatine phosphokinase [CPK], LDH) in the serum and creatinine excretion has been utilized in attempts to monitor muscle breakdown. Careful symptomatic review and clinical examination remain the most reliable and useful ways to follow the patient. Most patients can reliably report their functional neuromuscular status, and a careful clinical exam can substantiate this in a roughly quantitative way.

The patient who does not respond is a more difficult problem. Treatment may be continued with very high dosage (1300–7200 mg of dexamethasone per day), but the logic for this is, at best, shaky (80). Definition of a "nonresponder" or "prednisone failure" is arbitrary. Failure may be declared if there has been progression of weakness despite a daily prednisone dose of 60–100 mg for 6 weeks. In the face of severe or worsening disability at this point immunosuppressive therapy may be initiated. Various drugs are used, and no one agent is clearly superior. More important than the agent is the necessity for careful dosage and monitoring of the patient for therapeutic and toxic effects. Methotrexate, aza-

thioprine, and cyclophosphamide have been used. One of these agents is usually used in combination with prednisone. In one series of 16 patients a comparison of patients treated with prednisone and azathioprine (2 mg/kg/day) demonstrated no difference in the 2 groups over a 3-month period (81). The observation remains preliminary and does not answer the question of whether the long-term course is affected, if immunosuppression alone would be equally effective or if immunosuppression is of benefit to corticosteroid failure. The dosage of azathioprine may have been too low.

Literature review suggests that in P/DM in children immunosuppression is of benefit to patients classed as steroid failure (82, 83). The early use of methotrexate may minimize the amount of steroid required to achieve a response (84). There are some patients who deteriorate despite apparently adequate prednisone and immunosuppressive treatment. Again, arbitrary limits may be set to declare failure of chemotherapy, and alternative therapies may be considered. Thymectomy has been used as a treatment with reported benefit, but this remains an unproven therapy at present (85).

In the past few years, plasmapheresis has been undertaken in an attempt to modify the course of the disease. There is anecdotal evidence for its effectiveness. It is reasonable to utilize it as a therapy in the extreme case (86, 87), but its efficacy is not established. In order to establish meaningful guidelines for its use a carefully designed, controlled study is required to determine its effectiveness and at what stage in the disease it should be utilized.

Pathogenesis

The current treatment for P/DM is predicated upon the hypothesis that P/DM is an autoimmune disease. The evidence for this is equivocal. Many aspects of the immune response have been examined and conflicting observations are published. This may, in part, reflect heterogeneity of the clinical material used for study and technical limitations and differences in the tests used.

Antimyosin antibodies have been demonstrated in P/DM, but they also occur in denervation and dystrophic processes and are not cytotoxic for muscle (88, 89). Deposition of IgG, IgM, and C_4 in the blood vessel walls has been reported in P/DM of childhood and in some adult cases (90, 91). The significance of this finding is uncertain. It is suggested that this change occurs in adult cases of DM but not PM (91). Often the vascular deposits are not clearly related to areas of muscle damage.

Immunoglobulin levels have been reported as increased and decreased (92). Hypocomplementemia has been reported as rare (93) and fairly common (94).

Antinuclear antibodies which react with thymus derived antigens have been reported in P/DM. To date, though, no antibody has been identified which is clearly specific for P/DM (95–97) and which would serve as a diagnostic test.

Circulating lymphocytes which have been sensitized to muscle antigens are present in some P/DM patients. Migration inhibition tests and lymphocyte transformation tests have both been utilized. In vitro cytotoxicity for cultured muscle cells has been reported, but others have not observed this effect (98–100).

A commonly postulated trigger or initiating event for an autoimmune process is viral infection, which may damage tissues and expose self antigens or modify the antigens and immunological response. Despite many attempts, identification of viral inclusions or viral recovery from muscle is very unusual (101).

These observations may support the concept that an abnormal immune response is a significant etiologic factor. A more definitive understanding, though, must await clarification of the role of various lymphocyte subpopulations and the ways in which they modify the immunological response.

MALIGNANT HYPERTHERMIA SYNDROME

Malignant hyperthermia (MH) was first recognized as a syndrome in 1960 (102). The proband was a young man who required anesthesia. He was aware of a strongly positive family history for anesthetic-related deaths, and he warned his surgeon of this preoperatively. He developed fever and rigidity after induction of anesthesia but survived with cessation of the anesthesia and cooling with ice packs.

The syndrome has subsequently received considerable attention, particularly in the anesthesiology literature, as it is considered to be the most common cause of anesthetic-induced death. An equivalent condition occurs in certain strains of pigs and this has served as a useful animal model of the human disease (103–105). The condition in pigs is often stress induced and has been a major economic problem in the industry. Increased awareness of the condition, identification of family members who are at risk, and the availability of an effective therapy for the prevention or treatment of the acute episode have resulted in a decreased mortality from this condition, but it remains a significant clinical problem (104).

Clinical Presentation and Treatment

Typically the acute episode occurs unexpectedly shortly after induction of anesthesia. Succinyl chloride may induce a severe rigidity, which is not relieved by additional succinyl chloride, and the rigidity may prevent intubation. Usually cessation of all anesthetic agents at this time is sufficient to allow recovery. Subsequent fever and elevation of serum CK may support the diagnosis of MH, but confirmation of the diagnosis is made by appropriate in vitro tests as discussed below.

In some patients the initial response may be minimal and go unrecognized. The anesthetist may first note the onset of tachycardia, rapidly increasing body temperature, widespread muscle rigidity, and poor oxygenation of the blood. Untreated, the temperature will rapidly reach 44°C or more, and there will be severe respiratory and metabolic acidosis, ventricular arrhythmias, and respiratory failure. Massive myoglobinuria, acute renal failure, hyperkalemia, acute consumptive coagulopathy, and pulmonary edema may develop.

Successful treatment of the acute episode requires early recognition of the abnormal muscle response, immediate termination of the anesthesia, rapid cooling of the patient, adequate ventilation and oxygenation, and administration of appropriate fluids and electrolytes. These measures by themselves are not adequate. Dantrolene sodium is now the drug of choice for the treatment of the acute episode. It is administered intravenously in an initial dose of 1–2 mg/kg, but up to 10 mg/kg may be required (106). Procaine has also been used, but the dosages required may cause severe depression of myocardial function, and for this reason dantrolene sodium is the superior agent (107). Glucocorticoids in high dosage (methylprednisolone 10 mg/kg) may also be of benefit in treating the acute episode (108). The treatment is complex, and a protocol should be developed and available in each anesthesia department (106).

Surveys in the first decade in which the disease was recognized reported a mortality rate of 70% once an episode was established. Increased recognition and prompt initiation of treatment have resulted in a substantial reduction of mortality (104, 109).

Pathogenesis

The present evidence indicates that the basic defect in malignant hyperthermia results from excessive amounts of Ca^{2+} accumulating in the sarcoplasm of the muscle cell. In normal muscle, in vitro, caffeine is known to enhance the release of Ca^{2+} from the sarcoplasmic reticulum. The resulting increase of myoplasmic Ca^{2+} then induces a contracture (110). In MH the in vitro response to caffeine is exaggerated, and the contracture is increased (111). This abnormal contracture response of MH muscle can also be elicited with other agents such as halothane or succinyl chloride, which precipitate the in vitro crisis. The changes in MH also closely paralleled those observed in the animal model (105).

Ordinarily, neuromuscular transmission results in depolarization of the muscle plasma cell membrane and transverse tubular system with subsequent release of Ca^{2+} from the sarcoplasmic reticulum into the myoplasm of the muscle cell. Ca^{2+} interacts with the troponin of the actin-troponin complex and allows the interaction of actin and myosin and the development of tension and shortening of the sarcomere. Ca^{2+} also activates myosin adenosinetriphosphatase (ATPase), which is a vital part of the contractile process. Relaxation is initiated by the active uptake of Ca^{2+} into the sarcoplasmic reticulum where it remains sequestered.

In MH this mechanism appears to be defective. With muscle stimulation there is an exaggerated response, and excessive amounts of Ca^{2+} are released from the sarcoplasmic reticulum and accumlulate in the myoplasm. As a result the muscle generates excessive and prolonged tension. The sarcoplasmic reticulum appears to be abnormal and vulnerable to the effect of a variety of anesthetic agents, but most particularly halothane and succinylcholine.

The precise cause of the increased myoplasmic Ca^{2+} levels is not known. Entry of Ca^{2+} from outside the muscle cell may occur in vivo, but the abnormal contracture response occurs in vitro in the absence of external Ca^{2+} (112). Enhanced release of Ca^{2+} from the sarcoplasmic reticulum appears the most likely mechanism. Impaired uptake of Ca^{2+} by the sarcoplasmic reticulum remains a possibility but to date has not been documented (106). It also has been proposed that MH may result from an abnormality of the excitation-contraction coupling mechanism, but the data are more reasonably interpreted as an exaggerated release of Ca^{2+} from the sarcoplasmic reticulum following depolarization of the transverse tubule (113).

The abnormality of MH may not be restricted to derangement of the sarcoplasmic reticulum and muscle contracture. There may also be abnormalities of the mitochondria, and increased heat production occurs at sites other than muscle (114, 115). The presence of increased myoplasmic calcium may accelerate adenosine triphosphate (ATP) hydrolysis by myosin ATPase as well as by the overactivity of calcium pumps attempting to lower calcium levels. Other sources of heat produced by Ca^{2+} include uncoupling of oxidative phosphorylation, increased breakdown of glycogen, and peripheral vasoconstriction with subsequent decrease in heat loss. It is also recognized that in some cases MH occurs without rigidity (116).

The muscle rigidity itself may contribute significantly to heat production. It may impair blood supply to the muscle and aggravate the acidosis. The muscle damage results in release of potassium and myoglobin into the blood.

Identification of MH Population

The clinical presentation of the proband is usually totally unexpected. Awareness of MH, early recognition, and treatment of the acute episode have decreased the mortality figure for the acute episode and have led to evaluation of other family members who are at risk. MH appears to be transmitted as an autosomal dominant trait (117, 118) in many pedigrees, but it may be a multigene defect (106). MH patients frequently have high serum CK levels interictally. Although this finding is quite nonspecific, it is useful as an initial screening test.

Confirmation of the diagnosis continues to rely upon in vitro testing of muscle obtained at biopsy. Small muscle strips are incubated in physiological solution under defined conditions. Carefully measured doses of caffeine are then introduced, and the amplitude of twitch response and increase of resting tension are recorded. In MH the responses are exaggerated. Similar changes may be induced with halothane, and the two agents may have an additive effect. Laboratories differ in details of technique, and it is essential that the laboratory have well-standardized normal values (111, 118–120). Other tissues may be involved such as heart, autonomic nervous system, platelets, pancreas, and bone. In the future, platelets or red blood cells may prove useful in diagnosing individuals who are at risk for MH.

Confirmation of the diagnosis in a suspected MH proband or identification of affected relatives of a proven case may be easily established if the twitch response to caffeine or halothane is clearly abnormal. However, in a number of cases (106), the caffeine test gives intermediate values, and the diagnosis cannot be conclusively confirmed (Fig. 2).

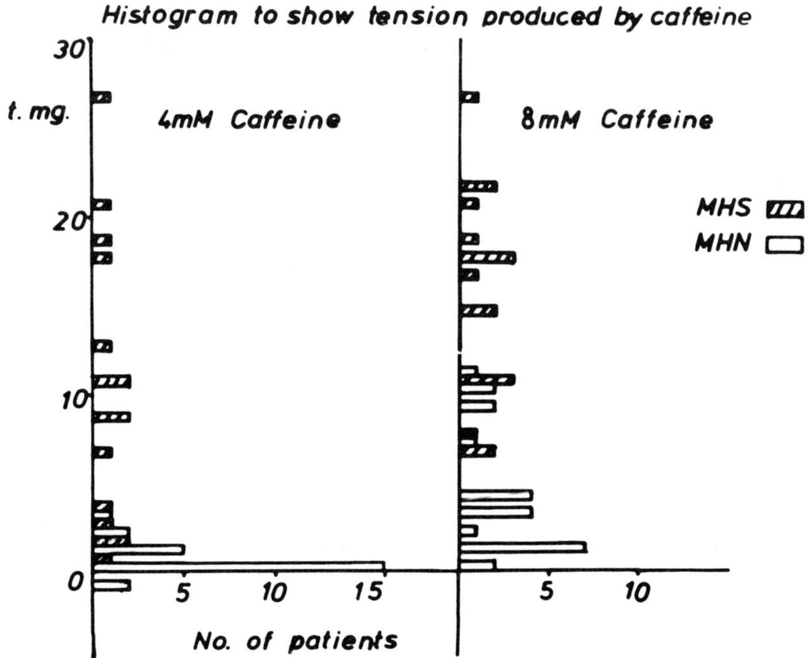

Figure 2. These histograms are showing the distribution of both MHS and normal (MHN) results of the caffeine contracture test. (MHS diagnosed by a positive halothane contracture). Note that at both 4 mmol/L and 8 mmol/L caffeine causes a greater increase in tension of the MHS muscle than MHN, but there is significant population overlap at both concentrations. (Reprinted with permission from Ellis FR: Malignant hyperpyrexia. In *Inherited Disease and Anesthesia*. Edited by Ellis FR. New York, Elsevier/North Holland, 1981.)

Muscle biopsy and in vitro testing are impractical as screening tests for MH in large populations. Reviews of the clinical experience have identified some factors which should be considered to identify at-risk individuals. The family history of anesthetic-related death is important and should never be overlooked or dismissed as insignificant. The MH population has an increased incidence of ptosis, squint, kyphoscoliosis, hernia, and pes cavus. Many probands present because they undergo anesthesia for surgical procedures to correct these abnormalities or because of trauma (106). In addition to these musculoskeletal abnormalities focal hypertrophy of muscles may be noted, and there may be a history of severe muscle cramps. CK levels may be useful as an additional screening test for this population.

Awareness of the condition in an affected family, elevated CK values, and abnormal caffeine twitch test allow identification of high-risk patients, and suitable precautions can be taken if anesthesia is required. This may include premedication with dantrolene, use of local anesthesia, or selected general anesthetic agents such as nitrous oxide.

Structural changes have been reported in muscle biopsies obtained from MH patients. The changes are quite variable and non-specific. There are reports of central core abnormalities in some pedigrees, but this observation has been disputed (121–123). MH-like episodes have also been reported in cases of Duchenne muscular dystrophy (124).

The variability of response to the in vitro pharmacological testing, muscle pathology, and CK levels, suggest that the syndrome presents in a population which is not entirely homogeneous, and that a battery of tests should be used in assessing these cases (112). Variability is also recognized in the clinical setting. Patients with MH may undergo anesthesia uneventfully on one or many occasions with the same agents that subsequently precipitate a MH episode. A small proportion of MH cases do not develop rigidity as part of the episode.

Recently, it has been suggested that MH may be part of a general stress syndrome in which environmental factors, including anxiety, may precipitate an episode or cause sudden death (125, 126). Stress-induced episodes are recognized in the swine model, and similar events in members of MH pedigrees have been observed (125).

MH results when an individual has a genetically determined metabolic abnormality which can be triggered by certain environmental factors and events. Anesthesia is the most frequently identified precipitating cause, and there is a high mortality rate if the event is not dealt with immediately and effectively. Identification of at-risk members in a pedigree requires muscle biopsy and in vitro testing to confirm the diagnosis. No practical screening test is presently available for large populations. The basic abnormality is increased Ca^{2+} concentration in the myoplasm, but the precise basis for this remains undefined.

REFERENCES

1. Bradley WG, Hudgson P, Gardner-Medwin D, et al: Myopathy associated with abnormal lipid metabolism in skeletal muscle. *Lancet* 1:495–498, 1969

2. Engel AG, Angelini C: Carnitine deficiency of human skeletal muscle with associated lipid storage myopathy: a new syndrome. *Science* 179:899–902, 1973

3. DiMauro S, DiMauro PMM: Muscle carnitine palmityl-transferase deficiency and myoglobinuria. *Science* 182:929–931, 1973

4. Lithell H, Boberg J: Determination of lipoprotein lipase activity in human skeletal muscle tissue. *Biochim Biophys Acta* 528:58–68, 1978

5. Pykälistö OJ, Vogel WI, Bierman EL: The tissue distribution of triglycerol lipase, monoacylglycerol lipase and phospholipase A in fed and fasted rats. *Biochim Biophys Acta* 369:254–263, 1974

6. Aas M: Organ and subcellular distribution of fatty acid activating enzymes in rat. *Biochim Biophys Acta* 231:32–47, 1971

7. Groot PHE, Hülsmann WC: The activation and oxidation of octanoate by rat skeletal muscle mitochondria. *Biochim Biophys Acta* 316:124–135, 1973

8. Pande SV: A mitochondrial carnitine acylcar-

nitine translocase system. *Proc Natl Acad Sci USA* 72:883–887, 1975

9. Middleton B: 3 Ketoacyl CoA thiolase of mammalian tissues. *Methods Enzymol* 35:128–136, 1975

10. Thorpe C, Matthews RG, Williams CH: Acyl coenzyme A dehydrogenase from pig kidney. Purification and properties. *Biochemistry* 18:331–337, 1979

11. Bremer J, Bjerve KS, Christopherson BO, et al: Factors controlling the metabolism of fatty acids in the liver. In *Regulation of Hepatic Metabolism.* Edited by Lundquist F, Tygstrup N. New York, Academic Press, 1974, pp 159–179

12. Fritz IB, Kopec, Brosnan JT: Localization of carnitine palmityl transferases on inner membranes of mitochondria, and their possible role in the regulation of fatty acyl group translocation. In *Regulation of Hepatic Metabolism.* Edited by Lundquist F, Tygstrup N. New York, Academic Press, 1974, pp 482–497

13. Hoppel CL, Tomec RJ: Carnitine palmityltransferase. Location of two enzymatic activities in rat liver mitochondria. *J Biol Chem* 247:832–841, 1972

14. DiMauro S, Trevisan C, Hays A: Disorders of lipid metabolism in muscle. *Muscle Nerve* 3:369–388, 1980

15. Boudin G. Mikol J, Guillard A, et al: Fatal systemic carnitine deficiency with lipid storage in skeletal muscle, heart and kidney. *J Neurol Sci* 30:313–315, 1976

16. Vandyke DH, Griggs RC, Markesberry W, et al: Hereditary carnitine deficiency of muscle. *Neurology* 25:154–159, 1975

17. Willner JH, DiMauro S, Eastwood A, et al: Muscle carnitine deficiency: genetic heterogeneity. *J Neurol Sci* 41:235–246, 1979

18. Hart ZH, Chang CH, DiMauro S, et al: Muscle carnitine deficiency and fatal cardiomyopathy. *Neurology* 28:147–151, 1978

19. Engel AG, Santa T, Stonnington HH, et al: Morphometric study of skeletal muscle ultrastructure. *Muscle Nerve* 2:229–237, 1979

20. Engel AG, Siekert RG: Lipid storage myopathy responsive to prednisone. *Arch Neurol* 27:174–181, 1972

21. Bradley WG, Tomlinson BE, Hardy M: Further studies of mitochondrial and lipid storage myopathies. *J Neurol Sci* 35:201–210, 1978

22. Isaacs H, Heffron JJA, Badenhorst M, et al: Weakness associated with the pathological presence of lipid in skeletal muscle: a detailed study of a patient with carnitine deficiency. *J Neurol Neurosurg Psychiatry* 39:1114–1123, 1976

23. Molstad P, Bohner T: Transport of L-carnitine induced by prednisolone in an established cell line (CCL27): a possible explanation of the therapeutic effect of glucocorticoids in muscle carnitine deficiency syndrome. *Biochim Biophys Acta* 585:94–99, 1979

24. Angelini C, Govoni E, Bragaglia MM, et al: Carnitine deficiency of skeletal muscle: report of a treated case. *Neurology* 26:633–637, 1976

25. Hosking GP, Cavanagh NPC, Smyth DPL, et al: Oral treatment of carnitine myopathy. *Lancet* 1:853, 1977

26. Seneger RC, Bakkeren JA, Trijbelo JM, et al: Successful treatment in a noncarnitine deficient lipid storage myopathy. *Eur J Pediatr* 135:205–209, 1980

27. Karpati G, Carpenter S, Engel AG, et al: The syndrome of systemic carnitine deficiency. *Neurology* 25:16–24, 1975

28. Carnelio F, DiDonata S, Peluchetti P, et al: Fatal cases of lipid storage myopathy with carnitine deficiency. *J Neurol Neurosurg Psychiatry* 40: 170–178, 1977

29. Mikhail MM, Mansour MM: The relationship between serum carnitine levels and nutritional status of patients with schistosomiasis. *Clin Chim Acta* 71:207–214, 1976

30. Böhmer T, Bergrem H, Eiklid K: Carnitine deficiency induced during intermittent hemodialysis for renal failure. *Lancet* 1:126–128, 1978

31. DeGrandis D, Mezzina C, Fiaschi A, et al: Myasthenia due to carnitine treatment. *J Neurol Sci* 46:365–371, 1980

32. DiDonato S, Cornelio F, Balestrini MR, et al: Mitochondria-lipid-glycogen myopathy, hyperlactacidemia and carnitine deficiency. *Neurology* 28: 1110–1116, 1978

33. Koenigsberger MR, Pellock JM, DiMauro S, et al: Juvenile mitochondrial myopathy, short stature, lactic acidosis: a clinical, ultrastructural and biochemical study (abstract). *Fifth National Meeting of the Child Neurology Society.* Monterey, Calif., 1976

34. DiMauro S, Mendell JR, Sahenk Z, et al: Fatal infantile mitochondrial myopathy and renal dysfunction due to cytochrome-c-oxidase deficiency. *Neurology.* In press, 1982

35. VanBiervliet JPAM, Briernvis L, Ketting D, et al: Hereditary mitochondrial myopathy with lactic acidemia a De Toni-Fanconi Debré syndrome and a defective respiratory chain in voluntary striated muscles. *Pediatr Res* 11:1088–1093, 1977

36. Angelini C, Philippart M, Barrone C, et al: Multisystem triglyceride storage disorder with impaired long chain fatty acid oxidation. *Ann Neurol* 7:5–10, 1980

37. Chanarin I, Patel A, Slavin G, et al: Neutral lipid storage disease: a new disorder of lipid metabolism. *Br Med J* 1:553–555, 1975

38. Miranda A, DiMauro S, Eastwood AB, et al: Lipid storage ichthyosis and steatorrhea. *Muscle and Nerve* 3:1–13, 1979

39. Slavin G, Wills EG, Richmond JE, et al: Morphological features in a neutral lipid storage disease. *J Clin Pathol* 28:701–710, 1975

40. DiMauro S, Eastwood AB: Disorders of glycogen

and lipid metabolism. In *Advances in Neurology,* vol 17. Edited by Griggs RC, Moxley RT. New York, Raven Press, 1977, pp 123–142

41. Layzer RB, Havel RJ, McIlroy MB: Partial deficiency of carnitine palmityltransferase. *Neurology* 30:627–633, 1980

42. DiDonato S, Cornelio F, Pacini I, et al: Muscle carnitine palmityl transferase deficiency: report of a case with enzyme deficiency in cultured fibroblasts. *Ann Neurol* 4:465–467, 1978

43. Patten BM, Wood JM, Harati Y, et al: Familial recurrent rhabdomyolysis due to carnitine palmityl transferase deficiency. *Am J Med* 67:167–171, 1979

44. Scholte HR, Jennekens FGI, Bouvy JJBJ: Carnitine palmityl transferase II deficiency with normal carnitine palmityl transferase I in skeletal muscle and leukocytes. *J Neurol Sci* 40:39–51, 1979

45. Engel WK, Vick NA, Glueck J, et al: A skeletal muscle disorder associated with intermittent symptoms and a possible defect in lipid metabolism. *N Engl J Med* 282:697–704, 1970

46. Medgser TA, Dawson WN, Masi AT: The epidemiology of polymyositis. *Am J Med* 48:715, 1970

47. Bohan A, Peter JB, Bowman RL, et al: A computer assisted analysis of 153 patients with polymyositis and dermatomyositis. *Medicine* 56:255–286, 1977

48. Bohan A, Peter JB: Polymyositis and dermatomyositis. *N Engl J Med* 292:344–347, 1975

49. Callen JP: Dermatomyositis. *Int J Dermatol* 18: 423–433, 1979

50. Jerusalem T: Die bioptische-histologische Differential diagnose der Polymositis und der progressiven Muskeldystrophies. *Dtsh Z Nervenheilk* 191:125–141, 1967

51. Bosch EP, Gowans JDC, Munsat T: Inflammatory myopathy in oculopharyngeal dystrophy. *Muscle Nerve* 2:73–77, 1979

52. Dubowitz V, Brooke MH: *Muscle Biopsy: A Modern Approach.* London, WB Saunders, 1973

53. Banker BQ, Victor M: Dermatomyositis (systemic angiopathy) of childhood. *Medicine* 45:261–289, 1966

54. Oshima Y, Becker LE, Armstrong DL: An electron microscopic study of childhood dermatomyositis. *Acta Neuropathol (Berl)* 47:189–196, 1979

55. Callen JP: Sarcoidosis appearing initially as polymyositis. *Arch Dermatol* 115:1336–1337, 1979

56. Alpert JN, Groff AE, Bastian FO, et al: Acute polymyositis caused by sarcoidosis: report of a case and review of the literature. *Mt Sinai J Med (NY)* 46: 486–488, 1979

57. Itoh J, Akiguchi I, Midorikawa R, et al: Sarcoid myopathy with typical rash of dermatomyositis. *Neurology* 30:1118–1121, 1980

58. Nassonova VA, Ivanova MM, Akhnazarova VD, et al: Eosinophilic fasciitis. *Scand J Rheumatol* 8:225–233, 1979

59. Stark RJ: Eosinophilic polymyositis. *Arch Neurol* 36:721–722, 1979

60. Hendrickx GFM, Verhage J, Jennekens FGI, et al: Dermatomyositis and toxoplasmosis. *Ann Neurol* 5:393–395, 1978

61. Pollock JL: Toxoplasmosis appearing to be dermatomyositis. *Arch Dermatol* 115:736–737, 1979

62. Topi GC, D'Alessandro L, Catricala C, et al: Dermatomyositis-like syndrome due to toxoplasma. *Br J Dermatol* 101:589–591, 1979

63. Phillips PE, Kassan SS, Kagen LJ: Increased toxoplasma antibodies in idiopathic inflammatory muscle disease. *Arthritis Rheum* 22:209–214, 1979

64. Ostensen M, Husby G, Aarli J: Polymyositis with acute myolysis in a patient with rheumatoid arthritis treated with penicillamine and ampicillin. *Arthritis Rheum* 23:375–377, 1980

65. Simpson NB, Golding JR: Dermatomyositis induced by penicillamine. *Acta Derm Venereol (Stockh)* 59:543–544, 1979

66. Kass E, Straume S, Mellbye OJ, et al: Dermatomyositis associated with BCG vaccination. *Scand J Rheumatol* 8:187–191, 1979

67. Talbott JH: Acute dermatomyositis/polymyositis and malignancy. *Semin Arthritis Rheum* 6:305–306, 1977

68. Callen JP, Hyla JT, Bole GG, et al: The relationship of polymyositis and dermatomyositis to internal malignancy. *Arch Dermatol* 116:295–298, 1980

69. Banker BQ: Dermatomyositis of childhood ultrastructural alterations of muscle and intramuscular blood vessels. *J Neuropathol Exp Neurol* 34:46–75, 1975

70. DeVere R, Bradley WG: Polymyositis: its presentation, morbidity and mortality. *Brain* 98:637–666, 1975

71. Riddoch D, Morgan-Hughes JA: Prognosis in adult polymyositis. *J Neurol Sci* 26:71–80, 1975

72. Songcharoen S, Raju ST, Pennebaker JB: Interstitial lung disease in polymyositis and dermatomyositis. *J Rheumatol* 7:353–360, 1980

73. Salmeron G, Greenberg, DS, Lidsky MD: Polymyositis and diffuse interstitial lung disease. *Arch Int Med* 141:1005–1010, 1981

74. Reid JM, Murdoch R: Polymyositis and complete heart block. *Br Heart J* 41:628–629, 1979

75. Henderson A, Cumming WJK, Williams DO, et al: Cardiac complications of polymyositis. *J Neurol Sci* 47:425–428, 1980

76. Cohn H, Lynfield YL: Myocardial infarction in dermatomyositis. *Cutis* 23:672–675, 1979

77. Rowland LP, Clark C, Olarte M: Therapy for dermatomyositis and polymyositis. *Adv Neurol* 17:63–97, 1977

78. Carpenter JR, Bunch TW, Engel AG, et al: Survival in polymyositis: corticosteroids and risk factors. *J Rheumatol* 4:207–214, 1977

79. Pearson CM, Bohan A: The spectrum of polymyo-

sitis and dermatomyositis. *Med Clin North Am* 61: 439–457, 1977

80. Fessel WJ: Megadose corticosteroid therapy in systemic lupus erythematosus. *J Rheumatol* 7:486–500, 1980

81. Bunch TW, Worthington JW, Combs JJ, et al: Azathioprine with prednisone for polymyositis. *Ann Intern Med* 92:365–369, 1980

82. Fischer TJ, Rachelefsky GS, Klein RB, et al: Childhood dermatomyositis and polymyositis: treatment with methotrexate and prednisone. *Am J Dis Child* 133:386–389, 1979

83. Niakan E, Pitner SE, Whitaker JW, et al: Immunosuppressive agents in corticosteroid-refractory childhood dermatomyositis. *Neurology* 30:286–291, 1980

84. Pirofsky B, Bordana EJ: Immunosuppressive therapy in rheumatic disease. *Med Clin North Am* 61: 419–437, 1977

85. Behan PO, Currie S: In *Clinical Neuroimmunology*. London, Saunders, 1977, p 155

86. Dau PC: Plasmapheresis in idiopathic inflammatory myopathy. *Arch Neurol* 38:544–552, 1981

87. Brewer EJ, Giannini EH, Rossen RD, et al: Plasma exchange therapy of a childhood onset dermatomyositis patient. *Arthritis Rheum* 23:509–512, 1980

88. Fairfax AJ, Gyöschel-Stewart V: Myosin auto antibodies detected by immunofluorescence. *Clin Exp Immunol* 28:27, 1977

89. Caspary EA, Gubbay SL, Steven GN: Circulating antibodies in polymyositis and other muscle wasting disorders. *Lancet* 2:941, 1964

90. Whitaker JN, Engel WK: Vascular deposits of immunoglobulin and complement in idiopathic inflammatory myopathy. *N Engl J Med* 286:333–338, 1972

91. Heffner RR, Barron SA, Jenis EH, et al: Skeletal muscle in polymyositis. *Arch Pathol Lab Med* 103: 310–313, 1979

92. Dawkins, RL: Review. Experimental autoallergic myositis, polymyositis and myasthenia gravis. *Clin Exp Immunol* 21:185–201, 1975

93. Lisak RP, Zweiman B: Serum immunoglobulin levels in myasthenia gravis, polymyositis and dermatomyositis. *J Neurol Neurosurg Psychiatry* 39:34–37, 1976

94. Behan WMN, Behan PO: Complement abnormalities in polymyositis. *J Neurol Sci* 34:241–246, 1977

95. Reichlin M, Mattioli M: Description of a serological reaction characteristic of polymyositis. *Clin Immunol Immunopathol* 5:12–20, 1976

96. Wolfe JF, Adelstein E, Sharp GC: Antinuclear antibody with distinct specificity for polymyositis. *J Clin Invest* 59:176–178, 1977

97. Nishikai N, Reichlin M: Heterogeneity of precipitating antibodies in polymyositis and dermatomyositis. Characterization of the Jo-1 antibody system. *Arthritis Rheum* 23:881, 1980

98. Haas DC: Absence of cell mediated cytotoxicity to muscle cultures in polymyositis. *J Rheumatol* 7: 671–676, 1980

99. Currie S, Saunders M, Knowles N, et al: Immunological aspects of polymyositis: the in vitro activity of lymphocytes on incubation with muscle antigen and muscle cultures. *Am J Med* 46:63–84, 1971

100. Kakulas BA, Shute GH, Leclerc ALF: In vitro destruction of human fetal muscle cultures by peripheral blood lymphocytes from patients with polymyositis and lupus erythematosus. *Proc Aust Assoc Neurol* 8:85–92, 1971

101. Gamboa ET, Eastwood AB, Hays J, et al: Isolation of influenza virus from muscle in myoglobinuric polymyositis. *Neurology* 29:1323–1335, 1979

102. Denborough MA, Lovell RRH: Anesthetic deaths in a family. *Lancet* 2:45, 1960

103. Williams CH, Shanklin MD, Hedrick HB, et al: The fulminant hyperthermia stress syndrome: genetic aspects, hemodynamic and metabolic measurements in susceptible and normal pigs. In *Second International Symposium on Malignant Hyperthermia*. Edited by Andrete JA, Britt BA. New York, Grune and Stratton, 1977, pp 113–140

104. Britt BA: *Malignant Hyperthermia*. Boston, Little Brown, 1979, p xiii

105. Jones EW, Nelson TE, Anderson, JL, et al: Malignant hyperthermia of swine. *Anesthesiology* 36: 42–51, 1972

106. Ellis TR: Malignant Hyperpyrexia. In *Inherited Diseases and Anesthesia*. Edited by Ellis TR. New York, Elsevier/North Holland, 1981, pp 163–199

107. Clarke IMC, Ellis TR: An evaluation of procaine in the treatment of malignant hyperthermia. *Br J Anaesth* 47:17–21, 1975

108. Ellis TR, Clarke INC, Appleyard TN, et al: Malignant hyperpyrexia induced by nitrous oxide and treated with dexamethasone. *Br Med J* 4:270–271, 1974

109. Britt BA, Kalow W: Hyperrigidity and hyperthermia associated with anesthesia. *Ann NY Acad Sci* 151:947–958, 1968

110. Kalow W, Britt BA, Terreau ME: Metabolic error of muscle metabolism after recovery from malignant hyperthermia. *Lancet* 2:895–898, 1970

111. Kalow W, Britt BA, Richter A: The caffeine test of isolated human muscle in relation to malignant hyperthermia. *Can Anaesth Soc J* 24:678, 1977

112. Moulds RFW, Denborough MA: Biochemical basis of malignant hyperpyrexia. *Br Med J* 2:241–244, 1974

113. Nelson TE, Denborough MA: Studies on normal human skeletal muscle in relation to the pathopharmacology of malignant hyperpyrexia. *Clin Exp Pharmacol Physiol* 4:315–322, 1977

114. Denborough MA, Hird FJR, King JO, et al: Mitochondrial and other studies in Australian Landrace pigs affected with malignant hyperthermia. *Pro-*

ceedings of the International Symposium on Malignant Hyperthemia, Toronto 1971. Springfield, Ill., Charles C Thomas, 1971, pp 229–237

115. Cheah KS, Cheah AM: The trigger for PSE condition in stress susceptible pigs. *J Sci Food Agric* 27:1137–1144, 1976

116. Kalow W, Britt BA, Chan FT: Epidemiology and inheritance of malignant hyperthermia. In *Malignant Hyperthermia.* Edited by Britt BA. Boston, Little Brown, 1979, pp 119–139

117. Denborough MA, Forster JFA, Lovell RRH, et al: Anesthetic deaths in a family. *Br J Anaesth* 34:395–396, 1962

118. Britt BA, Locher WG, Kalow W: Hereditary aspects of malignant hyperthermia. *Can Anaesth Soc J* 16:89–98, 1969

119. Ellis TR, Harriman DGF, Keaney NP, et al: Halothane-induced muscle contracture as a cause of hyperpyrexia. *Br J Anaesth* 43:721–722, 1971

120. Kalow W, Britt BA, Peters P: Rapid simplified techniques for measuring caffeine contraction for patients with MH. In *Second International Symposium on Malignant Hyperthermia.* Edited by Aldrette JA, Britt BA. New York, Grune and Stratton, 1977, pp 339–350

121. Denborough MA, Dennett X, Anderson RMcD: Central core disease and malignant hyperpyrexia. *Br Med J* 1:272, 1973

122. Frank JP, Harati Y, Butler IJ, et al: Central core disease and malignant hyperthermia syndrome. *Ann Neurol* 7:11–17, 1980

123. Harriman DGF: Preanesthetic investigation of malignant hyperthermia: microscopy. In *Malignant Hyperthermia.* Edited by Britt BA. Boston, Little Brown, 1979, pp 97–117

124. Ward CF: Muscular dystrophy and malignant hyperthermia similar signs. *Anesthesiology* 51:184–185, 1979

125. Wingard DW: Familial stress syndrome. In *Inherited Disease and Anesthesia.* Edited by Ellis TR. New York, Elsevier/North Holland, 1981, pp 201–211

126. Huckell VF, Staniloff, NM, McLaughlin P, et al: Cardiovascular manifestations of normal thermic malignant hyperthermia. In *Malignant Hyperthermia.* Edited by Adrett JA, Britt BA. New York, Grune and Stratton, 1977, pp 373–377

2
Multiple Sclerosis

Donald H. Silberberg

The search goes on because the cause, pathogenesis, and effective treatment of multiple sclerosis (MS) remain enigmas. Fortunately, an increasingly sophisticated armamentarium is available to both the research scientist and the clinician. The problems of deciding whether or not a proferred treatment is effective works to keep the clinician among the ranks of researchers. For purposes of writing this review, I have assumed that the reader has available the preceding volume of this series (1).

CLINICAL FEATURES

MS remains the most common neurological disease affecting young adults in temperate climates. Although the tremendously variable nature of its symptoms and course makes prognostication very difficult for an individual patient, clinicians must nevertheless attempt to provide some guidance regarding the prospects for continued employment, the need for family and community support, and the eventual course of the disease. The many published retrospective reviews which are available have an inherent error in an underrepresentation of milder cases. Many were conducted before the availability of more modern diagnostic techniques, such as cerebrospinal fluid (CSF) gammaglobulin determinations and evoked potential testing.

Clinical Course

McAlpine's classic series (2) has been reinforced and refined by a computer-processed analysis of 349 patients collected from 1957-1976 and followed for an average of 9 years at the Neurological Center in Lyon (3). Their data reinforced the notion that MS may be regarded as a single entity. Approximately 70% of patients who developed MS did so between 20 and 40 years of age. Typically, the onset was at 30, with complete remissions. By the age of 34, the remissions began to leave residual disability, and at 38 years the progressive phase began. These are mean ages, and the standard deviation is 10 years. Progressive deterioration from onset was found in 18% of the patients. In those patients who developed progressive disease after an earlier course of remissions and exacerbations, it appeared that the shorter the interval between the first two relapses, the sooner the progressive phase began. Increases in CSF gammaglobulin seemed to be more closely related to the age distribution of the patients than to prognosis.

The degree of disability in this series was expressed in McAlpine's terms (2) as no disability (grade 0-1), moderate disability (still ambulatory, grades 2-3), and severe disability (nonambulatory, grades 4-6). There was a strong correlation between the age of onset and the interval to moderate disability. This interval averaged 8 years in the youngest patients, with an age of onset at 20, but only 1 year in patients age 50 at onset. Severe disability developed after 14.3 years in the young and after 4.8 years in older patients. Within 15 years 10% died, suggesting a mean survival time of around 30 years.

Patients with benign MS constituted 14% of all patients; they showed no disability after 10 years and moderate disability after 15 years. Patients with hyperacute MS comprised 8% of the total; they were severely disabled within less than 5 years. Hyperacute disease was three times more common among patients with a progressive rather than with a remitting onset. Overall, late onset, a short interval between the first two relapses, and the occurrence of the progressive phase were all associated with a poor outcome.

The problem with counseling a particular patient rests with the fact that all of these generalizations represent the average of grouped data with wide confidence limits. Nothing permits accurate prognostication for an individual patient other than the generalization that any disability which has been present for 2 years or more is likely to remain permanently.

The possible effects of pregnancy on MS are a frequent concern. An analysis in Milan of 119 patients with MS who became pregnant indicated that a lower number of relapses than expected occurred during pregnancy, but a higher number occurred during the puerperium, the 3 months following delivery. During the total post-partum year, a lower number of relapses occurred than expected. The relatively negative effects of the puerperium were partially compensated for by the favorable course of the disease during pregnancy and during the postpartum year. No significant effect on the total course of the illness was observed, as compared with a control group of 349 patients (4).

Clinical Manifestations

The assessment of impaired intellectual functioning among patients with MS presents difficult problems. Some patients become depressed, and their performance suffers. Other patients make use of denial mechanisms to cope with the uncertainty of their situation, and this may lead the clinician to assume that the patient is exhibiting dementia. True impairment of intellectual functioning may occur as an early manifestation of MS, although the general impres-sion is that if intellect suffers, it is in proportion to the extent of cerebral white matter involvement. However, a study of 55 patients with a mean age of 41 and a reported length of illness averaging 10 years found that half the subjects exhibited cognitive impair-ment. Levels of neurological involvement, the degree of physical impairment, and depres-sions were not predictive of cognitive impairment. Half of the patients who were judged on neurological examination to have intact mentation were impaired, as detected by testing with the Minnesota Multiphasic Personality Inventory, the Halstead Category Test, and the Wechsler Adult Intelligent Scale Comprehension, Similarities and Vocabulary subtests (5). Perhaps better correlations with sites of anatomical involvement by plaques will become apparent with more sophisticated computer assisted tomographic brain scan and positron emission tomographic brain scan studies in the future. It is of interest that the verbal IQ and performance IQ as determined via the Wechsler Adult Intelli-gence Scale Test are more resistant to impairment than are the Minnesota Multi-phasic Personality Inventory or Halstead Category Test (6).

The experienced clinician appreciates the wide range of signs and symptoms which may be produced by MS. Reports of electroen-cephalogram (EEG)-confirmed narcolepsy/cataplexy in a monozygotic twin with MS (7) and of 3 patients exhibiting paroxysmal itching (8) must be added to the list.

Diagnostic Tests

An attempt to verify the usefulness of the so-called erythrocyte-unsaturated fatty acid (E-UFA) test as a specific diagnostic test for MS was negative (9). This test is based on a reported decrease in the electrophoretic mobility of erythrocytes from MS patients induced by unsaturated fatty acids, such as linoleic acid. Under the same conditions, the mobility of cells from normal donors was reportedly increased. A careful study of blood from 22 patients with MS in different phases of their disease, and 17 patients with other neurological diseases and 3 healthy subjects showed that the mobility of red blood cells was either accelerated or inhibited in the presence of linoleic acid, both in the MS patients as well as in the control group. The increase or inhibition of the absolute mobility was small and randomly distributed.

In a similar vein, in a prospective survey jejunal biopsy samples from 11 patients with MS on normal diets were compared with those from controls matched for age and sex. Quantitative histology, morphometry, and electron microscopy showed no difference between the two groups. This is offered as evidence that it is unlikely that gluten sensitivity plays a role in the etiology of MS (10).

Evoked Potentials and Neurophysiological Alterations

Further experience with various techniques for the elicitation and measurement of visual evoked responses has demonstrated that the sensitivity of this technique for detecting subclinical physiological alterations in the visual pathways is affected little by the method used for providing the visual stimulation (11, 12). The choices are among a diffuse flash stimulus, central foveal stimulation by alternation between bright and dark in a rectangle subtending a very small area within the central visual field, and pattern stimulation by alternating checkerboard patterns. The most sensitive indicator remains the latency of the major occipital positive peak, regardless of the method of stimulation. It is now clear that a prior bout of retrobulbar neuritis does not necessarily lead to a sustained prolongation of the visual evoked response latency. When prolongation does occur, it does not necessarily remain as a permanent finding (11).

Of further interest is the observation that there is little correlation between abnormalities of the visual evoked potential (VEP) and a psychophysical test which measures visual acuity by asking subjects to discern the minimum contrast necessary to detect the presence of dark and bright bands (13). The reason for this lack of concordance between a test of acuity and the measurement of VEP latency is not clear.

The measurement of the critical frequency of photic driving (CFPD) appears to be somewhat more sensitive than pattern reversal VEP for detecting abnormalities in the visual pathways of patients with MS (14). The CFPD is the highest frequency of photic driving in response to repetitive flash stimulation using averaging techniques. Of 22 patients tested with CFPD, 20 showed abnormalities (91%), while 19 of 25 patients (76%) showed abnormal latencies in one or both eyes on visual evoked response testing. Of 20 patients who had both tests performed, 19 showed abnormalities in at least one eye on one of the tests (95%). The technique for testing CFPD can be added to any laboratory which examines evoked potentials, requires a minimum of patient cooperation, and seems to be valid for patients whose best corrected vision is too poor for the proper assessment of visual evoked responses. Thus it appears to be a potentially important addition to the electrodiagnostic armamentarium for the detection of abnormalities of the visual pathway.

Patients with MS commonly complain of tingling and other sensory disturbances which may occur spontaneously or in response to movement. A neurophysiological study of sensory fibers traversing an experimentally produced central demyelinated lesion showed existence of spontaneously and mechanically induced trains of action potentials propagating in both directions from the lesion. A similar phenomenon may occur in plaques of demyelination in the corresponding sensory pathways in MS (15).

OPTIC NEURITIS

A prospective study of the risk of developing MS following a bout of optic neuritis indicated that examination of the CSF gave prognostic information. Re-evaluation of 48 patients was carried out 7-10 years after their initial neurological, neuro-ophthalmological, and CSF studies. Of these, 27 patients (56%) had developed probable MS and 9 (19%) possible MS. Among 20 patients who initially had increased CSF IgG, above 10% total protein, 19 developed probable or possible MS. However, 17 of 28 patients with an initially normal CSF IgG value also developed MS. Fourteen of the patients with optic neuritis reported some neurological symptom in their past medical history, but all had a normal neurological examination. Five patients had suffered earlier from an episode of optic neuritis in the contralateral eye. Twenty-eight patients presented with isolated optic neuritis—that is, no history of neurological symptoms nor of a previous episode of optic neuritis. Of these patients, 71% developed MS during this period of follow-up, as compared with 75% of the entire group of 48 patients. As these figures indicate, normal CSF did not rule out the possibility of dissemination (16).

EPIDEMIOLOGY

Epidemiology continues to play an important role in the attempt to understand MS. The clinical characteristics, the incidence rate, the mortality rate, and the prevalence rate within different population groups serve as the basic comparators from which new ideas may be drawn.

Within this natural laboratory, the Orkney and Shetland Islands north of Scotland are unique for having the highest prevalence of MS known. The high prevalence is probably at least partly due to the fact that these small populations (approximately 17,000 each) have been studied intensively, and the latest reports, based on prevalence days in 1970 and 1974 (17-24) are the third and fourth surveys of these islands since 1954. The prevalence of patients with probable MS was 258 per 100,000 in the Orkney Islands and 152 per 100,000 in the Shetland Islands. These studies are most notable for the inability of the investigative group to uncover any features which distinguished the patients with MS from the non-MS control population. There was a remarkable similarity between the patients and controls with respect to diet, social class, occupation, housing, exposure to animals, schooling, travel, infectious diseases, and other aspects of medical history. The frequency of the human leukocyte antigen (HLA) haplotypes A3, B7, and DW2 in the patients and controls was compared, but no significant differences were found, in contrast with the findings of many other studies. No consistent pattern of raised antibody titers or presence or absence of antibody was noted in patients as compared with the control groups. The patients had had common childhood infections, including measles, at a later age than inhabitants of Europe and the United States; in fact, 6 patients developed measles after they had developed MS.

An interesting correlation was the observation that HLA-B7 correlated with high titers of measles antibody in healthy controls; controls with haplotype B7, DW2, and the B-cell 4 alloantigen had significantly higher titers of measles and rubella antibody than controls without those haplotypes. This of course suggests that in normals, viral antibody titers are influenced by HLA haplotypes, another piece of evidence that a determinant in the HLA complex may govern the immune response and in turn be related to MS.

A study of the population of northeast Scotland has confirmed the fact that the area has the highest prevalence rate in the world for any population of comparable size. In 1973, the prevalence was 144 per 100,000 population (25). One in every three hundred and six individuals 40-59 years of age was affected.

An interesting study of 70 cases of MS seen at the Capital Hospital in Beijing, China, indicates many similarities to the clinical characteristics of MS in the West. The female to male ratio was 1.8:1; the average age of onset was 30.6 years, with an age range of 10-64 years. As in other reports from Asia, the most frequent sites of lesions based on clinical symptoms were the spinal cord and optic nerve (26). Similarly, a report of 54 patients with MS from northwest India describes features which are mostly in keeping with western experience, except for a predominance of visual involvement as a presenting sign, and 5 patients with concomitant bilateral visual impairment and transverse myelopathy (neuromyelitis optica) (27).

Family Studies

A detailed study of 30 sets of twins confirmed the results of previous twin studies and added new information. In 24 of the pairs, a firm clinical diagnosis was made on each twin. Among these 24 pairs, 6 of 12 monozygotic twins were concordant for clinical MS, compared with 2 of 12 dizygotic twins. Those with MS who were members of monozygotic twin pairs showed wide differences in age of onset and in the clinical severity of their disease, suggesting that the factors influencing the clinical behavior of MS, once it is established, are not under significant genetic control. Unexplained neurological signs were found in 3 asymptomatic twins, and a high proportion of clinically normal twins had abnormalities of CSF immunoglobulins. These findings suggest a high incidence of subclinical MS in this population (28).

Genetic Markers

The observed anomalies in IgG production by MS patients led to a study of genetic markers of IgG. A hemagglutination inhibition technique was used to detect Gm phenotypes, and a particular phenotype, Gm1,17;21, was significantly overrepresented among MS patients as compared with patients with other neurological diseases and with normal individuals. The immune response genes, which are linked to the structural loci for immunoglobulin allotypes (Gm), are probably on chromosome 14. Increasing evidence indicates that the genes from the major histocompatibility complex (on chromosome 6) and those coding for the constant region of immunoglobulin heavy chains somehow interact to produce an immune response. Studies to evaluate the interactive effect of HLA and Gm loci in MS are needed (29).

IMMUNOLOGICAL ALTERATIONS IN MS

It is certain that immunological alterations occur in patients with MS. It is far less certain whether or not those alterations play a role in the cause or evolution of the disorder. The possibility remains that any or all of the abnormalities that have been discovered are epiphenomena, which follow tissue destruction occurring on another basis. The hope and expectation is that, even if immunological alterations do not prove to be the primary

problem, a better understanding of these events may lead to discovery of the cause. The rapidly moving field of modern immunology provides an expanding array of approaches, and the field remains a fertile one for investigation of MS. What follows are a few highlights from recent reports.

The concepts of humoral and cell-mediated immunity as systems that are in any way mutually exclusive is fast disappearing. However, the methods used in the study of cell-mediated, that is, lymphocyte and monocyte-macrophage reactivities, are often quite distinct from those used to characterize soluble factors in either blood or spinal fluid, so that this traditional distinction will be maintained within this review.

Humoral Reactivity

Serum Alterations
There is as yet no agreement as to whether antibodies to any brain component circulate in serum or spinal fluid of MS patients to any greater extent than in patients with other neurological diseases, or than in normals. For example, a study of complement-dependent lysis of liposomes containing several purified brain gangliosides demonstrated activity in the sera of 30%-40% of 23 MS patients but in only 1 of 10 patients with other neurological diseases. This is potentially interesting because one of the gangliosides tested, GM_4 (sialosylgalactosyl ceramide) is a major component of human myelin (30). In contrast, CSF and serum specimens from 4 clinically definite MS patients were studied for any evidence of interaction with extracts of MS brain tissue, normal human brain tissue, purified bovine myelin, bovine myelin basic protein (MBP), and isolated bovine oligodendrocytes. Sensitive techniques were used, and no evidence of antibody activity was shown. Isoelectric focusing of the serum or CSF was followed by attempts to detect antibody by antigen immunofixation and autoradiography. These techniques were capable of demonstrating virus antibody levels (31). In a similar vein, an attempt to detect anti-oligodendrocyte antibodies in serum by a binding test with ^{125}I-protein A

from *Staphylococcus aureus* showed no difference between patients with MS and other neurological diseases, although both were significantly higher than the binding that occurs in controls (32). ^{125}I-protein A binds specifically to the Fc portion of most mammalian IgG subclasses and provides a measure of the number of IgG molecules bound per cell.

Another study reported finding that sera from several patients with MS and with other neurological diseases and from normals bound to isolated adult bovine oligodendrocytes, as did CSF from patients with MS and with other neurological diseases. These studies suggested that the binding of IgG to oligodendrocytes was not necessarily an antigen-antibody reaction but may have been due to nonspecific Fc-mediated binding (33).

Brain Immunoglobulins in MS

The distinction between brain and CSF immunoglobulins is somewhat arbitrary, since much evidence points to brain synthesis of a high proportion of the immunoglobulins found in CSF in patients with MS. A previously described empirical formula for calculating the rate of synthesis of IgG in the central nervous system (CNS) was validated by injecting radiolabelled IgG and albumin and following their passage from blood to CSF over 21 days in 9 patients with clinically definite MS. IgG synthesis rates calculated by the isotope exchange method were in excellent agreement with those calculated by the empirical formula, from a low rate of 5 mg per day to a high of 120 mg per day among the patients tested. A double radiolabelled IgG experiment in 2 of the patients showed that the blood-brain barrier of patients with MS processed normal serum IgG in the same way as IgG derived from MS serum (34). Using these techniques, it was possible to demonstrate that administration of corticosteroids was capable of reducing the rate of CNS IgG synthesis. This reduction persisted for months after cessation of treatment. However, CSF IgG oligoclonal bands persisted, indicating that CNS immune reactions among treated patients were not eradicated (35). These studies were carried out in chronic progres-

sive, severely disabled patients, which made it virtually impossible to demonstrate significant changes in neurological function, a subject of many other previous studies.

The first direct evidence that IgG participates locally in myelin breakdown in MS is based on an examination of macrophages in actively demyelinating lesions in 2 patients dying of MS. The peroxidase-antiperoxidase immunocytochemical technique was used to demonstrate IgG. In one case, in which the tissue was rapidly fixed in chilled fixative, macrophages, located among myelinated nerve fibers at plaque margins but not elsewhere in the plaque, revealed surface IgG in the form of caps restricted to one or both poles of the cell. These caps were absent in sections stained for albumin. Capping implies microprecipitation of cell membrane components with reactive substances such as particulate antigens, plant lectins, and anti-IgG antibody. In this study, the fact that IgG capping was observed only in macrophages located close to myelin sheaths suggests that the extracellular binding material close to the cell surface may be some component of myelin. The IgG caps may represent antibody which is cytophilic for macrophages, directed against an antigen expressed in plaque margins and associated with myelin sheaths (36). As pointed out by the authors, the possible interest of this observation is enhanced by previous work which demonstrated that only the IgG1 and IgG3 subclasses of IgG are cytophilic for human macrophages and monocytes, and that the oligoclonal IgG of both CSF and brain in MS belongs mainly to the LgG1 subclass.

CSF

Oligoclonal Patterns. Further characterization of the phenomenon of the occurrence of multiple discrete IgG molecules with CSF IgG (the oligoclonal pattern seen on electrophoresis) has yielded information of both clinical and research interest. It is already recognized that patients with acute aseptic meningitis, subarachnoid hemorrhage, polyneuropathy, syphilis, and cerebral tumors may show an oligoclonal pattern in their CSF. Now, 12 selected patients with acute cerebrovascular disease, cerebral infarction, or transient ischemic attacks showed an oligoclonal CSF pattern during the course of their disease. The pattern disappeared in 6 patients; only 3 patients had elevated CSF IgG levels or an abnormal synthesis rate of IgG in the nervous system. As detailed below, an extension of this study showed that the oligoclonal bands contained antibodies to several viruses (37). These studies suggest that acute destruction of brain tissue may release substances which induce polyclonal B–lymphocyte activation and antibody synthesis in the CNS and emphasize the nonspecificity of the oligoclonal CSF pattern. Its clinical usefulness rests on the very high incidence of this pattern in CSF in MS, as compared with a much lower incidence in other disorders. Unfortunately, the study just cited does not describe the frequency of this abnormality in cerebrovascular disease, since the number of patients tested in order to find those with an oligoclonal pattern was not stated.

The more sensitive technique of isoelectric focusing has made possible the demonstration of a change in the oligoclonal pattern in MS CSF with time. A serial study of 10 MS patients showed an increase in the number of bands in 4 patients (and in 3 of 5 subacute sclerosing panencephalitis [SSPE] patients), and fluctuations in band intensity were also noted. The SSPE pattern could be made to resemble the MS pattern through the addition of normal polyclonal IgG to the SSPE CSF, suggesting that in addition to oligoclonal IgG, polyclonal IgG is synthesized locally within the CNS in MS (38).

Isoelectric focusing was also used to compare the pattern of IgG eluted from three different plaques and a white matter pool of an MS brain, and three regions of an SSPE brain. Eluates from individual MS plaques had distinct IgG patterns; in contrast, those from separate SSPE brain areas had essentially identical IgG patterns. The identical patterns in the three areas of SSPE brain suggest a common response to the same antigen. The different IgG patterns among the MS plaques suggest a variable response to the same antigen in each plaque, a response to different antigens in different plaques, or different degrees of nonspecific antibody synthesis in different plaques (39).

Antibody Reactivity to Brain Components. A solid phase radioimmunoassay was used to detect antibodies to MBP in the CSF of 48 patients with MS, and 30 patients with SSPE. Precautions were taken to insure that the assay measured a true antigen-antibody reaction, rather than nonspecific adherence of IgG to MBP, and testing was carried out at identical IgG concentrations. In MS, the levels of antibody were highest in patients with acute exacerbations and lower in patients in remission. The reaction with MBP was consistently more pronounced in SSPE than in MS. The presence of antibody indicates that an autoimmune reaction occurs but does not answer the question of whether it is secondary to the presence of free MBP, which occurs as a result of tissue breakdown, or whether it is part of the primary process that leads to myelin breakdown (40).

Concentrated CSF from patients with MS and with other neurological diseases were tested for antibodies against oligodendrocytes by indirect immunofluorescence on frozen brain sections and by complement fixation against isolated bovine oligodendrocytes. When tested on human brain sections, CSF from 8 out of 10 (80%) of MS patients showed some degree of staining of brain by immunofluorescence; 8 of 21 (40%) of other neurological diseases showed the same. Similar studies using MS and control sera on bovine brain showed staining by 87% of MS sera, 60% of those with other neurological diseases and 45% of patients with psychiatric diseases (41). These studies, in conjunction with earlier results from the same laboratory (42), indicate that anti-oligodendrocyte antibodies in serum and CSF occur more commonly among patients with MS than with other neurological diseases but are not specific indicators for MS.

Idiotype Determinations. It is now recognized that the gamma globulins are a family of molecules with different specificities. Immune responses to antibody molecules themselves may play a role in the modulation of immune responsiveness. Many studies center on the idiotypic determinant, which is that portion of the gamma globulin molecule that has specific binding activity for the antigen towards which that antibody molecule is directed. Naturally existing anti-idiotypic antibodies occur, and such antibodies may be prepared in experimental systems for the identification and quantification of specific antibody molecules. Anti-idiotypic antibodies have been prepared against the CSF IgG from patients with MS by immunizing rodents (43-45). In another study, mouse anti-CSF IgG hybridoma monoclonal antibodies were produced against the immunoglobulins present in the CSF of a patient with MS. One hybridoma antibody recognized an idiotypic determinant which constituted approximately 1% of the immunoglobulin present in the CSF (46). In each of these studies, the anti-idiotypic antibody demonstrated that the idiotype-bearing antibody used as the antigen was present in approximately tenfold higher concentrations in the CSF than in the serum of the donor patient.

In each instance, the idiotype could not be detected in CSF or serum samples from other patients with MS, optic neuritis, or with other neurological diseases. However, the idiotype recognized by the hybridoma antibody reacted with a Theiler murine encephalomyelitis virus stain WW, which had been isolated from mice after inoculation with periplaque white matter from the brain of a histologically confirmed case of MS (46). This is in distinction to many previous studies which have shown that predominant CSF IgG populations in MS patients often react with measles virus (see below). By contrast, this hybridoma anti-idiotypic antibody failed to react with measles and several other viral agents, hence the reactivity with the WW virus must be further explored. It is of further interest that the idiotype described persisted in the MS patient from which it was derived at increasing concentrations over a 6-year observation period.

Although these studies are in accord with the other evidence that a source of IgG production exists within the CNS of most MS patients, the concentrations of IgG with the particular idiotypes in the serum cannot be explained by the production of this IgG within the CNS and CSF alone. That would imply diffusion of idiotype-positive IgG from CSF to blood against a gradient of that IgG. This suggests that the production of the IgG that is enriched in the CSF is not restricted to the CNS only, but is a more general response of the immune system (44).

Complexes. The presence of immune complexes in the serum of MS patients has attracted interest for at least three reasons. The first is that these antigen-antibody complexes might offer the opportunity to extract the antigen towards which the antibody is directed, and thus investigation of its possible involvement in the pathogenesis of MS. The second is recognition that the occurrence of immune complexes itself seems to be implicated in the pathogenesis of a number of other disorders of presumed autoimmune etiology, such as serum sickness in man, lupus nephritis, rheumatoid arthritis, and others. One mechanism for the production of pathology is that complexes may result in complement activation. The third reason for interest is for their potential use as genetic markers (see below).

Complexes have now been found in 50% of CSF samples from 32 MS patients taken during an active phase of their disease (47). There was no correlation between the presence of immune complexes and disease duration, severity, or degree of activity. In view of the evidence for the existence of antibody to MBP (48), some of these complexes may represent MBP-MBP antibody complexes.

The phenotypes of the complement factor C3 were evaluated in 60 patients with MS, and the results correlated with the occurrence of circulating immune complexes in those patients. A significantly increased frequency of the C3F-gene was found among patients and was closely associated with the occurrence of circulating immune complexes.

Perhaps this points to a genetically determined immunological abnormality which predisposes to MS and must be taken into consideration along with those factors known to be involved, such as HLA haplotype (49).

Cell-Mediated Alterations

Immunoregulation
The availability of monoclonal antibodies which can be used to sort and quantitate different types of T lymphocytes has made it possible to characterize the peripheral lymphocytes in patients with MS, compared with normals and age-matched control subjects with other neurological diseases. In contrast with normal individuals and the controls with other neurological diseases, the patients with MS had a reduced percentage of total T cells. More importantly, there was a selective decrease in a suppressor T-cell subset in most patients with active MS, but rarely in patients with inactive MS and in none of the normals or controls with other neurological diseases (50, 51). Serial analysis of patients with MS showed a correlation between the absence of the suppressor subset and disease activity. Thus, there appeared to be a loss of peripheral suppressor cells in many patients with active MS.

This supports previous findings using other techniques. However, it may be difficult to compare such analyses done by different techniques, since it appears that there is little correlation between T-cell subsets defined by these monoclonal antibodies and those defined by, for example, Fc receptors (52).

These determinations of the distribution of T-cell subsets suggest the possibility that alterations in the regulation of antibody production might in some way be implicated in MS. Other studies have focused on the functional consequences of such alterations, such as the suggestion that the changes of T-cell subsets in MS are related to changes in the functional ability to modulate immunoglobulin production by normal B cells. However, the MS B cells partly escaped regulation by their own T cells, suggesting an associated B-cell hyperactivity (53). Similarly, studies of pokeweed mitogen-stimulated IgG synthesis

showed that MS cell cultures provided less suppression than those from normal individuals. However, the lower levels of suppression did not appear to be the result of T-suppressor cell dysfunction alone (54). Our understanding of this complex field is in its infancy; it is an area of increased research activity and promise.

Reactivity to Brain Antigens

Efforts continue to detect reactivity of peripheral blood or CSF cell populations with brain components in MS. For example, peripheral blood lymphocytes from 24 of 26 patients with clinically well-defined MS in remission showed sensitization to MS brain extracts as assayed by enhancement of the early erythrocyte rosette test. Such an increase in the number of early rosettes was not found when the lymphocytes of MS patients were exposed to extracts of control brains. In contrast, the sensitized cells were found in the circulation in only 2 of 11 patients with MS during acute exacerbations. A longitudinal study of 1 patient who was studied before, during, and after a relapse, revealed the disappearance in the blood of the sensitized T cells during the relapse and their subsequent reappearance after recovery. Of 36 patients with other neurological diseases, 2 responded solely to MS brain, 2 responded to both MS and control brain, and 3 responded only to control brain. None of 10 healthy controls showed sensitization to any brain extract (55). Similarly, peripheral blood lymphocytes from all of 35 patients with MS produced a significant rise in active E-rosette formation after incubation with preparations of purified bovine, gangliosides, or cerebrosides. Only 3 of 26 patients with other neurological diseases were stimulated in a similar fashion. Fifteen healthy subjects did not respond to either antigen in this test (56).

Using a similar technique, increased peripheral blood sensitivity to isolated bovine oligodendrocytes was found in 49% of 104 MS patients, 23% of 62 patients with other neurological diseases, and 8% of 26 normal individuals (57). Unfortunately, these studies do not answer the question of whether the increased peripheral blood lymphocyte sensitivity is simply a response to antigen released by another destructive process, or whether their sensitization has something to do with the production of the lesions. A related study in CSF lymphocytes addresses the same question, but does not answer it. Elevated levels of MBP and enhanced CSF lymphocyte reactivity to MPB were observed in patients with MS and with other inflammatory diseases of the nervous system. There was no particular correlation between the magnitude of the in vitro response and the amount of MBP-like material in the CSF (58).

Perhaps related to cellular reactivity to brain antigens is the fact that circulating T lymphocytes from patients with MS adhere preferentially to myelin in brain sections. This is done to a greater extent than lymphocytes from normal individuals (59). Although the mechanism for this phenomenon is obscure, it may relate to leukocyte adherence to measles-infected epithelial cells in vitro. Further studies of this phenomenon suggest that the leukocyte adherence which underlies adherence to measles-infected cells is partially dependent on those determinants expressed on the target cell, which may resemble glial antigens (60).

Past studies of antibody-dependent cellular cytotoxicity (ADCC) in MS have provided conflicting information. In a study employing a rat glial tumor as the target, gliotoxic ADCC activity in MS patients was significantly higher than was seen with normals or patients with other neurological diseases. Patients with chronic progressive MS displayed the most significantly raised ADCC activity against glial cells, while patients who were inactive had almost normal ADCC activity (61). Further studies will be needed to verify this observation and to determine whether or not ADCC plays a role in the pathogenesis of MS.

Interferon

In addition to its property as an antiviral molecule, interferon can generate resistance to acute and persistent virus infections by producing an antiviral state at the cellular level and also by modulating immune responses in the whole organism. This led to studies of interferon production in MS, with conflicting results. The in vitro interferon responses of peripheral blood leukocytes to measles virus, Newcastle's disease virus, and to other substances often used to induce interferon synthesis, (polyinosinicpolycytodilic [poly I:C] and concanavalin A) were studied in 57 patients with clinically definite MS, and 34 normal donors. The interferon responses of the MS patients appeared to be deficient to each of these stimuli, as compared with peripheral blood leukocytes from normals (62). In contrast to these findings, in a similar study, 72 patients with clinically definite MS in various stages were compared with a similar number of normal control individuals for their responsiveness and interferon production after infection with various strains of measles and SSPE viruses. No defect was detected in the ability of the MS patients' lymphocytes to produce interferon or activate natural killer cells. Enhanced natural killer activity was also induced by an exogenous interferon preparation and by poly I:C to the same extent in patients and controls, and there was no deficiency in either spontaneous cell-mediated cytotoxicity, nor in antibody-dependent cell-mediated cytotoxicity (63).

CSF Cell Characterization

An aid to characterizing mixed populations of cells in blood or spinal fluid is the development of fluorescence-activated cell sorters, which can measure discrete bands of emitted fluorescence, as well as measure simultaneously small-angle light-scatter for each cell as it passes rapidly through a focused laser beam. This technology has been used to characterize the cell-cycle phase of lymphocytes from CSF obtained from patients with MS, in comparison with age-matched patients with noninflammatory or no disease of the CNS and patients with meningitis. Stimulated cells in the first stage of the proliferative cycle (G_1 phase) were found in all categories of MS. In addition, increased numbers of cells in the second stage of the cycle (S phase) were seen in specimens from patients with MS, most of whom had active disease, but no increases were seen in controls, including the patients with meningitis. This indicates that stimulated lymphocytes are present in the CSF during all phases of MS, and that stimulation becomes more intense during an acute exacerbation (64). By use of this technique, rapid quantification of T-cell and B-cell subpopulations in spinal fluid and classification of stimulated cells will become possible, even with normal spinal fluid cell counts.

THE SEARCH FOR A VIRAL ETIOLOGY

Canine Viruses

Interest continues in the possibility that canine distemper virus (CDV) or some other canine virus might play a role in MS. An epidemiological study in Switzerland analyzed the evolution of the incidence of canine distemper encephalitis in dogs and compared it with the rate of MS in the same areas. Canine distemper encephalitis became a rare disease after the second half of the 1960s, while the MS incidence rate has remained approximately the same, suggesting that a causal link between canine distemper infection in dogs and MS in man seems unlikely (65).

It is difficult to detect CDV-specific antibodies in human sera by means of standard assays because measles-virus antibodies cross-react with CDV antigens. However, with the development of an immune precipitation technique in combination with polyacrylamide-gel electrophoresis, it is now possible to characterize immune reaction of a host against each individual structural protein of the virus in question. Using this technique, serum and spinal fluid samples from a group of MS patients and controls was carried out. No CDV-specific antibodies were found in the samples tested. Using this technique, both SSPE and MS patients had a higher activity towards measles virus components than did controls (66). Similar studies using radioimmunoassay (67), and enzyme-linked immunoabsorbent assay [ELISA] (68) showed an association of CDV antibody levels with the occurrence of measles-virus antibodies, but were not able to distinguish specifically between them.

Neutralizing antibodies were measured for the most common canine viruses in addition to CDV, and no differences were found between MS patients and controls (69).

Coronaviruses

Two coronaviruses were isolated from brain material obtained at autopsy from 2 MS patients (70). Coronaviruses represent an attractive candidate for a role in the etiology of MS, since viruses of this group cause a demyelinating-remyelinating disease in mice. However, subsequent work indicated that the coronavirus isolates were most closely related to a murine coronavirus (A59) and to a human coronavirus [OC43] (71). The prevalence of antibodies to three strains of MS and matched controls showed no differences (72). The possible role of coronaviruses in MS remains an open question.

Nucleic Acid Probes

As they become available, the more sensitive nucleic acid probes provide increasingly sensitive ways to search for viral material in MS tissues. Molecular hybridization experiments employ a radioactive complementary DNA (cDNA) probe transcribed in vitro from the RNA of the virus in question, or radiolabelled purified DNA can be used. Using these techniques, no measles nucleotide sequences were found in the brains of 4 MS patients (73). A similar search for human cytomegalovirus and herpes simplex virus was negative in testing the brains of 5 MS patients (74). These results do not necessarily indicate that these viruses are not involved in MS; the genetic information, if present, may be below the sensitivity of the detection of these hybridization techniques.

Other Viral Antibody Studies

Sera and CSF from 87 patients with clinically definite MS, 50 with probable MS, 26 patients with probable inflammatory neural disease, and 140 with noninflammatory neural disease were analyzed for antiviral antibodies. A variety of methods was used to assay for antibodies to rubella, mumps, measles, influenza I (Strain 6/94), herpes simplex, cytomegalovirus, varicella zoster, and vaccinia viruses. The MS patients had higher serum antibody titers to measles virus, and a higher proportion had CSF antibodies to measles, rubella, and vaccinia viruses. A greater percentage of patients with MS had viral antibodies to more than one virus, and there was a correlation between the duration and severity of MS with the occurrence of multiple CSF antibodies. The presence of CSF antibody was also correlated with the height of the corresponding serum titer, although a high serum titer did not necessarily insure the presence of CSF antibody. Oligoclonal bands were present in the CSF of equal proportions of patients with MS and without CSF viral antibody. There was no tendency for certain antibodies to be associated (75-77). These data support the occurrence of local antibody synthesis within the CNS but do not implicate any particular virus. A similar study in 25 patients with MS included detection of antibodies to mumps. When thin-layer polyacrylamide-gel isoelectric focusing was followed by antigen immunofixation, antibody activity was also found in polyclonal IgG zones (78).

These studies address the important question as to whether preprogrammed antibody-forming lymphocytes enter the CNS and then produce antibody either because of nonspecific polyclonal activation in situ, or because of a failure of normal regulation, or alternatively, were originally primed by exposure to viruses which invaded the nervous system. This latter alternative fits with the fact that the most frequently observed specificity of the predominant CSF immunoglobulin populations are against potentially neurotropic viruses, such as measles, mumps, rubella, varicella, and herpes, but not against ubiquitous pneumotropic viruses, such as influenza. The fact that a particular idiotypic determinant was present for at least 6 years in 1 patient (46) suggests either aberrant B-cell regulation, or in that case the presence of ongoing stimulation by WW virus, an antigenically related virus, or even a nonviral immunogen.

However, quantitation of measles-specific IgG in the CSF of 41 patients with MS showed that less than 5% of the total IgG was measles virus specific (79). Little similar data exists for other viruses, but one would expect similar results, indicating that only a minor proportion of the total CSF IgG can be accounted for as viral antibody of known specificities.

BIOCHEMICAL ALTERATIONS

The breakdown of myelin in and around MS plaques has been attributed to the action of proteolytic enzymes, particularly those with an acid pH optimum, some of which are elevated in and around the plaques, or even in normal-appearing white matter. Some of these enzymes are capable of breaking down MBP and thus possibly lead to the release of immunogenic fragments. A proposed source of the increased levels of proteolytic enzymes is invading lymphocytes and macrophages (80). However, an increase in lysosomal hydrolase activity, including proteinases, occurs wherever tissue destruction and cell death occur. Hence other possible sources of increased proteinase activities include oligodendrocyte degeneration per se, or the ensuing response by surrounding astrocytes.

Recent evidence suggests that at least some of the increased lysosomal enzyme activity can be attributed to proliferation of or increased activity of astrocytes within and around MS plaques (81-83). This does not detract from the possibility that lymphocyte or macrophage-produced proteinases might not also occur and participate in the evolution of the MS plaque; however, most of the enzyme activity can be accounted for by the observed astrocytosis.

Another enzyme appears to be useful as a marker of the reduction in the number of oligodendrocytes within a plaque. Glycerol phosphate dehydrogenase (GPDH) in the nervous system has been found exclusively in oligodendrocytes by immunocytochemical methods (84). This finding was used to design a study that demonstrated that chronic MS plaques from which the oligodendrocytes have disappeared, show a dramatic loss of GPDH (85). The loss of this enzyme paralleled the decline of other enzymes, which in white matter appear to be localized in the oligodendrocyte cell body.

One of the major problems of all clinical and research studies, which seek to make correlations with the clinical course of MS, is our lack of an objective method for following disease activity. The level of CSF MBP provides a measure of disease activity, but its use is limited to those situations in which serial lumbar punctures are warranted. It now appears that measurement of serum glutamate may be of value as a correlate of disease activity. In a study of serum amino acids, serum samples were collected randomly over a period of 6 months from 99 different MS patients of varying disability and from 50 normal control individuals. Subsequently, serum samples were collected at 2-month intervals from 24 MS patients over a period of 3 years. A significant elevation in serum glutamate occurred in association with relapses. The levels rose gradually within a month or two prior to the onset of clinical relapse, reached a peak during the relapse, and then slowly declined (86).

THERAPY

Treatment of the patient with MS remains as the paramount enigma for the clinician. The physician is faced with the appeals of many desperate patients, who may or may not improve after a relapse, or may or may not cease their relentless progression and are enticed by new treatments, many of which have a well-thought-out rationale. It is the treatments designed to modify the course of MS which present the problems. Most efforts to provide symptomatic relief are much easier to evaluate and less risky to implement. As background for the section on Attempts to Modify the Course of MS, the reader is reminded of the necessity for controlled double blind trials in order to evaluate a new treatment (87). The high rate of spontaneous remission, the frequency with which patients who have been experiencing a progressive course spontaneously plateau, and the potential for an enormous placebo effect of any treatment make interpretation of uncontrolled trials virtually impossible.

Attempts to Modify the Course of MS

The various bits of evidence suggesting that immune alterations play a role in the pathogenesis of MS have given impetus to a variety of efforts to modify immunologic events in patients with MS. Approaches include techniques for enhancing the immune response, for suppressing the immune response, and for removing humoral factors from the peripheral circulation.

Immunosuppression

In one prospective double-blind trial, the effects of administration of the combination of antilymphocyte globulin (ALG), prednisolone, and azathioprine in 15 patients was compared with the effects of placebo on another 15 patients with MS. The 2 groups were matched for disability and sex and were treated for 15 months. The lymphocyte response to phytohemagglutinin was suppressed in the patients treated with ALG, prednisolone, and azathioprine. This combination produced no effect on the IgG concentrations in CSF. After 6 and 11 months of treatment, 2 of the immunosuppressed male patients developed complications (intercurrent infection and gastric irritation, respectively). The first died 4 months later, and the other died 1 year later.

Their results show a marginal effect in decreasing the frequency of relapses; significance at the $P = 0.06$ level was seen among women only. Similarly, the women who were immunosuppressed appeared to progress somewhat more slowly, as measured by disability scores before and after the treatment period. The inclusion of the men who died during the trial resulted in a higher rate of deterioration among the immunosuppressed males, since the 2 who died were included in their calculations as having the highest disability score [10 on the Kurtzke scale] (88).

In another study (89), the effects of azathioprine administered daily at a dosage of 2 mg/kg body weight to 56 randomly chosen patients with MS was compared in an open study with a control group of 51 randomly selected MS patients who were instructed to follow a diet of low-fatty acids with sunflower oil and sunflower margarine. The results of this prospective study, during which azathioprine was continued on average for 732 days, as compared with the control group, who were followed for 792 days, suggested to the investigators that long-term azathioprine therapy partially alleviated the further progress of MS, in comparison with the nontreated control group. This favorable effect was statistically most apparent for those patients who had had MS for less than 2 years; for those affected longer, no such beneficial effect was demonstrated. Treatment with azathioprine did not lower the relapse rate, which averaged approximately 1 per year per patient in both groups. Patients in either group were treated with prednisone for varying periods. The statement is made that prednisone treatment was maintained in some cases over several months, and in others became continuous.

This study has several drawbacks which weaken the conclusions. The most important problem is that the study was not carried out in a double-blind manner; both the patients and the examining physicians knew which patients were receiving what. The possible bias introduced by the open nature of the study overshadows the other problems which include the fact that some patients were treated with prednisone, and that the patients treated with azathioprine were on average more severe cases and had been affected for a longer period of time. However, their results may be interpreted as being sufficiently suggestive to warrant a double-blind study of azathioprine alone in comparison with administration of a placebo.

The use of cyclophosphamide has also been advocated for the treatment of MS. The most recent study which promotes its use describes the effects of treatment with a short course of intensive immunosuppression via high doses of cyclophosphamide and prednisone on 39 patients with chronic progressive MS (90). The follow-up period was from 1-5 years, with a mean of 2½ years. Progression of the disease ceased in 27 patients for varying periods of time, with a mean of 2 years. In 13 patients the progression ceased during the whole follow-up period. This was interpreted as a favorable response, which was most likely to occur in patients who were DRw2 positive, whose disease started at an early age (28 years), whose disease duration before treatment was short (6 years), whose progression was fast, and whose disability before treatment was low.

In contrast, another study compared 21 patients with moderately advanced MS, treated with a short-term intensive course of cyclophosphamide as compared with a nontreated control group of 21 patients retrospectively matched for disability. Of the 21 who had received cyclophosphamide, 5 had a chronic progressive course; 7 of the control group had a progressive course. Patients were excluded who had experienced an acute exacerbation within 3 months prior to entry into the study. This was done to eliminate those patients who might be expected to improve following an exacerbation but who might appear to have improved as the result of cyclophosphamide administration. In this study, no significant difference between the treatment and control groups could be detected during a follow-up period of 2 years (91).

There is growing interest in the use of plasmapheresis as a possible new therapy for MS. Two uncontrolled studies, which describe treatment with a combination of plasmapheresis, prednisone, and azathioprine, describe modest improvement which is attributed to the plasmapheresis and medications (92, 93). Many other clinicians throughout the United States have undertaken plasma exchange in MS. Although plasmapheresis is a procedure with a convenient rationale—presumably to eliminate autoantibodies, toxic substances, neuroelectric blocking factors, or significant subpopulations of lymphocytes—there is as yet no evidence that the plasmapheresis results are an improvement over the natural course of untreated MS. A double-blind control study is sorely needed (94).

A review of the risks of long-term treatment with immunosuppressants is sobering (95). A recent report describes 33 cases of leukemia in patients who had undergone immunosuppressive therapy of more than 1 year's duration for chronic inflammatory disease (96).

Immune Enhancement

Most attempts to influence the course of MS

by stimulating the immune response have not been successful. Levamisole has no effect (97-99). Three trials of transfer factor, a human leukocyte extract, reported no beneficial effect. No change in disability, evoked potentials or CSF abnormalities were observed in 30 patients treated for 3 months in Glascow (100). Less rapid deterioration failed to show in 48 patients from Copenhagen (101) and 58 patients from New York (102) who were treated for 16 and 12 months, respectively. Transfer factor is a soluble leukocyte extract which contains a number of components, one of which has the capacity to transfer cell-mediated (but not humoral) immunity from an immune donor to a nonimmune recipient. It appears to be antigen-specific and free of unwanted side effects. Transfer factor has been in clinical use for a number of years and has an established role in the treatment of patients with immunodeficiencies, such as chronic muco-cutaneous candidiasis and the Wiskott-Aldrich syndrome. The attempts to treat MS with transfer factor relate to the assumption that MS is due to a subtle defect in host defenses, which results in persistent infection.

Ideally, if transfer factor were to help patients with MS, it should be obtained from individuals who are immune to the putative environmental agent which causes MS. In an effort to achieve this, a 2-year prospective double-blind trial in Australia utilized transfer factor pooled from leukocytes of cohabiting relatives selected for high responsiveness to measles and parainfluenza III viruses. Fifty-eight patients were treated for 2 years with placebo or with transfer factor. The patients were matched with respect to sex ratio, disability, duration of disease, ratio of moderate to severe cases, and HLA phenotype (103). The results indicated that transfer factor retarded but did not reverse progression of the disease; a significant difference between treatment and placebo groups was not apparent until 18 months after the start of the trial; and treatment appeared to be effective only in those patients with mild to moderate disease activity. Despite a large range of immuno-logical tests, no transfer of immune function was demonstrated.

Symptomatic Therapy

Dorsal Column Stimulation

Spinal cord stimulation by means of epidural electrodes in 19 patients with MS reportedly had its most beneficial response on bladder function: 75% of 16 patients with bladder symptoms improved, and 7 of 11 patients with severe bladder disturbance improved (104). These authors concluded that a favorable response is heavily dependent upon the type of stimulation received, which is detailed in a companion report (105). These and another recent report (106) are reviewed in an excellent editorial (107), which reviews the history of dorsal column stimulation and the many pitfalls in interpreting results.

REFERENCES

1. Silberberg DH: Multiple sclerosis. In *Current Neurology*, vol 3. Edited by Appel, SH. Boston, Houghton, Mifflin, 1981, pp 43-65

2. McAlpine D: Course and prognosis. In *Multiple Sclerosis, a Reappraisal*, 2nd ed. London, Churchill, 1972, pp 197-223

3. Confavreux C, Aimard G, Devic M: Course and prognosis of multiple sclerosis assessed by the computerized data processing of 349 patients. *Brain* 103:281-300, 1980

4. Ghezzi A, Caputo D: Pregnancy: a factor influencing the course of multiple sclerosis. *Eur Neurol* 20:115-117, 1981

5. Peyser JM, Edwards KR, Poser CM, et al: Cognitive function in patients with multiple sclerosis. *Arch Neurol* 37:577-580, 1980

6. Marsh GG: Disability and intellectual function in multiple sclerosis. *J Nerv Ment Dis* 168:758-762, 1980

7. Schrader H, Gotlibsen OB, Skomedal GN:

Multiple sclerosis and narcolepsy/cataplexy in a monozygotic twin. *Neurology* 30:105-108, 1980

8. Yamamoto M, Yabuki S, Hayabara T, et al: Paroxysmal itching in multiple sclerosis—a report of 3 cases, *J Neurol Neurosurg Psychiatry* 44:19-22, 1981

9. Cuypers J, Reddemann H: Evaluation of the erythrocyte-UFA (E-UFA) mobility test for the diagnosis of multiple sclerosis. *J Neurol Neurosurg Psychiatry* 43:995-998, 1980

10. Bateson MC, Hopwood D, MacGillivray JB: Jejunal morphology in multiple sclerosis. *Lancet* 1:1108-1110, 1979

11. Oepen G, Brauner C, Doerr M, et al: Visual evoked potentials (VEP) elicited by checkerboard versus foveal stimulation in multiple sclerosis—a clinical study in 235 patients. *Arch Psychiatr Nervenkr* 229:305-313, 1981

12. Wilson WB, Keyser RB: Comparison of the pattern and diffuse-light visual evoked responses in definite multiple sclerosis. *Arch Neurol* 37:30-34, 1979

13. Bodis-Wollner I, Hendley CD, Mylin LH, et al: Visual evoked potentials and the visuogram in multiple sclerosis. *Ann Neurol* 40-47, 1979

14. Cohen SN, Syndulko K, Tourtellotte WW, et al: Critical frequency of photic driving in the diagnosis of multiple sclerosis; a comparison to pattern evoked responses. *Arch Neurol* 37:80-83, 1980

15. Smith KJ, McDonald WI: Spontaneous and mechanically evoked activity due to central demyelinating lesion. *Nature* 286:154-155, 1980

16. Nikoskelainen E, Frey H, Salmi A: Prognosis of optic neuritis with special reference to cerebrospinal fluid immunoglobulins and measles virus antibodies. *Ann Neurol* 9:545-550, 1981

17. Poskanzer DC, Prenney LB, Sheridan JL, et al: Multiple sclerosis in the Orkney and Shetland Islands. 1. Epidemiology, clinical factors, and methodology. *J Epidemiol Community Health* 34:229-239, 1980

18. Poskanzer DC, Sheridan JL, Prenney LB, et al: Multiple sclerosis in the Orkney and Shetland Islands. 2. The search for an exogenous aetiology. *J Epidemiol Community Health* 34:240-252, 1980

19. Poskanzer DC, Terasaki PI, Prenney LB, et al: Multiple sclerosis in the Orkney and Shetland Islands. 3. Histocompatibility determinants. *J Epidemiol Community Health* 34:253-257, 1980

20. Poskanzer DC, Sever JL, Sheridan JL, et al: Multiple sclerosis in the Orkney and Shetland Islands. 4. Viral antibody titres and viral infections. *J Epidemiol Community Health* 34:258-264, 1980

21. Poskanzer DC, Sever JL, Terasaki PI, et al: Multiple sclerosis in the Orkney and Shetland Islands. 5. The effect on viral titres of histocompatibility determinants. *J Epidemiol Community Health* 34:265-270, 1980

22. Roberts DF, Roberts MJ, Poskanzer DC: Genetic analysis of multiple sclerosis in Orkney. *J Epidemiol Community Health* 33:229-235, 1979

23. Roberts DF, Papiha SS, Poskanzer DC: Polymorphisms and multiple sclerosis in Orkney. *J Epidemiol Community Health* 33:236-242, 1979

24. Taylor R, Illsley R, Poskanzer DC: Multiple sclerosis in the Orkney and Shetland Islands. 6. The effects of migration and social structure. *J Epidemiol Community Health* 34:271-276, 1980

25. Shepherd DI, Downie AW: A further prevalence study of multiple sclerosis in north-east Scotland. *J Neurol Neurosurg Psychiatry* 43:310-316, 1980

26. Baoxun Z, Xiuqin L, Yupu G, et al: Multiple sclerosis. A clinical study of 70 cases. *Chin Med J* [*Engl*] 93:260-264, 1980

27. Chopra J, Radhakrishnan K, Sawhney B, et al: Multiple sclerosis in north-west India. *Acta Neurol Scand* 62:312-322, 1980

28. Williams A, Eldridge R, McFarland H, et al: Multiple sclerosis in twins. *Neurology* 30:1139-1147, 1980

29. Pandey JP, Goust JM, Salier JP, et al: Immunoglobulin-G heavy chain (Gm) allotypes in multiple sclerosis. *J Clin Invest* 67:1797-1800, 1981

30. Arnon R, Crisp E, Kelley R, et al: Antiganglioside antibodies in multiple sclerosis. *J Neurol Sci* 46:179-186, 1980

31. Shorr J, Rostrom B, Link H: Antibodies to viral and non-viral antigens in subacute sclerosing panencephalitis and multiple sclerosis demonstrated by thin-layer polyacrylamide gel isoelectric focusing, antigen immunofixation and autoradiography. *J Neurol Sci* 49:99-108, 1981

32. Steck AJ, Regli F: Oligodendrocyte-binding antibodies in multiple sclerosis: ^{125}I-protein A studies. *Neurology* 30:540-542, 1980

33. Ma BI, Joseph BS, Walsh MJ, et al: Multiple sclerosis serum and cerebrospinal fluid immunoglobulin binding to Fc receptors of oligodendrocytes. *Ann Neurol* 9:371-377, 1981

34. Tourtellotte WW, Potvin AR, Fleming JO, et al: Multiple sclerosis: measurement and validation of central nervous system IgG synthesis rate. *Neurology* 30:240-244, 1980

35. Tourtellotte WW, Baumhefner RW, Potvin AR, et al: Multiple sclerosis de novo CNS IgG synthesis: Effect of ACTH and corticosteroids. *Neurology* 30:1155-1162, 1980

36. Prineas JW, Graham JS: Multiple sclerosis: capping of surface immunoglobulin G on macrophages engaged in myelin breakdown. *Ann Neurol* 10:149-158, 1981

37. Rostrom B, Link H: Oligoclonal immunoglobulins in cerebrospinal fluid in acute cerebrovascular disease. *Neurology* 31:590-596, 1981

38. Mattson DH, Roos RP, Arnason BGW: Isoelectric focusing of IgG eluted from multiple sclerosis and subacute sclerosing panencephalitis brains. *Nature* 287:335-337, 1980

39. Mattson DH, Roos RP, Arnason BGW: Comparison of agar gel electrophoresis and isoelectric focusing in multiple sclerosis and subacute sclerosing panencephalitis. *Ann Neurol* 9:34-41, 1981

40. Panitch HS, Hooper CJ, Johnson KP: CSF antibody to myelin basic protein—measurement in patients with multiple sclerosis and subacute sclerosing panencephalitis. *Arch Neurol* 37:206-210, 1980

41. Traugott U, Raine CS: Anti-oligodendrocyte antibodies in cerebrospinal fluid of multiple sclerosis and other neurologic diseases. *Neurology* 31:695-700,1981

42. Traugott U, Snyder S, Raine CS: Oligodendrocyte staining by multiple sclerosis serum is nonspecific. *Ann Neurol* 6:13-20, 1979

43. Baird LG, Tachovsky TG, Sandberg-Wollheim M, et al: Identification of a unique idiotype in cerebrospinal fluid and serum of a patient with multiple sclerosis. *J Immunol* 124:2324-2390, 1980

44. Naglekerken LM, Aalberse RC, vanWalbeek HK, et al: Preparation of antisera directed against the idiotype(s) of immunoglobulin G from the cerebrospinal fluid of patients with multiple sclerosis. *J Immunol* 125:384-389, 1980

45. Ebers GC, Zabriskie JB, Kunkel HG: Oligoclonal immunoglobulins in subacute sclerosing panencephalitis and multiple sclerosis: a study of idiotypic determinants. *Clin Exp Immunol* 35:67-76, 1979

46. Gerhard G, Taylor A, Wroblewska Z, et al: Analysis of a predominant immunoglobulin population in the cerebrospinal fluid of a multiple sclerosis patient by means of an anti-idiotypic hybridoma antibody. *Proc Natl Acad Sci USA* 78:3225-3229, 1981

47. Deicher H, Meyerzuschwabedissen H, Baruth B, et al: Cerebrospinal fluid immune complexes in multiple sclerosis. *Experientia* 35:1249-1250, 1979

48. Panitch HS, Huffer DA, Johnson KP: Antibodies to myelin basic protein in multiple sclerosis: Clinical conditions. *Neurology* 28:394, 1978

49. Jans H, Sorensen H: C3 polymorphism and circulating immune complexes in patients with multiple sclerosis. *Acta Neurol Scand* 62:237-243, 1980

50. Reinherz MD, Weiner HL, Hauser SL, et al: Loss of suppressor T-cells in active multiple sclerosis. *N Engl J Med* 303:125-129, 1980

51. Bach MA, Phan-Dinh-Tuy F, Tournier E, et al: Deficit of suppressor T cells in active multiple sclerosis. *Lancet* 2:1221-1228, 1980

52. Reinherz EL, Moretta L, Roper M, et al: Human T-lymphocyte subpopulations defined by Fc receptors and monoclonal antibodies. *J Exp Med* 151:969-974, 1980

53. Goust JM, Hoffman PM, Pryima J, et al: Defective immunoregulation in multiple sclerosis. *Ann Neurol* 8:526-533, 1980

54. Kelley RE, Ellison GW, Myers LW, et al: Abnormal regulation of in vitro IgG production in multiple sclerosis. *Ann Neurol* 9:267-272, 1981

55. Turner A, Cuzner ML, Davison AN, et al: On the role of sensitized lymphocyte T in the pathogenesis of multiple sclerosis. *J Neurol Neurosurg Psychiatry* 43:305-309, 1980

56. Offner H, Konat G: Stimulation of active E-rosette forming lymphocytes from multiple sclerosis patients by gangliosides and cerebrosides. *J Neurol Sci* 46:101-104, 1980

57. Traugott U, Scheinberg LC, Raine CS: Lymphocyte responsiveness to oligodendrocytes in multiple sclerosis. *J Neuroimmunol* 1:41-51, 1981

58. Lisak RP, Zweiman B, Whitaker JN: Spinal fluid basic protein immunoreactive material and spinal fluid lymphocyte reactivity to basic protein. *Neurology* 31:180-182, 1981

59. Dore-Duffy P, Goertz V, Rothman BL: Lymphocyte adherence to myelinated tissue in multiple sclerosis. *J Clin Invest* 66:843-846, 1980

60. Barna BP, Goren H, Jacobs B, et al: Analysis of leukocyte adherence to measles-infected cells in multiple sclerosis. *Ann Neurol* 9:28-33, 1981

61. Mar P: Antibody-dependent cellular cytotoxicity in multiple sclerosis. *J Neurol Sci* 47:285-303, 1980

62. Neighbour PA, Miller AE, Bloom BR: Interferon responses of leukocytes in multiple sclerosis. *Neurology* 31:561-566, 1981

63. Santoli D, Hall W, Kastrukoff L, et al: Cytotoxic activity and interferon production by lymphocytes from patients with multiple sclerosis. *J Immunol* 126:1274-1278, 1981

64. Noronha ABC, Richman DP, Arnason BGW: Detection of in vivo stimulated cerebrospinal fluid lymphocytes by flow cytometry in patients with multiple sclerosis. *N Eng J Med* 303:713-718, 1980

65. Vandevelde M, Meier C: Multiple sclerosis and canine distemper encephalitis. *J Neurol Sci* 47:255-260, 1980

66. Stephenson JR, Meulen Volker ter, Kiessling W: Search for canine-distemper-virus antibodies in multiple sclerosis. *Lancet* 2: 772-781, 1980

67. Arnadottir T: Measles and canine distemper virus antibodies in patients with multiple sclerosis determined by radioimmunoassay. *Acta Neurol Scand* 62:81-90, 1980

68. Madden DL, Wallen WC, Houff SA, et al: Measles and canine distemper antibody—presence in sera from patients with multiple sclerosis and matched control subjects. *Arch Neurol* 38:13-15, 1981

69. Appel MJ, Glickman LT, Raine CS, et al: Canine viruses and multiple sclerosis. *Neurology* 31:944-959, 1981

70. Burks JS, DeVald BL, Jankovsky LD, et al: Two coronaviruses isolated from central nervous system tissue of two multiple sclerosis patients. *Science* 209:933-934, 1980

71. Gerdes JC, Klein I, DeVald BL, et al: Coronavirus isolates SK and SD from multiple sclerosis patients are serologically related to murine coronaviruses A59 and JHM and human coronaviruse OC43, but not to human coronavirus 229E. *J Virol* 38:231-238, 1981

72. Madden DL, Wallen WC, Houff SA, et al: Coronavirus antibodies in sera from patients with multiple sclerosis and matched controls. *Arch Neurol* 38:209-210, 1981

73. Stevens JG, Bastone VB, Ellison GW, et al: No measles virus genetic information detected in multiple sclerosis derived brains. *Ann Neurol* 8:625-627, 1980

74. Aulakh GS, Albrecht P, Tourtellotte WW: Search for cytomegalovirus and herpes simplex virus genetic information in multiple sclerosis. *Neurology* 30:530-532, 1980

75. Johnson KP, Likosky WH, Nelson BJ, et al: Comprehensive viral immunology of multiple sclerosis. I. Clinical, epidemiological and CSF studies. *Arch Neurol* 37:537-542, 1980

76. Cremer NE, Johnson KP, Fein G, et al: Comprehensive viral immunology of multiple sclerosis. II. Analysis of serum and CSF antibodies by standard serologic methods. *Arch Neurol* 37:610-615, 1980

77. Forghani B, Cremer NE, Johnson KP, et al: Comprehensive viral immunology of multiple sclerosis. III. Analysis of CSF antibodies by radioimmunoassay. *Arch Neurol* 37:616-619, 1980

78. Rostrom B, Link H, Laurenzi MA, et al: Viral antibody activity of oligoclonal and polyclonal immunoglobulins synthesized within the central nervous system in multiple sclerosis. *Ann Neurol* 569-574, 1981

79. Mehta PD, Thormar H, Wisniewski HM: Quantification of measles-specific IgG—its presence in CSF and brain extracts of patients with multiple sclerosis. *Arch Neurol* 37:607-609, 1980

80. Cammer W, Bloom BR, Norton WT, et al: Degradation of basic protein in myelin by neutral proteases secreted by stimulated macrophages — A. Possible mechanism of inflammatory demyelination. *Proc Natl Acad Sci USA* 75:1554-1558, 1978

81. McKeown SR, Allen IV: The cellular origin of lysosomal enzymes in the plaque in multiple sclerosis: a combined histological and biochemical study. *Neuropathol Appl Neurobiol* 4:471-483, 1978

82. Allen IV, Glover G, McKeown SR, et al: The cellular origin of lysosomal enzymes in the plaque of multiple sclerosis. II. A histochemical study with combined demonstration of myelin and acid phosphatase. *Neuropathol Appl Neurobiol* 5:197-210, 1979

83. Hirsch HE, Parks ME: A thiol proteinase highly elevated in and around the plaques of multiple sclerosis. *J Neurochem* 32:505-513, 1978

84. Leveille PJ, McGinnis JF, Maxwell DS, et al: Immunocytochemical localization of glycerol-3-phosphate dehydrogenase in rat oligodendrocytes. *Brain Res* 196:287-307, 1980

85. Hirsch HE, Blanco CE, Parks ME: Glycerol phosphate dehydrogenase: reduced activity in multiple sclerosis plaques confirms localization in oligodendrocytes. *J Neurochem* 34:760-762, 1980

86. Westall FC, Hawkins A, Ellison GW, et al: Abnormal glutamic acid metabolism in multiple sclerosis. *J Neurol Sci* 47:353-364, 1980

87. Brown JR, Beebe GW, Kurtzke JF, et al: The design of clinical studies to assess therapeutic efficacy in multiple sclerosis. *Neurology* 29 (II): 1-23, 1979

88. Mertin J, Knight S, Rudge P, et al: Double-blind, controlled trial of immunosuppression in treatment of multiple sclerosis (preliminary communication). *Lancet* 2:949-957, 1980

89. Patzold U, Pocklington P: Azathioprine in multiple sclerosis—a 3-year controlled study of its effectiveness. *J Neurol* 223:97-119, 1980

90. Hommes OR, Lamers KJB, Reekers P: Effect of intensive immunosuppression on the course of chronic progressive multiple sclerosis. *J Neurol* 223:177-191, 1980

91. Theys P, Gosseye-Lissoir F, Ketelaer P, et al: Short-term intensive cyclophosphamide treatment in multiple sclerosis. A retrospective controlled study. *J Neurol* 225:119-134, 1981

92. Dau PC, Petajan JH, Johnson KP, et al: Plasmapheresis in multiple sclerosis: preliminary findings. *Neurology* 30:1023-1028, 1980

93. Weiner HL, Dawson DM: Plasmapheresis in multiple sclerosis: preliminary study. *Neurology* 30:1029-1033, 1980

94. van den Noort S, Waksman BH: Plasma exchange: aid to therapy of multiple sclerosis. *Neurology* 30:111, 1980

95. Weiner LP: Recent trends in MS therapy—reporting results (discussion). In *Progress in Multiple Sclerosis Research*, edited by Bauer, HJ, Poser, S, Ritter, G. Berlin, Springer-Verlag, 1980, pp. 411-412

96. Mougeot-Martin M, Krulik M, Harousseau J-L, et al: Leucemies aigues survenues au decours d'une maladie de Beheet et d'une sclerose en plaques traitees par immunosuppresseurs. *Ann Med Interne (Paris)* 129:175-198,1978

97. Dau PC, Johnson KP, Spitler LE: The effect of levamisole on cellular immunity in multiple sclerosis. *J Clin Exp Immunol* 26:302-309, 1976

98. Cendrowski W, Czlonkowska A: Levamisole in multiple sclerosis; with special reference to immunological parameters. A pilot study. *Acta Neurol Scand* 57:354-359, 1978

99. Myers LW, Ellison GW, Levy J, et al: Evaluation of levamisole as a treatment for multiple sclerosis. *Neurology* 27:363, 1977

100. Behan PO, Melville ID, Durward WF, et al: Transfer factor therapy in multiple sclerosis. *Lancet* 1: 988-989, 1976

101 Fog T, Raun N, Pederson L, et al: Long-term transfer factor treatment for multiple sclerosis. *Lancet* 1: 851-853, 1978

102. Collins RC, Espinoza LR, Plank CR, et al: A double-blind trial of transfer factor vs. placebo in multiple sclerosis patients. *Clin Exp Immunol* 33:1-11, 1978

103. Basten A, McLeod JG, Pollard JD, et al: Transfer factor in treatment of multiple sclerosis. *Lancet* 2:931-933, 1980

104. Illis LS, Sedgwick EM, Tallis RC: Spinal cord stimulation in multiple sclerosis. Clinical results. *J Neurol Neurosurg Psychiatry* 43:1-14, 1980

105. Jobling DT, Tallis RC, Sedgwick EM, et al: Electronic aspects of spinal-cord stimulation in multiple sclerosis. *Med Biol Eng Comput* 18:48-56, 1980

106. Hawkes CH, Wyke M, Desmond A, et al: Stimulation of dorsal column in multiple sclerosis. *Br Med J* 280:889-891, 1980

107. Dorsal column stimulation in multiple sclerosis (editorial). *Br Med J* 280:1287-1288, 1980

3
Hereditary Ataxias

Sandro Sorbi and John P. Blass

The hereditary spinocerebellar ataxias continue to arouse increasing research interest. The number of articles cited in review chapters in this series has increased from 36 in 1979 to 80 in 1980 and 114 in this article.

DESCRIPTION AND CLASSIFICATION

The term "hereditary ataxia" has been used in different ways by different authors to refer to a group of disorders characterized by degenerations of the cerebellar peduncles, cortex, motor long-fiber tracts, and proprioceptive fibers (1). In the last few years, new entities have been recognized and variants of classical syndromes reported (2). In an overview of the third phase of the Quebec Cooperative Study, Barbeau (3) suggested that "Until biochemical markers are identified and can be tested in the field, it is far more prudent to give these variants either a family name or a geographic name."

This wise course assumes only that patients in a family or in a geographic isolate who have the same syndrome probably derive from a common ancestor, and all have the same gene defect. It avoids hidden assumptions inherent in the use of older eponyms. It specifically bypasses the risky presumption that hereditary syndromes defined by clinical criteria are necessarily biologically and genetically homogeneous. Modern neurogenetic research has shown that reality is, in fact, often more complex (4).

Classical Syndromes

Whatever the faults of the classical eponymic spinocerebellar syndromes, they are part of classical neurology. Reports on these entities and their variants continue to appear.

Clinical Observations

During the past year Friedreich's ataxia (FA) has been observed for the first time in a girl from an Indonesian family of North Sumatra (5). Two of her sisters and a brother died of a disease with the same symptoms. Another brother, surviving, was reported to have the same illness. They had the classic symptoms: ataxia, kyphoscoliosis, positive Babinski's and Romberg's signs, dysmetria, adiadochokinesis, and absence of knee and ankle jerks.

Dysarthria was studied in patients with FA (6). Two speech factors have been observed, general dysarthria and a phonatory stenosis. Five reports appeared on cardiac abnormalities in FA. Torsade de pointes, as the only cardiac involvement, has been described in a patient (7). Hypertrophic cardiomyopathy (HCM) has been found in 50% of 22 patients with FA and in the 29% of obligate heterozygotes [parents] (8). The authors suggest that HCM is inherited in a pattern different from FA and that it can appear in heterozygotes free of the typical neurological symptoms of FA. Hypertrophic idiopathic subaortic stenosis has been reported in parents of FA patients (9). Lipofuscin granules and deposits of iron were observed in the myocardial fibers

---

Note—These studies were supported by the Winifred Masterson Burke Relief Foundation, the Will Rogers Institute, the National Foundation (No. 6–215), the Dystonia Foundation, and the National Institutes of Health (NS15125 NS16994, and AA03883).

of 3 cases (10). In 15 FA patients, symmetric, concentric hypertrophic cardiomyopathy was the predominant (67%) abnormality in contrast with previous reports proposing that the asymmetric septal hypertrophy is the usual type of cardiomyopathy in this disorder (11).

A report appeared on an FA patient in whom the large neurons of the dorsal root ganglia were selectively involved (12), and a degeneration of pacinian corpuscles was observed in another 5 patients (13). These authors suggest that if the large-fiber degeneration is of the dying-back type, the alterations of pacinian corpuscles would be useful as a predictive test in young at-risk siblings (Fig. 1).

Behr's syndrome with marked static and locomotor ataxia has been reported in a family (14). Three members of a non-consanguineous family were reported affected by Gillespie's syndrome (15), confirming autosomal recessive inheritance of this entity.

Clinical Laboratory Observations

Hereditary ataxias have been associated with a large variety of metabolic abnormalities of lipids, amino acids, purines, and oxidative metabolism (1). The most wide-ranging clinical laboratory examination of patients with hereditary ataxias has been done over the last 6 years by the Quebec Cooperative Studies. These workers hypothesize that the primary factor of "the pathophysiology of most symptoms in Friedreich's ataxia and possibly of many other forms of hereditary ataxias appears to be interference with the incorporation of linoleic acid into the phosphatidylcholine component of high density lipoproteins" (3). They report also abnormalities in cerebrospinal fluid (CSF) monoamine metabolism in 23 patients (16), but studying clinical, neurophysiological, and biochemical data from another 18 patients indicated that "no single clinical or laboratory finding is typical of Friedreich's ataxia" (17).

Ataxia in Systemic Disorders

Reports continue to appear associating spino-cerebellar symptoms with different systemic disorders. A macroglobulinemic patient had ataxia unrelated to cerebral infarction or blood hyperviscosity (18). His cerebellar symptoms improved with chlorambucil treatment for the myeloproliferative disorder. Sensory ataxia was reported in the course of systemic lupus erythematosus (19), improving gradually on treatment of the systemic disease with prednisone.

New Syndromes

Despite the number of variants of the more or less classic hereditary ataxias described in the literature, almost 10 patients or families have been reported as transitional or new original forms. A new neurocutaneous syndrome was described (20) in which familial spastic paraplegia, peroneal neuropathy, and crural hypopigmentation are inherited in a dominant pattern. A similar neurocutaneous syndrome with disordered pigmentation was reported in 3 siblings, but presumably in a recessive pattern (21).

Lima and Coutinho (22) described a family of non-Azorean origin affected by an autosomal dominant inherited ataxia resembling Machado-Joseph disease. This family from Freixo-de-Espada-a-Cinta, a small village in northeastern Portugal, comprises 16 affected people in 5 generations. The authors suggested that in the absence of a recognized genetic marker, the diagnosis of Machado-Joseph disease can be made by the following clinical criteria: (1) autosomal dominant inheritance; (2) major neurological picture including cerebellar ataxia and pyramidal signs (type II), associated in variable degrees with a dystonic-rigid extrapyramidal syndrome (type I) or peripheral amyotrophy (type III); (3) minor clinical signs such as progressive external ophthalmoplegia, dystonia, intentional facial and lingual fasciculation-like movements, and bulging eyes.

Association of hereditary ataxia and tapetal-retinal degeneration has been observed in 2 Italian siblings (23) and in a 16-year-old Swiss boy with FA (24). Because of the more than 200 observations of this association, Bourguin and associates (24) accept the theory of Franceschetti and Klein (25) that a unique recessive pleiotropic gene is responsible for the degeneration of both central

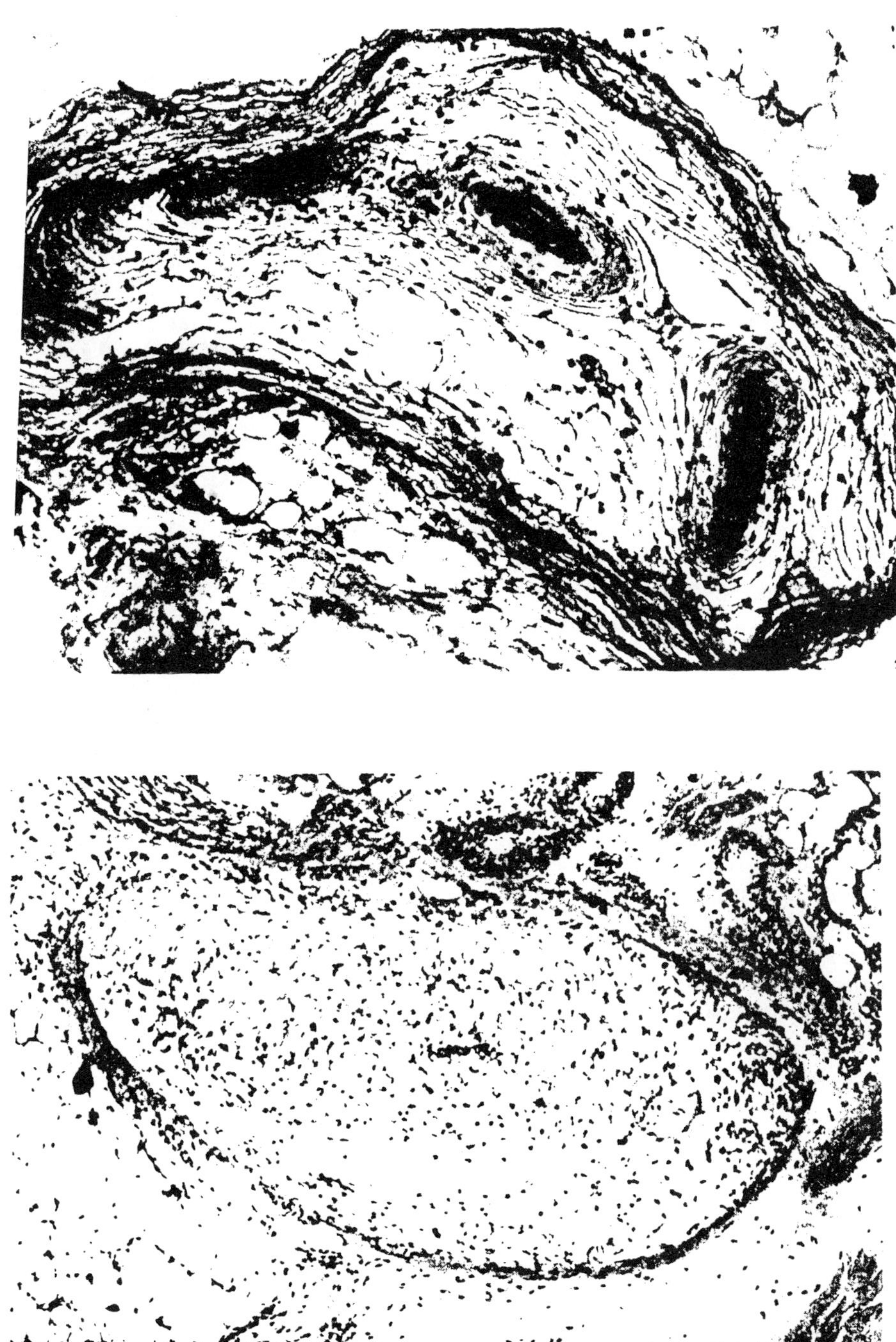

Figure 1. Degenerated pacinian corpuscle in spinal Friedreich's ataxia (FA). The *upper figure* shows a pacinian corpuscle of a normal control. The *three whorls* may belong to three corpuscles or be one refolded corpuscle cut three times. The *lower figure* is from a patient with FA. (Reprinted with permission from Marolda M, et al: Diagnostic significance of pacinian corpuscle degeneration in Friedreich's ataxia. *Acta Neurol (Napoli)* 35:373–381, 1980

nervous system (CNS) and neurosensory retinal cells.

Schott (26) described 2 brothers who, during their fourth decade, presented with isolated down-beat nystagmus and later developed a progressive cerebellar ataxia. Both up- and down-beat nystagmus have previously been reported in ataxias. In this case, however, the ataxia developed after the nystagmus. While interesting, this hardly appears to represent a new syndrome.

Ichthyosis, hepatosplenomegaly, and cerebellar degeneration have been reported in 3 brothers as a new disease (27). The family pedigree was consistent with either autosomal or X-linked recessive inheritance. The occurrence of skin changes in an otherwise normal brother suggests the presence of two discrete disorders segregating in the sibship, such as an X-linked ichthyosis and an autosomal recessive storage disease (27). Bouchard and colleagues (28) described a family of which 7 members suffer from a progressive ataxia, tremor, and severe distal amyotrophy with onset in the first decade. They fit the clinical criteria for the Charcot-Marie-Tooth disease. However, they lacked pes cavus, and there was severe atrophy of the cerebellum on computerized tomography (CT) scan, and electronystagmograms resembled those of FA. In addition, the tremor in 4 of these patients was consistent with a lesion in the rubro-olivo-dentatorubral loop. The authors suggest that those patients have a combination of spinal and olivo-cerebellar degeneration with a neuronal type of autosomal recessive peroneal muscular atrophy.

Classification

The complexities of classifying patients with hereditary ataxias have been belabored elsewhere (1, 3), including last year's article in this series. Every patient is unique, and every new patient or new family with a hereditary ataxia can be defined as a new syndrome if the clinical distinctions are drawn finely enough. We question whether that degree of erudition is useful, for the patients or for science. Two simple classification schemes obviate these issues. One is that proposed by Barbeau—to use family or geographic names to characterize variants of hereditary ataxias (3). Another simple classification is to divide them into primarily spinal ataxias, primarily cerebellar ataxias, and more diffuse ataxic encephalopathies (29). These systems of classification are not mutually exclusive. They are descriptive and involve a minimum of assumptions about the genetics and other biology of these disorders. Biochemical identification of the genetic defects may allow an etiologic classification. However, it is worth remembering that detailed biochemical information about the primary genetic defects in the lipidoses has not made the classification of those disorders simple.

MOLECULAR ABNORMALITIES

Biochemical studies continue to extend the already diverse list of metabolic abnormalities associated with hereditary ataxias as well as to refine previous measurements.

Ataxia Telangiectasia (AT)

This multifaceted syndrome continues to rouse intense interest. The clinical heterogeneity of this disorder has been emphasized again (30, 31). Typical features include progressive cerebellar ataxia, oculocutaneous telangiectasia, immune defects with underdevelopment of the thymus and repeated infections, endocrine abnormalities, elevated risk of cancers (notably lymphoreticular), and untoward response to standard doses of ionizing radiation (30). The variability can be marked even in the same family. Bodensteiner and coworkers (32) described 2 siblings—a boy in whom dystonia masked ataxia and his affected sister who had the usual ataxia. Jason and Gelfand (31) suggest that the most consistent diagnostic signs are oculomotor abnormalities, elevated α-fetoprotein, and increased chromosomal breakage.

Attempts to define the nature of the deficits in cellular immunity in AT continue. With a recently recognized lymphokine, neutrophil-migration factor, abnormalities were found in T cells but not B cells in mitogenic stimulation and mixed lymphocyte culture reactivity (33). Cocultivation of plasma and lymphocytes from AT patients with those of normal individuals increased chromosomal damage in the normal cells (34). Identification of the responsible factors would be a major step in clarifying the pathophysiology of AT. Lymphoblastoid cells from AT patients had longer generation times than controls, because they had a longer S-period (35). The AT cells spent about 60% of the cycle in the deoxyribonucleic acid (DNA) synthesis compared to about 40% for controls.

Cancers of various forms are a major risk for AT patients—about 1200 times that of age-matched controls (36). During the last year, there were reports of the first patient with AT to also have renal cell carcinoma, hepatoma, and a mixed malignant hepatic tumor (37) and of the 20th patient with AT and acute lymphoblastic leukemia (38). Although this latter patient had a number of poor prognostic risk factors, his response to chemotherapy was relatively gratifying. Chromosomal instability is another characteristic of AT, and it may relate to the high incidence of malignancies (39, 40). Aurias and coworkers (39) reported a high incidence of inversions and translocations of chromosomes 7 and 14, and Al Saadi and coworkers (40) suggested that abnormal clones due to such chromosomal aberrations escape immunological surveillance (Fig. 2). As noted before, immunological function in AT is not great, either. From a clone, which escaped immunologicial surveillance, to a malignant proliferation is an easy step in terms of current theories.

It is tempting to try to relate the various functional deficits in AT to abnormalities in DNA (and therefore chromosomal) metabolism. Several groups reported during the last year that AT cells are resistant to DNA damage induced by bleomycin (41–43). Houldsworth and Lavin (44) showed that the onset of inhibition of DNA synthesis after ionizing radiation is delayed in AT cells; the extent of inhibition is less than in controls, and recovery to near normal levels, though transient, is more rapid in AT cells. However, Fornace and Little (45) found normal repair

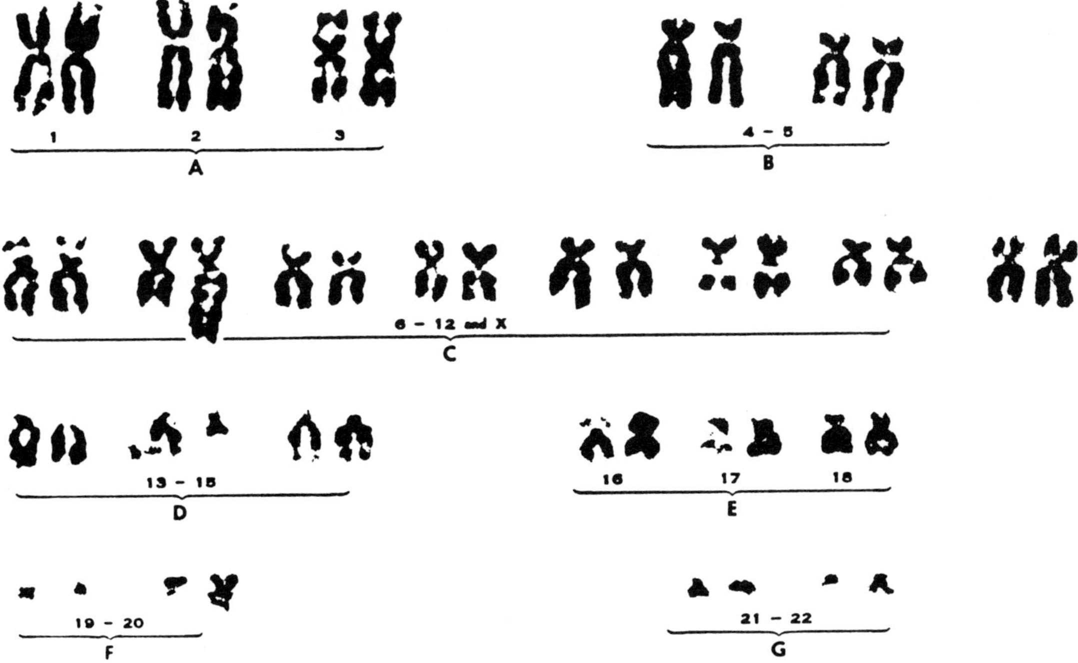

Figure 2. Translocation in ataxia telangiectasia (AT). This karyotype, showing a 7/14 translocation, is from the major lymphocyte clone of a patient with AT. (Reprinted with permission from Al Saadi A, et al. Evolution of chromosomal abnormalities in sequential cytogenetic studies of ataxia telangiectasia. *Hum Genet* 55:23–29, 1980.)

of breaks in single-stranded DNA in AT fibroblasts, and AT cells showing normal susceptibility to damage induced by *N*-methyl-N^1nitro-*N*-nitrosoguanidine and 4-nitroquinoline-l-oxide (41–43). The data are consistent with a defect in AT in the system that normally prolongs the time during which strand breaks can be repaired, replication initiation inhibited, and chromatin structure returned to its normal state. Edwards and Taylor (46) suggest that these changes may be due to unusual levels of adenosine diphosphate $(ADP\text{-ribose})_n$, a suppressor of DNA synthesis. It would not be surprising if intensive studies of this rare hereditary ataxia lead to breakthroughs in understanding human DNA repair and the mechanisms of malignant transformation.

Amino Acids

Previous studies have shown that several well-characterized disorders of amino acids are associated with ataxias (20). The relation between amino acid metabolism and ataxias is of particular interest, since seven major types of cerebellar neurons use amino acids as neurotransmitters (47).

Perry and coworkers (48) measured levels of 36 amino acids in multiple regions of autopsy brains from 11 patients with various spinocerebellar disorders. Aspartate and glutamate levels were low in several areas, notably cerebellar cortex; γ-aminobutyric acid (GABA) was low in cerebellar cortex and dentate nucleus. These authors suggested that decreased aspartate may relate to selective loss of climbing fibers, decreased glutamate to loss of either mossy fibers or granule cells and their parallel fibers, and decreased GABA to loss of either inhibitory neurons or Purkinje's cells. They even suggested that the different patterns of amino acid loss might provide a basis for classifying these patients into subgroups. This latter suggestion is hard to evaluate on the basis of 1 study of 11 patients.

Furthermore, there are other problems which limit the interpretation of amino acid levels in autopsy human brain. Perry and coworkers (48) review the studies—including classical studies from their laboratory—

demonstrating that levels of amino acids change rapidly *postmortem* though in some cases to levels which are then stable for hours. Differences between patients and controls in amino acid levels in autopsy brain might reflect differences in levels in vivo, but they might also reflect differences in the magnitude of the artifacts induced by studying autopsy brain. There is no evidence that these changes are primary rather than consequences of the disease. There is no evidence—at least as yet—for primary disorders of amino acid metabolism in the vast majority of patients with hereditary ataxias. For instance, there is no evidence for abnormal amino acid transport or metabolism in fibroblasts from all but the few patients with classical aminoacidopathies (49).

Despite these caveats, the findings of Perry and coworkers (48) are most interesting. They confirm and substantially extend previous reports or abnormalities of amino acids in spinal cord or brain of ataxic patients. These changes in amino acids might be critical in the pathophysiology even if they are not primary. For instance, glutamate, GABA, and aspartate in the brain derive from glucose. In patients with disorders of carbohydrate metabolism, alterations in these amino acids may mediate the abiotrophy.

Carbohydrate Metabolism

The frequent occurrence of defective carbohydrate metabolism in hereditary ataxias is becoming solidly established. Tolis and coworkers (50) found impaired glucose tolerance in patients from 16 families and in obligate and potential heterozygotes as well, confirming and extending previous results. The carbohydrate intolerance was not typical diabetes. Prolactin and growth hormone (51) as well as insulin (50) levels are normal, and glycosylated hemoglobin does not accumulate (52). As Barbeau has pointed out (3), the existence of abnormalities in clinically normal heterozygotes intermediate between values for the patients and controls indicates that they are in a global sense genetic. Presumably, they link in some way to the primary genetic defect.

Multiple Biotin-Dependent Carboxylase Deficiency

Intermittent ataxia at age 18 months was the presenting abnormality in 1 of 3 siblings who had neurological disease, *Candida* dermatitis, keratoconjunctivitis, and alopecia (53, 54). This patient had intermittent lactic acidosis and excreted excessive amounts of β-hydroxypropionate, β-hydroxyisovalerate, β-methylcrotonylglycine, and methylcitrate. Treatment with 10 mg a day of oral biotin reduced the abnormal urinary metabolites, consistent with deficiency of several biotin-responsive carboxylases, a known syndrome. The lactic acid accumulation is presumably secondary to deficiency of the biotin-dependent pyruvate carboxylase. One of her two siblings, with the same disorder, came to autopsy and had atrophy of the superior vermis of the cerebellum, strikingly similar to that observed in chronic alcoholism (53).

There has been no reported systematic survey of the incidence of abnormalities of pyruvate carboxylase in patients with hereditary ataxias; so one can only speculate about whether such defects might relate to the abnormalities in carbohydrate oxidation discussed before. It is interesting that the clinical pattern of severe pyruvate carboxylase deficiency is similar to that of severe deficiency of the pyruvate dehydrogenase complex. White cells have been used to demonstrate deficiencies of pyruvate carboxylase (and pyruvate dehydrogenase). Cowan and coworkers (54) have now demonstrated that in the multiple biotin-dependent carboxylase deficiency, there are deficits in T-cell mediated and B-cell mediated immunity. Thus, this defect is not only *in* but also *of* white cells. Among the fascinating questions these studies raise is whether decreased resistance to infection might be a mechanism in some of the neurological damage in other disorders of carbohydrate or energy metabolism.

Pyruvate Dehydrogenase Complex (PDHC)

Studies of the PDHC in ataxias using older methods continue to give confusing and largely negative results (3, 55–59). Bertagnolio and coworkers (56) found low activity of PDHC in a group of 5 patients with spinal FA if the cultured fibroblasts were disrupted by homogenization in glycerol but not if they were sonicated. The latter method gave lower activities. However, Barbeau and coworkers (57, 58) continue to find no consistent abnormalities in FA fibroblasts or platelets, using similar methods. Constantopoulos and coworkers (59) restudied one of the ataxic patients in whose fibroblasts PDHC deficiency had been reported previously by Blass and coworkers (20) and found entirely normal activity in his platelets. Evans (60) found PDHC activity in muscle biopsies from 9 patients with progressive ataxias. Two of four with FA had PDHC significantly below normal controls, but similarly low activities occurred in muscle from a patient with polymyositis, from a patient with polyneuropathy, and from a patient with phosphorylase deficiency. Subsequent studies by Evans (61) document that even experimental damage to nerve can alter pyruvate metabolism by the innervated muscle and emphasize the problems in choosing controls in studying diseased muscle. The consensus of all these workers was that if deficiencies of PDHC occur in vivo in these patients, they are probably secondary.

Technical advances in studying human PDHC may clarify some of the outstanding problems. In an important paper, Sheu, Hu, and the late Merton Utter (62) reported values for PDHC in cultured fibroblasts that were 5- to 100-fold higher than reported by previous workers. They achieved these activities by preincubating the cells with dichloroacetate (DCA), a reagent which inhibits the covalent inactivation of PDHC by phosphorylation. We (63) have modified their technique to measure PDHC spectrophotometrically in a coupled enzyme assay in which the production of acetyl-CoA is followed with pigeon liver anylamine acetyltransferase (64, 65). This technique has allowed demonstration of an abnormality in PDHC activation in fibroblasts from 2 patients with subacute necrotizing encephalomyelopathy of Leigh (Fig. 3). These observations on Leigh disease confirm and extend similar observations of DeVivo and cowork-

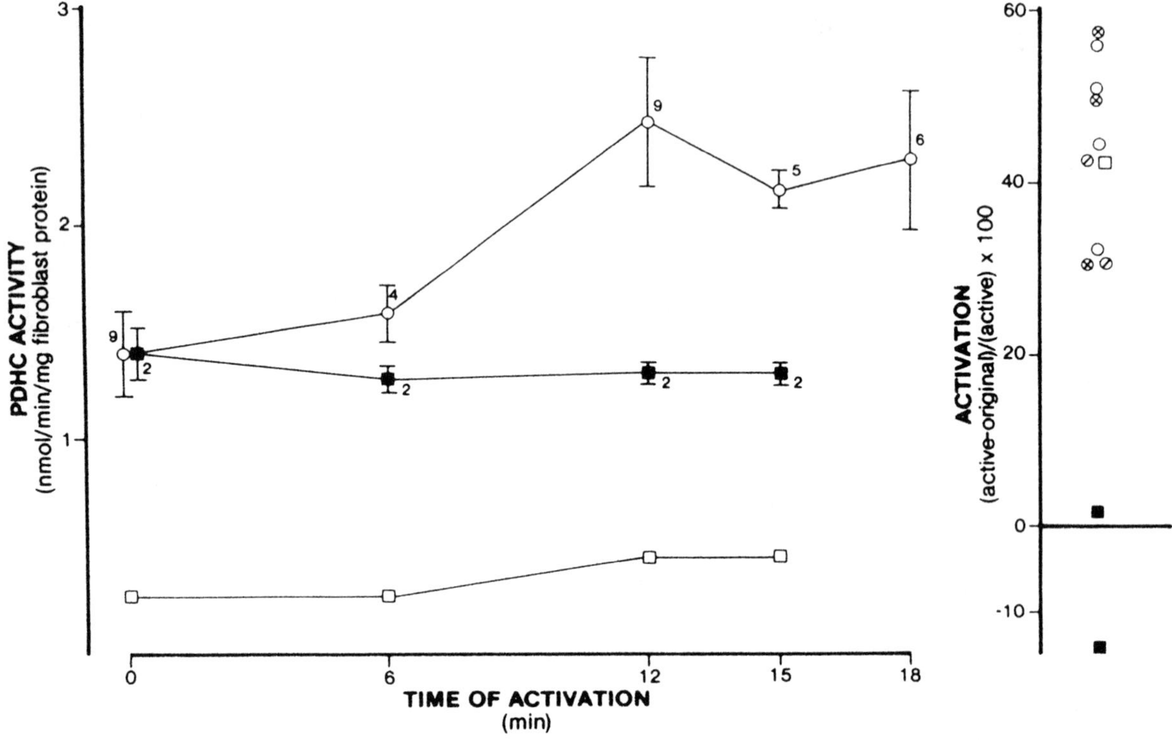

Figure 3. Pyruvate dehydrogenase complex (PDHC) activity in Leigh disease fibroblasts. Activity in disrupted fibroblasts was measured spectrophotometrically using arylamine acetyltransferase, after activation by incubation for varying times with dichloroacetate (63). Values are shown for 2 patients with Leigh disease (*black squares*) and 1 with well-demonstrated PDHC-deficiency (*white squares*) as well as controls (*circles*). The *numbers* indicate the number of control lines studied for each point. For details, see Sorbi and Blass (63-65).

ers (114). They may relate to hereditary ataxias, since the adult form of Leigh disease resembles a hereditary ataxia clinically (66). This technique is being used to restudy fibroblasts from the patients in whom Constantopoulos and Barranger did not find a PDHC deficiency. Preliminary results indicate that they do, indeed, have an abnormality of PDHC activity. DiDonato (personal communication) has used a different technique to activate PDHC in fibroblasts and found low activity of PDHC in 1 of 5 patients with hereditary ataxia.

These observations with newer methods suggest again that some, but not most, patients with hereditary ataxias have deficiencies of PDHC and that some, but not most, of the PDHC deficient patients fit within the Quebec criteria for FA (3). These newer methods appear easier and more reproducible than the older, partly because higher activities are easier to measure and partly because previous techniques examined PDHC in variable states of activation (62, 63). Indeed, most of the earlier studies presumably looked at the residual activity of the largely inactivated (i.e., phosphorylated) enzyme. One hopes that these newer techniques will allow more definitive conclusions about the frequency of PDHC deficiency in hereditary ataxias and their clinical correlations.

Lipoamide Dehydrogenase (LAD)

Kark and coworkers (67–71) have continued a series of papers supporting the hypothesis that some ataxic patients have deficiencies of LAD, an enzyme which is a component of several dehydrogenases including PDHC and the ketoglutarate dehydrogenase complex. They reported abnormal heat lability of LAD in disrupted platelets from 7 patients (69), suggesting a change in LAD structure or conformation. They claimed to be able to detect carriers and the preclinical state by kinetic analyses of LAD activity in crude platelet homogenates (70). One partial confirmation of the existence of abnormalities of LAD in some ataxic patients is the report of Melancon and coworkers (72). They found an elevated K_m for lipoamide for LAD in sera from 3 of 9 patients with FA. However, the kinetic anomalies reverted to normal on treatment with lecithin, and Melancon and coworkers (72) concluded that they were presumably secondary. Stumpf and Parks (73) found no abnormality of LAD activity or kinetics in patients with ataxias, in agreement with earlier studies of platelets and fibroblasts by the Quebec group (3). Robinson and coworkers (74) found that the clinically normal heterozygote parents of a child with severe LAD deficiency had activities of LAD in the range reported by Kark and coworkers to be associated with hereditary ataxia. Critical reexamination of the LAD assays used to demonstrate putative deficiencies indicated that they were flawed—that used in sera because it was not specific for this enzyme, and that used in cells because it involves studying kinetically anomalous properties of the enzyme (75). Kark and coworkers (71) retracted a report (67) claiming that they could demonstrate the defect in LAD if the samples were assayed double-blind. The minimum condition for accepting a putative defect would seem to be that it be readily replicable in the laboratory which originally reports it. However, lack of substantial data does not prove the negative. It certainly remains possible that there are ataxic patients who also have a hereditary aberration in LAD.

Glutamate Dehydrogenase (GDH)

Since this enzyme intraconverts an intermediate of carbohydrate metabolism with an amino acid, it can be considered an enzyme of either carbohydrate or amino acid metabo-

lism. Barbeau and coworkers (76) confirmed low activities of GDH in some (but not all) patients—values were below the lowest control in leukocytes from 5 of 18 patients with spinal FA and in 2 of 8 with cerebellar ataxia (OPCA) [Gaspe type]. The group mean for the FA patients was low as well. However, if cells were disrupted in triton detergent rather than by sonication, the FA activity was comparable to controls. DiDonato (personal communication) has replicated the demonstration by Plaitakis and coworkers (77) of low GDH in some patients with OPCA but not in FA. As with the PDHC defects, the complexities probably reflect a combination of technical factors and different ways of classifying patients. Deficiencies of GDH can probably be added to the list of molecular defects associated with hereditary ataxia syndromes.

Lipid Metabolism

Willner and associates (78) reported a progressive spinocerebellar degenerative disorder in 9 patients from 4 unrelated Ashkenazi Jewish families. These patients had early onset of cerebellar signs and, with maturity, the development of upper and lower motor neurons disorders, marked dysarthria, and ataxia. Dementia or recurrent psychotic episodes occurred in 3 older patients, aged 26–37 years. In these patients were observed membrane-bound, lamellar-cytoplasmic inclusions in rectal ganglia, consistent with lysosomal ganglioside accumulation. Beta-hexosaminidase A was markedly deficient in all sources analyzed. This enzyme, partially purified from cultured skin fibroblasts, was heat labile. Parents had activity consistent with heterozygosity confirming autosomal recessive transmission of the β-hexosaminidase A deficiency gene. The results suggest that the patients were allelic for this mutation and may represent a genetic compound of this allele and the allele causing Tay-Sachs disease.

Huang and coworkers (79) reported a small reduction in the percentage of linoleic acid in phosphatidylcholine in red cell membranes of ataxic patients (from $22\% \pm 2\%$ to $19\% \pm 2\%$), but Walker and coworkers (80) found identical fatty acid profiles in lipids of high and low density lipoproteins in 10 patients with FA compared to carefully matched controls. Filla and coworkers (81) in southern Italy found a high incidence of dyslipoproteinemias in their patients with spinal FA. Of 16 patients, 1 had hypo-β-lipoproteinemia, 2 had low levels of high-density lipoprotein (HDL) cholesterol (presumably hypo-α-lipoproteinemia), 1 had type IIB hyperlipoproteinemia, and 1 had type IV hyperlipoproteinemia. This incidence of dyslipoproteinemias would be extraordinarily high in an unselected population of American ataxias.

Other Molecular Abnormalities

Hamida and coworkers (82) reported the results of electrophoresis of cerebrospinal fluid from 110 patients with various spinocerebellar degenerative diseases. They found an overall reduction in CSF proteins, an increase in prealbumin, and a reduction in γ-globulins in 82 cases.

Chamberlain and colleagues (83) reported that cells from FA patients were hypersensitive to ionizing radiation. They respond to radiation similarly to AT cells in terms of levels of single-stranded DNA, but their pattern of postirradiation DNA synthesis differs. FA cells showed an inhibition of DNA synthesis comparable to that in control cells, while AT cells showed no such inhibition. The authors suggested that defective DNA repair may play a part in the pathogenesis of the CNS changes in FA.

Studies of red cell membranes (84) did not demonstrate a generalized defect in membranes inferred by Barbeau and coworkers (3, 76) from indirect studies. As Chamberlain and coworkers (83) point out, lack of direct evidence does not prove the negative.

Genetic Linkage

Genetic linkage analysis for hereditary ataxias could be important for preclinical diagnosis and genetic counseling. The recent data on linkage studies are encouraging. Pederson and coworkers (85) reported the results of studying 31 genetic systems in 13 families from patients with spinocerebellar disorders (Fig. 4). They suggest that there are two forms of cerebellar ataxia: one linked to

human leukocyte antigen (HLA) loci with symptoms restricted to the cerebellum and spinocerebellar systems and another non-HLA linked form with symptoms from more widespread lesions of the central nervous system (CNS).

Morton and colleagues (86) reported significant HLA linkage to a locus on chromosome 6, loosely linked to HLA, at which at least 1 allele produces OPCA I. Whittington and coworkers (87), analyzing 5 families in which a form of spinocerebellar ataxia was present on chromosome 6. It appears to be loosely linked to the HLA locus, and the authors suggest that the most likely order is HLA-red cell glyoxylase (GLO)-spinocerebellar ataxia (SCA1) with SCA1 close to the centromere.

Moreover, Koeppen and colleagues (88) found, in 5 families with dominant ataxia, 5 subjects with linkage of ataxia to the HLA locus, 4 for ataxia-properidin factor B (Bf) and 2 for ataxia GLO-I. All three genetic markers studied are located on the short arm of chromosome 6. The authors concluded that these particular genetic markers are probably not useful for predicting the disease.

DIAGNOSTIC PROCEDURES

Standardization of the Clinical Examination

One of the most common difficulties encountered in the field of research in hereditary ataxias is the problem of quantification of symptoms and of the stage of disease. Campanella and coworkers (89, 90) reported a scheme in which most of the spinocerebellar symptoms are scored. Pourcher and Barbeau (91) presented a detailed scheme for quantifying most symptoms encountered in the various ataxic syndromes, as well as a new staging system, similar to the one commonly used in Parkinson's disease (Tables 1 and 2). They field-tested this new scheme in 47 ataxic patients and reported it easy to use and reliable. These authors added two more evaluation schemes to that proposed by Campanella and his associates (89, 90), permitting major subscores: cranial nerves, coordination, tone reflex, peripheral signs, and muscle strength. All scores are graded on a scale of 0–3, which is probably the one most

Table 1. Functional Staging of Ataxia

Stage 0:	Normal in at-risk subject
Stage 1:	Patient with minimal signs detected during family screening, but previously undetected and unsuspected by patient
Stage II:	Symptoms present, recognized by patient, but still mild. The patient is physically capable of leading an independent life, but work activities can be somewhat restricted
Stage III:	Symptoms are completely developed. The patient needs help or aids to move about and transfer
Stage IV:	Patient is confined to wheel chair
Stage V:	Patient is confined to bed

Note.—Reprinted with permission from Poucher E, Barbeau A: *Can J Neurol Sci* 7:339–344, 1980.

Table 2. Ataxia Clinical Rating Scale

*Items**	*Score*	*Items**	*Score*
Cranial Nerves	Maximum—18	**Coordination**	Maximum—42
Speech		Normal gait	
Nystagmus		Tandem gait	
Eye movements		Romberg	
Fundi		Finger to nose—right	
Tongue changes		Finger to nose—left	
Cough		Heel to knee—right	
		Heel to knee—left	
Tone	Maximum—18	Spiral—right	
Tone—right arm		Spiral—left	
Tone—left arm		Adiadochokinesia—right	
Tone—right leg		Adiadochokinesia—left	
Tone—left leg		Tapping—right hand	
Holmes test—right		Tapping—left hand	
Holmes test—left		Postural tremor	
Peripheral Signs	Maximum—18	**Reflexes** (Deviation from normal)	Maximum—24
Atrophy upper limbs		DTR—right biceps	
Atrophy lower limbs		DTR—left biceps	
Fasciculations		DTR—right knee	
Myoclonias		DTR—left knee	
Pes cavus		DTR—right Achilles	
Scoliosis		DTR—left Achilles	
Vibrations—right (seconds)		Babinski—right	
Vibrations—left (seconds)		Babinski—left	
Muscle Strength Decrease	Maximum—12		
Right arm			
Left arm			
Right leg			
Left leg			

Note.—Reprinted with permission from Poucher E, Barbeau A: *Can J Neurol Sci* 7:339–344, 1980.
*All items on 0–3 scale. 0 = normal; 1 = mild; 2 = moderate; and 3 = severe disability.

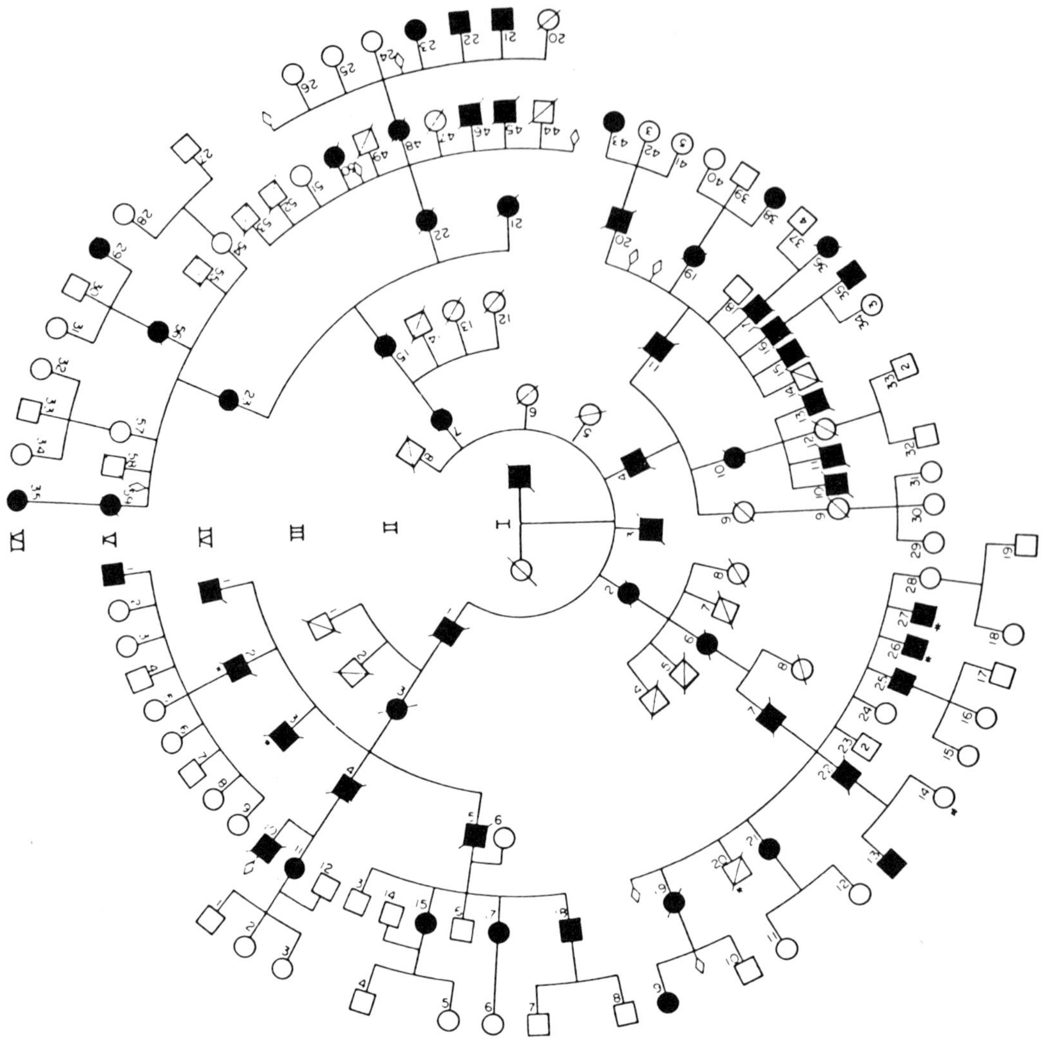

Figure 4. Pedigree of a human leukocyte antigen (HLA)-linked dominant cerebellar ataxia. Results with this and 2 other families with cerebellar ataxia yielded a lodscore of 2.128 at a recombination fraction ϕ of 0.05. In a fourth family, no HLA linkage was found. (Reprinted with permission from Pedersen L, et al: A linkage study of hereditary ataxias and related disorders. *Hum Genet* 54:371–383, 1980.)

familiar to clinicians: slight, moderate, and severe disability or deviation from normal.

Electrophysiological Techniques

Important advances continue to come from the application of electrophysiological techniques to the hereditary ataxias. Neil and coworkers (92) reported alteration in electroencephalogram (EEG) sleep tracings in OPCA. In these diseases, lesions of the pontine nuclei usually do not lead to alterations in sleep. However, all-night polygraphic recording of the EEG, horizontal electro-oculogram, and submental electromyogram (EMG) demonstrated subnormal rapid-eye movement (REM) and delta (slow-wave) sleep. Phasic eye movements were reduced out of proportion to tonic components of REM sleep. Osorio and Daroff (93) reported absence of REM and stage 4 sleep with an extremely short stage 3 and long stage 2 in 2 patients with a spinocerebellar degeneration. Both demonstrated a previously unreported sleep stage, which began after several hours of sleep and occupied 5%–7% of the total sleep time. The most common pattern in this stage consisted of high-voltage slow (4 Hz) waves during which tonic EMG activity was markedly increased. This substage usually persisted for about 1 minute but was interrupted by a brief (15–25 seconds) activated EEG of lower voltage and faster activity than in stage 1. There were no electrocardiographic or respiratory changes during any of these abnormal stages.

Most studies of evoked potentials continue to show abnormalities in hereditary ataxias. Bird and Crill (94) reported a study of pattern-reversal visual evoked potentials (PRVEP) in 19 patients with different forms of hereditary ataxias. All 5 patients with FA, 1 with dominant spastic paraparesis and 1 with recessive dentorubrospinal degeneration, had abnormal PRVEP latencies. Nine other patients had PRVEP latencies at or below the upper limit of normal. Montanini and associates (95) reported abnormal latencies in visual evoked potentials in another 15 patients with spinocerebellar degeneration. However, Fujita and coworkers (96) failed to confirm previous reports of abnormally prolonged latencies in short latency auditory evoked brain-stem potentials (BAERs) in patients with hereditary ataxias. Despite the discrepancies and variability among patients, the bulk of the evoked potential data indicate the existence of relatively widespread disease of the nervous system even in these patients with classic system degenerations. This is the expected result, since the abnormal gene is present in all cells in the body. How selective the vulnerability is depends partly on how hard one looks for damage.

Girotti and coworkers (97) used a new electrooculogram to confirm the existence of abnormal saccades in 2 patients with cerebellar ataxia, and Stanescu-Segal and Michiels (98) reported decreased amplitudes of electroretinograms in 6 patients with hereditary ataxias.

Sauer (99) confirmed the existence of abnormalities of peripheral sensory nerves in FA. In 15 of 17 patients, motor conduction velocity (MCV) was normal. The sensory nerve-action potential markedly decreased or disappeared in all cases. This picture, accordingly, corresponds to that of patients with the neuronal type of peroneal muscular atrophy. Moreover, all patients showed prolonged latencies of somatosensory evoked potential, due to a slowing of the conduction velocity via the spinobulbar tracts.

Richards and coworkers (100) reported EMG abnormalities in 17 patients. Reduced amplitude of the EMG in the medial hamstring was seen in the majority. Moreover, in patients with both types of spinal ataxia studied, dynamic strength was lower than normal when measured throughout maximum voluntary isokinetic knee movements.

THERAPY

More than a century has elapsed since Friedreich's original description of hereditary ataxias (2). Satisfactory therapy has not yet evolved (3, 29).

Dietary Therapy

Dietary therapy with precursors of neurotransmitters has been adopted for treatment of ataxia on four continents. Most intensive efforts have been with choline or choline derivatives as cholinergic agonists on the basis of experimental studies which indicate that cholinergic systems are exquisitely sensitive to derangements of carbohydrate metabolism (101).

Two of three studies with choline chloride were encouraging. Livingston and Mastaglia (102) reported improvements in upper limb coordination and other ataxic symptoms in a double-blind crossover trial, in 8 patients with spinal FA, 6 with sporadic cerebellar degeneration and 6 with cerebellar ataxia and lower limb spasticity. Clayton (103) reported beneficial effects in a 24-year-old patient in Australia. However, Philcox and Kies (104) found no beneficial effects in 6 patients with late onset, dominant ataxias.

Three reports appeared during the last year of beneficial effects of lecithin (phosphatidyl-choline). Giovannini and coworkers (105) reported beneficial effects of lecithin in 8 Italian patients with spinocerebellar degenerations. In a double-blind crossover study, Reding and coworkers (106) reported improvement on both lecithin and placebo in a boy with spinal ataxia but not in a woman with cerebellar ataxia. The placebo, a mixture of peanut butter and corn oil, could hardly have been worse. Peanut butter probably has the highest choline content of any constituent of the normal American diet. Melancon and coworkers (72) reported that 3 months of oral lecithin therapy not only improved motor performance in 9 patients with spinal FA but also reduced kinetic abnormalities in serum LAD activity. Despite the caveats about LAD discussed before, their observations provide biochemical support for the use of lecithin in such patients. Sorbi and coworkers (107) reported beneficial effects of phosphorylcholine in both spinal FA and OPCA in an open and as yet unconfirmed study.

Evidence for deficiency of neurotransmitter amino acids in ataxias logically suggest treatment with amino acid precursors. In experimental ataxia induced with 3-acetyl-pyridine, treatment with glutamate did improve gait in studies in Quebec (108, 109). We gave casein, the major protein of milk, to 3 patients because it contains high proportions of glutamate and aspartate. Treatment with up to 50 g a day had no significant effects, beneficial or harmful.

Medications

Another report appeared confirming the effectiveness of acetazolamide in hereditary intermittent ataxia (110). Unfortunately, we have found no benefit from this carbonic anhydrase inhibitor in half a dozen patients with different forms of nonintermittent ataxia.

Sobue and coworkers (111) reported effective treatment of 29 patients with hereditary ataxia with thyrotropin releasing hormone (TRH); 500 μg of TRH were injected, and eye movements were recorded within 90 minutes. The amplitude ratio of saccades normalized after TRH injection compared to saline controls. The authors proposed that the mechanism of TRH effect could be related to an improvement of abnormal noradrenaline metabolism in the cerebellum and brain stem. The clinical utility of this observation still has to be determined.

Physical Therapy and Rehabilitation

Physical therapy and rehabilitation have an important role to play in the care of these patients with chronic neurological disease, but only two papers appeared during the last year on this important subject. Pasetti and coworkers (112) studied 6 patients with spinal FA and concluded that care should emphasize psychological factors—specifically, stimulating mental activity and interpersonal relationships. They also stress the value of physical therapy analagous to that used for peripheral neuropathies and the need to follow the foot and spine deformities closely. Allard and coworkers (113), on the basis of studies of 21 patients with FA, emphasize the need to treat actively scoliosis of over 20° in growing children. They recommend bracing for curves of 30° or more and surgery for curves of 40° or more. The 30° and greater curves usually remained stable after growth ended. They also proposed a special seat for non-ambulatory patients, to retard lateral deviation of the spine.

Recommendations

Therapy for hereditary ataxias is currently in a confusing state. There is no good, established, effective therapy; not enough data to allow strong recommendations; and too many mildly encouraging reports to justify therapeutic nihilism. We tend to give lecithin (30 g a day of 25% lecithin) to patients with spinal ataxias or ataxic encephalopathies and a β-blocker (in doses which do not drive down the resting pulse) to patients with late onset cerebellar ataxias (20). In some but not all patients, results have been mildly encouraging to enthusiastic patients and physicians. Lecithin in particular appears to be associated with minimal side effects in the doses used. Even if it is only a placebo, it may have the beneficial psychological effects emphasized by Pasetti and coworkers (112).

SUMMARY

Hereditary ataxias are a challenging topic. They require at least some familiarity with classical neurological erudition in this field, as well as keeping up with a new set of data, which may ultimately prove just as complex if more in keeping with modern neurobiology. One may also hope—reasonably—that this steadily growing body of new knowledge will improve neurologists' ability to counsel and treat these patients. Probably this is an example of a common phenomenon in science—a developing field which becomes more complicated and controversial, until finally a new clarity and simplicity develop at a deeper level of knowledge.

REFERENCES

1. Blass JP: Spinocerebellar degeneration (hereditary ataxias). In *Molecular Basis of Neuropathology.* Edited by Davison A, Thompson RHS. London, Edward Arnold, 1981, pp 323–344

2. Friedreich N: Ueber degenerative atrophie der spinale hinter strange. *Virchows Arch [Pathol Anat]* 26:443–459, 1863

3. Barbeau A: Friedreich's ataxia 1980. An overview, *Can J Neurol Sci* 7:455–468, 1980

4. Blass JP, Omenn GS: Molecular neurogenetics. *Neurology* 31:172–173, 1981

5. Soerjadi MR, Sutanto AH, Saing B, et al: Friedreich's ataxia. *Paediatr Indones* 19:117–122, 1979

6. Joannette Y, Dudley JG: Dysarthric symptomatology of Friedreich's ataxia. *Brain Lang* 10:39–50, 1980

7. Robustelli Della Cuna F, Giustiniani S, Forni MC, et al: Una insolita manifestazione di interessamento cardiaco nella atassia di Friedreich: la torsione di punta. *G Ital Cardiol* 9:631–634, 1979

8. Malone S, Giunta A, Mansi D, et al: Cardiac abnormalities in Friedreich's ataxia patients and first degree relatives. *Acta Neurol (Napoli)* 35:354–366, 1980

9. Teti A, Carlomagno A, Mansi D, et al: Alterazioni cardiologiche nei familiari di pazienti con atassia di Friedreich. In *Sindromi Extrapiramidali E Sindromi Di Confine: Eredoatassie E Demenze.* Edited by Agnoli A, Bertolani G. Roma, D. Guanella, 1980, pp 46–55

10. Lamarche JB, Cote M, Lemieux B: The cardiomyopathy of Friedreich's ataxia — morphological observations in 3 cases. *Can J Neurol Sci* 7:389–396, 1980

11. Pasternac A, Krol R, Peticlerc R, et al: Hypertrophic cardiomyopathy in Friedreich's ataxia: symmetric or asymmetric? *Can J Neurol Sci* 7:379–382, 1980

12. Inoue K, Hirano A, Hasson J: Friedreich's ataxia selectively involves the large neurons of the dorsal ganglia. *Trans Am Neurol Assoc* 104:75–76, 1979

13. Marolda M, Filla A, Giordano-Lanza G, et al: I corpuscoli di Pacini nell'atassia di Friedreich. Studio preliminare. In *Sindromi Extrapiramidali E Sindromi Di Confine: Eredoatassie E Demenze.* Edited by Agnoli A, Bertolani G. Roma, D. Guanella, 1980, pp 40–45

14. Klein D: Vingt ans d'observations d'une famille atteinte de maladie de Behr (atrophie optique infantile compliquée heredo-familiale). *Rev Otoneuroophtalmol* 52:179–185, 1980

15. Crawfurd MDA, Hacourt RB, Shaw PA: Nonprogressive cerebellar ataxia, aplasia of pupillary zone of iris, and mental subnormality (Gillespie's syndrome) affecting 3 members of a non-consanguineous family in 2 generations. *J Med Genet* 16:373–378, 1979

16. Campanella G, Filla A, DeFalco F, et al: Friedreich's ataxia in the south of Italy — a clinical and biochemical survey of 23 patients. *Can J Neurol Sci* 7:351–358, 1980

17. D'Angelo A, DiDonato S, Nigro G, et al: Friedreich's ataxia in northern Italy. I. Clinical, neurophysiological and in vivo biochemical studies. *Can J Neurol Sci* 7:359-366, 1980

18. Spencer SS, Moench JC: Progressive and treatable cerebellar ataxia in macroglobulinemia. *Neurology* 30:536–538, 1980

19. Saheh M, Saroua-Pinhas I, Ohry A: Sensory ataxia as an initial symptom of systemic lupus erythematosus. *J Rheumatol* 7:420–422, 1980

20. Stewart RM, Tunell G, Ehle A: Familial spastic paraplegia, peroneal neuropathy and crural hypopigmentation: a new neurocutaneous syndrome. *Neurology* 31:754–757, 1981

21. Abdallat A, Davis SM, Farrage J, et al: Disordered pigmentation, spastic paraparesis and peripheral neuropathy in three siblings: a new neurocutaneous syndrome. *J Neurol Neurosurg Psychiatry* 43:962–966, 1980

22. Lima L, Coutinho P: Clinical criteria for diagnosis of Machado-Joseph disease: report of a non-Azorean Portuguese family. *Neurology* 30:319–322, 1980

23. Cotrufo R, Federico A, Melone MAB, et al: Associazione familiare di atassia cerebellare congenita, degenerazione tapetoretinica settoriale e insufficienza mentale. In *Sindromi Extrapiramidali E Sindromi Di Confine: Eredoatassie E Demenze.* Edited by Agnoli A, Bertolani G. Roma, D. Guanella, 1980, pp 56–64

24. Bourquin M, Korol S, Klein D: Hérédoataxie, dégénerescence tapéto-retinienne et signes dysmorphiques chez un garçon de 16 ans. *Klin MBL Augenheilk* 176:694–698, 1980

25. Franceschetti A, Klein D: Les manifestations tapé-
torétiniennes et leur importance clinique et géné-
tique dans les hérédo-ataxias. *Rev Otoneuroophtalmol* 20:109–117, 1948

26. Schott GD: Familial cerebellar ataxia presenting
with down-beat nystagmus. *J Med Genet* 17:115–
118, 1980

27. Harper PS, Marks R, Dykes PJ, et al: Ichthyosis,
hepatosplenomegaly, and cerebellar degeneration in
a sibship. *J Med Genet* 17:212–215, 1980

28. Bouchard JP, Bedard P, Bouchard R: Study of a
family with progressive ataxic tremor and severe
dystal amyotrophy. *Can J Neurol Sci* 7:345–359,
1980

29. Blass JP: Hereditary ataxias. In *Current Neurology*,
vol 3. Edited by Appel SH. New York, John Wiley,
1981, pp 66–91

30. Paterson MC, Smith PJ: Ataxia telangiectasia: an
inherited human disorder involving hypersensitivity to ionizing radiation and related DNA-
damaging chemicals. *Annu Rev Genet* 13:291–318,
1979

31. Jason JM, Gelfand EW: Diagnostic consideration
in ataxia telangiectasia. *Arch Dis Child* 54:682–686,
1979

32. Bodensteiner JB, Golblum RM, Goldman AS: Progressive dystonia masking ataxia in ataxia-telangiectasia. *Arch Neurol* 37:464–465, 1980

33. Whisbart RH, Kacena A, Golde DW, et al: Impaired cellular interactions involving lymphocytes
from patients with chronic lymphocytic leukemia
and ataxia-telangiectasia. *J Lab Clin Med* 96:114–
118, 1980

34. Shaham M, Becker Y, Cohen MM: A diffusable
clastogenic factor in ataxia telangiectasia. *Cytogenet Cell Genet* 27:155–161, 1980

35. Cohen MM, Simpson SJ: Growth kinetics of ataxia
telangiectasia lymphoblastoid cells. *Cytogenet Cell
Genet* 28:24–33, 1980

36. Weichselbaum RR, Little JB: Familial retino-
blastoma and ataxia telangiectasia. Human models
for the study of DNA damage and repair. *Cancer*
45:775–779, 1980

37. Yoshitomi F, Zaitsu Y, Tanaka K: Ataxia telangiectasia with renal cell carcinoma and hepatoma.
Virchows Arch A Path Anat Histol 389:119–125,
1980

38. Toledano SR, Lange BJ: Ataxia telangiectasia and
acute lymphoblastic leukemia. *Cancer* 45:1675–
1678, 1980

39. Aurias D, Dutrillauy B, Buriot D, et al: High
frequencies of inversion and translocations of
chromosomes 7 and 14 in ataxia telangiectasia.
Mutat Res 69:369–374, 1980

40. Al Saadi A, Palutke M, Krishna-Kumar G: Evolution of chromosomal abnormalities in sequential
cytogenetic studies of ataxia telangiectasia. *Hum
Genet* 55:23–24, 1980

41. Cramer P, Painter RB: Bleomycin-resistent DNA
synthesis in ataxia telangiectasia cells. *Nature* 291:
671–672, 1981

42. Scudiero DA: Decreased DNA repair synthesis and
defective colony-forming ability of ataxia telangiectasia fibroblasts cell strains treated with N-methyl-
N^1-nitro-N-nitrosoguanidine. *Cancer Res* 40:984–
990, 1980

43. Smith PJ, Paterson MC: Defective DNA repair and
increased lethality in ataxia telangiectasia cells exposed to 4-nitroquinoline-l-oxide. *Nature* 287:747–
749, 1980

44. Houndsworth J, Lavin MF: Effect of ionizing radiation on DNA synthesis in ataxia telangiectasia cells.
Nucleic Acids Res 8:3709–3720, 1980

45. Fornace AJ, Little JB: Normal repair of DNA
single-strand breaks in patients with ataxia telangiectasia. *Biochim Biophys Acta* 607:432–437, 1980

46. Edwards MJ, Taylor AMR: Unusual levels of
$(ADP\text{-}ribose)_N$ and DNA synthesis in ataxia telangiectasia cells following γ-ray irradiation. *Nature*
287:745–747, 1980

47. Llinas RR: The cortex of the cerebellum. *Sci Am*
232:56–71, 1975

48. Perry TL, Kish SJ, Hansen S, et al: Neurotransmitter amino acids in dominantly inherited cerebellar disorders. *Neurology* 31:237–242, 1981

49. Melancon SB, Grignon B, Ledru E, et al: The beta-
amino acid transport system in Friedreich's ataxia.
Can J Neurol Sci 7:441–446, 1980

50. Tolis G, Mehta A, Andermann E, et al: Friedreich's
ataxia and glucose tolerance. I. The effect of ingested glucose on serum glucose and insulin values
in homozygotes, obligate heterozygotes and potential carriers of the Friedreich's ataxia gene. *Can
J Neurol Sci* 7:397–400, 1980

51. Tolis G, Mehta A, Harvey G, et al: Friedreich's
ataxia and glucose tolerance. II. The effect of ingested glucose on serum growth hormone in homozygotes, obligate heterozygotes and potential carriers of the Friedreich's ataxia gene. *Can J Neurol Sci*
7:401–404, 1980

52. Draper P, Shapcott D, Langlois M, et al: Glycosylated hemoglobins in Friedreich's ataxia. *Can J
Neurol Sci* 7:405–408, 1980

53. Sander JE, Malomud N, Cowan MJ, et al: Intermittent ataxia and immuno deficiency with multiple
carboxylase deficiencies: a biotin-responsive disorder. *Ann Neurol* 8:544–547, 1980

54. Cowan MJ, Wara DW, Packman S, et al: Multiple biotin-dependent deficiencies associated with
deficits in T-cell and B-cell immunity. *Lancet* 2:
115–118, 1979

55. Blass JP: Pyruvate dehydrogenase deficiencies. In
Inherited Disorders of Carbohydrate Metabolism.
Edited by Burman D, Holton JB, Pennock CA.
Lancaster, England, MTP Press, 1980, pp 239–268

56. Bertagnolio B, Uziel G, Bottachi E, et al: Fried-

reich's ataxia in northern Italy. II. Biochemical studies in cultured cells. *Can J Neurol Sci* 7:409–412, 1980

57. Barbeau A, Davignon J: Biochemical changes in Friedreich's ataxia. *Trans Am Neurol Assoc* 104:53–54, 1979

58. Filla A, Butterworth RF, Barbeau A: Active pyruvate dehydrogenase in platelets from Friedriech's ataxia patients. *Can J Neurol Sci* 7:417–420, 1980

59. Constantopoulos G, Chang CSC, Barranger JA: Normal pyruvate dehydrogenase complex activity in patients with Friedreich's ataxia. *Ann Neurol* 8:636–639, 1980

60. Evans OB: Normal muscle pyruvate oxidation in spinocerebellar degenerations. *Ann Neurol* 1:93–94, 1981

61. Evans OB: Pyruvate oxidation by muscle fiber type following nerve crush. *Ann Neurol* 1:86, 1981

62. Sheu KFR, Hu CWC, Utter MF: Pyruvate dehydrogenase complex activity in normal and deficient fibroblasts. *J Clin Invest* 67:1463–1472, 1981

63. Sorbi S, Blass JP: Spectrophotometric measurement of pyruvate dehydrogenase complex activity in cultured human fibroblasts. *J Biochem Biophys Method* 5:169–175, 1981

64. Sorbi S, Blass JP: Spectrophotometric assay of pyruvate dehydrogenase in cultured human cells. *Trans Am Soc Neurochem* 12(1):170, 1981

65. Sorbi S, Blass JP: Abnormal activation of pyruvate dehydrogenase in Leigh disease fibroblasts. *Neurology,* 32:555–558, 1982

66. Plaitakis A, Whetsell WO, Cooper JR, et al: Chronic Leigh disease: a genetic and biochemical study. *Ann Neurol* 4:304–310, 1980

67. Kark RAP, Becker D, Perlman S: Reduced enzyme activities in inherited ataxia. *Ann Neurol* 8(3):342, 1980

68. Rodriguez-Budelli M, Kark RAP: Kinetic evidence for a structural abnormality of lipoamide dehydrogenase in two patients with Friedreich's ataxia. *Neurology* 28:1283–1296, 1978

69. Kark RAP, Rodriguez-Budelli M, Becker D, et al: Lipoamide dehydrogenase: rapid heat inactivation in platelets of patients with recessively inherited ataxia. *Neurology* 31:199–202, 1981

70. Kark RAP, Budelli MR, Perlman S, et al: Preclinical diagnosis and carrier detection in ataxia associated with abnormalities of lipoamide dehydrogenase. *Neurology* 30:502–508, 1980

71. Kark RAP, Becker DM, Perlman S: Retraction. *Ann Neurol* 9:514, 1981

72. Melancon SB, Fontaine G, Geoffroy G, et al: Correlation between serum lipoamide dehydrogenase activity and phosphatidylcholine therapy in Friedreich's ataxia. *Can J Neurol Sci* 7:413–416, 1980

73. Stumpf DA, Parks JK: Friedreich ataxia. II. Normal kinetics of lipoamide dehydrogenase. *Neurology* 29:820–826, 1979

74. Robinson BH, Sherwood WG, Kahler S, et al: Lipoamide dehydrogenase deficiency. *N Engl J Med* 304(1):53–54, 1981

75. Blass JP, Hinmman L, Soricelli A: Clinical assays of lipoamide dehydrogenase. *Neurology* 31:783–784, 1981

76. Barbeau A, Charbonneau M, Cloutier T: Leukocyte dehydrogenase activity in various hereditary ataxias. *Can J Neurol Sci* 7:421–424, 1980

77. Plaitakis A, Nicklas WJ, Desnick RJ: Glutamate dehydrogenase deficiency in three patients with spinocerebellar syndrome. *Ann Neurol* 7:297–303, 1980

78. Willner JP, Grabowski GA, Gordon RE, et al: Chronic GM_2 gangliosidosis masquerading as atypical Friedreich ataxia: clinical, morphological, and biochemical studies on one case. *Neurology* 31:787–798, 1981

79. Huang YS, Marcel YL, Vezina C, et al: Lecithin: cholesterol acyltransferase activity and fatty acid composition of erythrocyte phospholipids in Friedreich's ataxia. *Can J Neurol Sci* 7:429–434, 1980

80. Walker JL, Chamberlain S, Robinson N: Failure to detect abnormal fatty acid profiles in serum lipoproteins in Friedreich's ataxia. *Ann Neurol* 8:74–76, 1980

81. Filla A, Postiglione A, Rubba P, et al: Plasma lipoprotein concentration and erythrocyte membrane lipids in patients with Friedreich's ataxia. *Acta Neurol (Napoli)* 35:382–389, 1980

82. Hamida MB, El-Youndi C, Isautier C: Électrophorèse du liquide céphalorachidien au cours des hérédogénérescences spinocérebelleuses. Étude de III Observations. *Rev Neurol (Paris)* 136:25–32, 1980

83. Chamberlain S, Cramp WA, Lewis PP: Defects in newly synthesized DNA in skin fibroblasts from patients with Friedreich's ataxia. *Lancet* 1:1165, 1981

84. Wong P, Barbeau A: Protein kinase activity of human erythrocyte membranes in Friedreich's ataxia. *Can J Neurol Sci* 7:425–428, 1980

85. Pederson L, Platz P, Ryder LP, et al: A linkage study of hereditary ataxias and related disorders. *Hum Genet* 54:371–383, 1980

86. Morton NE, Laloued JM, Jackson JF, et al: Linkage studies in spinocerebellar ataxia (SCA 1). *Am J Med Genet* 6:251–257, 1980

87. Whittington JE, Keats BJB, Jackson JF, et al: Linkage studies on glyoxalase I (GLO), pepsinogen (PG), spinocerebellar ataxia (SCA1) and HLA. *Cytogenet Cell Genet* 28:145–150, 1980

88. Koeppen AH, Goedde HW, Hirt L, et al: Genetic *linkage in hereditary ataxia. Lancet* 1:92–93, 1980

89. Campanella G, Filla A, DeFalco FA, et al: Eredo atassie spino-cerebellari: problemi di valutazione clinica. In *Sindromi Extrapiramidali E Sindromi Di Confine: Eredoatassie E Demenze.* Edited by

Agnoli A, Bertolani, G. Roma, D. Guanella, 1980, pp 32–39

90. Filla A, Carlomagno S, DiIorlo G, et al: Studio epidemiologico delle eredoatassie spinocerebellari in Campania. In *Sindromi Extrapiramidali E Sindromi Di Confine: Eredoatassie E Demenze.* Edited by Agnoli A, Bertolani G. Roma, D. Guanella, 1980, pp 23–31

91. Pourcher E, Barbeau A: Field testing of an ataxia scoring and staging system. *Can J Neurol Sci* 7:339–344, 1980

92. Neil JF, Holzer BC, Spiker DG, et al: EEG sleep alterations in olivopontocerebellar degeneration. *Neurology* 30:660–662, 1980

93. Osorio I, Daroff RB: Absence of REM and altered NREM sleep in patients with spinocerebellar degeneration and slow saccades. *Ann Neurol* 7:277–280, 1980

94. Bird TD, Crill WE: Pattern-reversal visual evoked potentials in the hereditary ataxias and spinal degenerations. *Ann Neurol* 9:243–250, 1981

95. Montanini R, Ghezzi A, Braida A: Studio dei potenziali evocativi visivi nelle eredoatassie. In *Sindromi Extrapiramidali E Sindromi Di Confine: Eredoatassie E Demenze.* Edited by Agnoli A, Bertolani G. Roma, D. Guanella, 1980, pp 87–93

96. Fujita M, Hosoki M, Hiyazoki M: Brainstem auditory evoked responses in spinocerebellar degenerations and Wilson disease. *Ann Neurol* 9:42–47, 1981

97. Girotti F, Pederzoli M, Avanzini G, et al: Metodica elettrooculografica per la valutazione della dismetria in referimento alla evoluzione delle sindromi atassiche. In *Sindromi Extrapiramidali E Sindromi Di Confine: Eredoatassie E Demenze.* Edited by Agnoli A, Bertolani G. Roma, D. Guanella, 1980, pp 75–86

98. Stanescu-Segal B, Michiels J: Heredoataxia (spinocerebellar degenerations), ERG alterations, temporal aspects. *Ophtalmologica* 78:267–272, 1979

99. Sauer M: Somatosensible leitungsmessungen bei neurologischen systemrkrankungen. *Arch Psychiatr Nervenkr* 228:223–242, 1980

100. Richards C, Bouchard JP, Bouchard R, et al: A preliminary study of dynamic muscle function in hereditary ataxias. *Can J Neurol Sci* 7:367–378, 1980

101. Blass JP, Gibson GE, Duffy TE, et al: Cholinergic dysfunction: a common denominator in metabolic encephalopathies. In *Cholinergic Mechanisms: Phylogenetic Aspects, Central and Peripheral Synapses, and Clinical Significance.* Edited by Pepeu G, Ladinsky H. New York, Plenum Press, 1982, pp 921–928

102. Livingstone IR, Mastaglia FL: Choline chloride in the treatment of ataxia. *Br Med J* 6195:939, 1979

103. Cayton MR: Choline in treatment of ataxia. *Med J Aust* 2:402–403, 1980

104. Philcox DV, Kies B: Choline in hereditary ataxia. *Br Med J* 6190:613, 1979

105. Giovannini P, Ladinski H, Consolo S, et al: La lecitina nel trattamento delle sindromi atassiche. In *Sindromi Extrapiramidali E Sindromi Di Confine: Eredoatassie E Demenze.* Edited by Agnoli A, Bertolani G. Roma, D. Guanella, 1980, pp 65–75

106. Reding M, Blass JP, DiPonte P, et al: Lecithin in hereditary ataxias. *Neurology* 31:363–364, 1981

107. Sorbi S, Antuono P, Bracco L, et al: Atassie spinocerebellari: aspetti patogenetici e terapeutici. In *Atti Del Congresso Della Società Italiana Di Neurologia.* Catania, Italy, 1979, p 112

108. Butterworth RF, Landreiville F, Hamel E, et al: Effect of aspargine, glutamine, and insulin on cerebral amino acid neurotransmitters. *Can J Neurol Sci* 7:447–450, 1980

109. DiMichele G, Jolicoeur FB, Rondeau DB, et al: Effects of glutamate and aspartate on ataxic gait induced by 3-acetylpyridine in rats. *Can J Neurol Sci* 7:451–454, 1980

110. Wolf P: Familiare episodische ataxie. *Nervenarzt* 51:355–358, 1980

111. Sobue I, Yamamoto H, Konagaua M, et al: Effect of thyrotropin-releasing hormone on ataxia of spinocerebellar degeneration. *Lancet* 1:418–419, 1980

112. Pasetti C, Zotti AM, Villani A, et al: Valutazioni psichometriche e possibilita riabilitative nel morbo di Friedreich: considerazioni in merito allo studio di sei casi. In *Sindromi Extrapiramidali E Sindromi Di Confine: Eredoatassie E Demenze.* Edited by Agnoli A, Bertolani G. Roma, D. Guanella, 1980, pp 102–111

113. Allard P. Duhaime M, Raso JV, et al: Pathomechanics and management of scoliosis in Friedreich's ataxia patients. *Can J Neurol Sci* 7:383–388, 1980

114. DeVivo DC, Haymond MW, Obert KA, et al: Defective activation of the pyruvate dehydrogenase complex in subacute necrotizing encephalomyelopathy (Leigh disease). *Ann Neurol* 6:483–491, 1979

4
MOVEMENT DISORDERS

Robert E. Burke and Stanley Fahn

The movement disorders comprise an area of neurology in which therapeutic advances are being made and will be made at a steady pace. The clinician must be aware of new therapeutic options and controversies. The availability of specific therapeutic approaches makes diagnostic accuracy of paramount importance, so the clinician must also be aware of unusual presentations of classic movement disorders and new diagnostic entities. This chapter is devoted to recent diagnostic and therapeutic advances in these disorders, with an emphasis on present and future relevance to clinical practice.

PARKINSONIAN SYNDROMES

Parkinson's Disease

Parkinson's disease (PD) remains the best example of a movement disorder in which we have been able to develop therapy because of our understanding of the underlying biochemical alteration of dopamine deficiency. Recent advances in the treatment of PD have been rapid and diverse, ranging from the development of new ergot derivatives to new questions about the appropriate use of levodopa. The clinician needs an annual review to keep abreast of the many publications on treatment of PD, and much of this section is devoted to their review.

Although we have made advances in the treatment of PD, and the purpose of an annual review is to emphasize progress in an area, we nevertheless must avoid compla-

cency and realize that the therapeutic developments in PD have not brought answers to many fundamental questions about the disease (1). We remain in ignorance about the etiology of PD and its pathophysiological mechanisms. Our ignorance in these areas is reflected in our inability to alter the progressive course of PD, our uncertainty about its prognosis, and in controversies about symptomatic therapies. Some progress in our understanding of the etiology of PD has been made by recent studies of human leukocyte antigens (HLA) and antibodies to viruses in PD patients. We will review several recent epidemiological studies which offer some insight into the relative importance of environmental and genetic factors in the development of PD. Studies of motor control in normals and parkinsonian patients using electromyography (EMG) have been helpful in delineating the altered neurophysiology in PD, and they will be reviewed.

Etiology

There are two leading ideas about the cause of PD. One proposes that premature or accelerated aging affects pigmented neurons. This idea is based on the observation that many biochemical changes which occur in PD, such as depletion of cerebral dopamine, its metabolites, and tyrosine hydroxylase, also occur with aging. This interesting hypothesis remains unproven, and as Calne and Kebabian (1) point out, it does not readily lend itself to experimental analysis.

The second hypothesis is that PD is due to

either a viral infection or an abnormal immunological response to a viral infection. Marttila and coworkers (2) studied serum and cerebrospinal fluid (CSF) antibody titers to herpes simplex viruses (HSV) types 1 and 2 and to cytomegalovirus (CMV) using a microindirect hemagglutination test. They found that patients with idiopathic PD tended to have higher serum titers to HSV type 1 than controls. There were no differences in titers to HSV type 2 and CMV. However, there were no differences between the PD patients and controls in the CSF titers to HSV type 1. The authors point out that they have been unable to show evidence of HSV infection in PD brains using immuno-fluorescence staining and tissue culture. Furthermore, Elizan and coworkers (3) had found no difference in HSV titers in serum or CSF between PD patients and controls. Using complementary nucleic acids Wetmur and coworkers were unable to find evidence of HSV type 1 DNA in PD brains. These negative studies, and the lack of HSV type 1 antibody titer elevations in the CSF make uncertain the significance of the serum findings in the Marttila study. Thus, there is no convincing evidence to date for a viral etiology of idiopathic PD.

Elizan and coworkers (4) have studied the frequency of HLA antigens in 18 patients with postencephalitic parkinsonism. The patients were unrelated and residing in a chronic-disease hospital. Controls were 147 ethnically-matched individuals. The HLA-B14 antigen occurred in 44% of the patients and only 8% of the controls. No other significant differences were found in HLA-B, HLA-A, or HLA-C antigen frequencies. Although this association between HLA-B14 and posten-cephalitic parkinsonism may reflect a genetic susceptibility to the disease, there are other possible interpretations, as the authors point out. For example, an HLA type might be associated with ability to survive a particular disease and thus occur with higher frequency in surviving patients.

Epidemiology

The relative importance of genetic and environmental factors in the occurrence of idiopathic PD has been studied in Mediter-ranean people (5). Most prior studies of the prevalence of PD have been from Northern Europe, the United States, Australia, or New Zealand, using white populations of primarily Northern European descent. These studies have found a rather similar prevalence rate, exceeding 100 per 100,000, and it has been suggested that PD is rather uniformly distributed throughout the world. Rosati and coworkers (5) studied prevalence of PD on Sardinia, a western Mediterranean island, whose inhabitants are of mixed Southern European and North African descent. That Sardinians are genetically distinct from Northern Europeans is suggested by different HLA antigen frequencies in the two groups. Sardinians were found to have a prevalence rate of 65.6 per 100,000, which is much lower than that for Northern Europeans. This is unlikely to be due to deficient case reporting on the island. PD was evenly distributed between rural and urban areas on Sardinia, and there was no correlation between PD and occupation. The authors conclude that genetic factors are more important than environmental in the geographic distribution of PD.

Preliminary findings of a twin study of PD, however, do not suggest an important role for genetic factors. Duvoisin and coworkers (6) have studied 12 twins, confirmed to be monozygotic by study of erythrocyte anti-gens, serum protein homologies, and HLA typing. They found no twins concordant for PD. Histories revealed no differences between the twins in childhood illnesses, immunizations, injuries, infectious diseases, or toxin exposure. Interestingly, there appeared to be a difference in smoking habits; twins of probands had smoked heavily for longer. There also was an indication that consistent personality differences existed between patients and cotwins since early adult-hood, with patients being quieter, more introverted, or more serious.

The smoking behavior of PD patients was recently compared to age- and sex-matched neighbors (7). Prior studies which had shown an inverse relationship between smoking and PD suffered from use of patient controls, because there is a relationship between smoking, having an illness, and being a patient. Among 237 PD patients, 37% smoked, compared to 57% of the neighbors, a highly significant difference. The interpretation of this intriguing relationship is, of course, unclear. Although smoking may in some way prevent PD, it is also possible, as the Duvoisin and coworkers' study (6) suggests, that there are premorbid personality traits in PD patients which affect the likelihood of smoking.

Pathogenetic Mechanisms

Neurophysiology. Application of EMG to the study of motor control in simple, standardized paradigms of motor response has yielded useful information about altered physiology underlying bradykinesia, postural control, and tremor. Hallett and Khoshbin have studied ballistic movements in PD patients in a simple elbow-flexion task (8). Ballistic movements are defined as fast movements which are so brief that the agonist ceases firing before the end of the movement. Ballistic movements have a different pattern of motor unit behavior than slower ramp movements; they have a triphasic EMG pattern with a burst first in the agonist (Ag1), followed by a burst in the antagonist while the agonist is silent (An1), followed by a second burst in the agonist (Ag2). Normal individuals are able to make ballistic movements over varying distances with a single triphasic cycle. They increase the amount of muscle activity (EMG amplitude) during a burst to cover greater distances; they do not change the duration of the EMG burst. Hallett and Khoshbin found in bradykinetic PD patients that the amount of EMG activity during a burst was not increased, and consequently, to perform ballistic movements over greater distances, the patients had to repeat triphasic cycles, sometimes up to five cycles for a longer distance. Thus, PD patients have a normal triphasic cycle EMG pattern, with normal burst durations during a ballistic movement, but an abnormal low amplitude EMG during longer movements. These observations rather nicely correspond to the kinematic observations in PD patients made by Flowers (9), who noted that short ballistic movements are done with normal speed, but longer ones are done more slowly. These findings lead Hallett and Khoshbin to suggest that the basal ganglia may play a role in energizing a muscle for a particular movement—that is, selecting it for use and setting its absolute amplitude for activity.

Evarts and coworkers (10) studied reaction time and movement time in PD patients. Although a slow reaction time tends to correlate with slow movement time (i.e., bradykinesia), it may be impaired in the absence of bradykinesia and vice versa. In general, movement time is more profoundly impaired than reaction time.

Traub and coworkers (11) have studied postural reflexes in patients with PD. They found that when normal individuals are standing and pulling with arms against a resistance, a sudden increase in the resistance will elicit EMG activity in the gastrocnemius, which prevents the patient from being pulled off balance forward. The response occurs at 80 msec, the speed of a reflex response rather than a volitional one. The response occurs before the leg is moved, and therefore does not depend on muscle stretch, nor is it eliminated by intravenous local anesthetic which abolishes the ankle jerk reflex. The authors suggest that this anticipatory reflex is driven by central mechanisms, which are activated by afferent input from the stretched arm. This anticipatory reflex was absent or reduced in many PD patients, especially those with postural instability. The absence of this reflex, however, cannot be equated with clinical postural instability, because 8 of 18 patients with clinical instability had normal anticipatory reflexes. Also, 4 patients with progressive supranuclear palsy with clinical instability had normal anticipatory reflexes. The authors conclude that although this reflex may not be necessary or sufficient to maintain balance, it may be important in fine postural adjustments.

As the methodology for studying tremor in PD becomes more sophisticated, the issues have become more complex. It seems that there are as many questions raised as are answered. Lance and coworkers (12) studied tremor in PD patients with EMG techniques and found that action tremor at a frequency of 6-12 hertz (Hz) is common in PD.

Cogwheeling is usually elicited at these frequencies rather than at the lower frequencies of rest tremor. They proposed that the action tremor of PD may be an exaggeration of physiological tremor.

Recently, Findley and coworkers (13) have studied oscillatory motor phenomena (tremors, cogwheeling, and clonus) in PD patients using linear accelerometers, surface EMGs, and a digital computer to compute power spectra of accelerometer data. They found that there are several types of tremor which they defined by frequency analysis. The classic rest tremor of PD has a frequency of 4-5.3 Hz, and although it is typically present at rest, it is also present in some patients on posture holding. Many patients also have postural tremor, with a frequency of 6-6.2 Hz, which is typically present on posture holding but may be present at rest. These two tremors can be present simultaneously and independently in an individual patient, as shown by harmonically unrelated peaks in the power spectra of accelerometer data. More than 80% of patients had tremors at both frequencies. Typically, however, only one of them will be symptomatic in an individual patient.

Cogwheeling is elicited at two frequencies: 6 Hz, which corresponds to the postural tremor frequency, and 7.5-9 Hz, which corresponds to the frequency of physiological tremor. These two frequencies of cogwheeling may be simultaneously present in an individual patient. In this study, Findley and coworkers equate active cogwheeling (cogwheeling during movement initiated by the patient) with action tremor and note that active cogwheeling, like passive cogwheeling, occurs at two frequencies, 6 Hz and 7.5-9 Hz. Since only the higher frequency is likely to be an exaggeration of physiological tremor, the authors are only in partial agreement with Lance and coworkers (12), who proposed that the action tremor and cogwheeling of PD represent exaggerated physiological tremor.

Findley and coworkers (13) are thus classifying the tremor phenomena of PD into three frequency bands (4-5.3 Hz, 6 Hz, and 7.5-9 Hz), which have varied relationships to the phenomena which we have traditionally defined by bedside maneuvers: tremor at rest, postural tremor, action tremor, and cogwheeling. Whereas their approach may represent a more fundamental and precise approach to these phenomena, its reproducibility needs assessment, and it must be carefully translated into clinically observable phenomena.

Neurochemistry and Neuropharmacology. Although there is no doubt that dopamine is depleted in the brains of PD patients, and that levodopa ameliorates many of the symptoms of parkinsonism, the precise mechanism whereby levodopa achieves this benefit is unclear. Melamed and coworkers (14-16) have attempted to determine where in the striatum levodopa is decarboxylated to dopamine. They reject the idea that exogenous dopa is converted to dopamine only in the surviving dopaminergic nigrostriatal neurons. Exogenous levodopa can increase striatal dopamine levels even after near total destruction of nigrostriatal neurons (15). Furthermore, the efficacy of levodopa is not negatively correlated with initial severity of disease, and levodopa has efficacy in postencephalitic parkinsonism, in which there is often an extreme reduction of dopaminergic neurons. Possible alternative sites of decarboxylation could be in serotonergic or noradrenergic terminals, which contain dopa decarboxylase. However, the striatum contains few, if any noradrenergic terminals, and these authors have shown that lesions of serotonergic neurons do not reduce striatal dopa decarboxylase activity (14). Brain capillaries contain dopa decarboxylase, but the enzyme at this site is outside the blood-brain barrier and unlikely to influence cerebral dopamine levels. A final possible site of levodopa conversion to dopamine is within striatal neurons. Melamed and coworkers (16) have shown that kainic acid lesions, which affect only striatal efferent and interneurons, produce a 20% decline in striatal dopa decarboxylase activity, without affecting dopaminergic neurons. Striatal neurons are therefore a possible site of conversion of exogenous levodopa to dopamine in PD patients.

The discovery of dopamine agonist properties of ergot derivatives has led to the current concept that there are at least two dopamine receptors in brain: a D-1 receptor, which is associated with adenylate cyclase, and a D-2 receptor, which is not (17). This scheme is based on the observations that ergot derivatives such as bromocriptine inhibit prolactin release and have dopamine agonist properties in animal models of parkinsonism but do not stimulate dopamine-sensitive adenylate cyclase. The existence of different dopamine receptors creates the possibility that selective agents for them may improve our therapy for PD by providing benefit with fewer adverse effects. However, this possibility has not yet been realized in clinical practice. The relative roles of D-1 and D-2 receptors in parkinsonian symptoms and levodopa-induced adverse effects are not clearly defined. Schachter and coworkers (18) recently reported that the motor effects of dopamine agonists probably depend more on interaction with D-2 receptors, because ergots (e.g., bromocriptine and lisuride) are agonists only at D-2 receptors, and selective D-2 blockers (e.g., sulpiride and tiapride) block levodopa-induced motor improvement. However, cis-flupenthixol, which has D-1 antagonist effects in striatum, also appeared to block levodopa-induced improvement. Furthermore, the motor effects of levodopa, bromocriptine, and lisuride were similar despite different effects of these drugs on D-1 and D-2 receptors.

Involvement of dopaminergic systems in PD other than the well-described nigro-striatal system has been the subject of two recent studies. Javoy-Agid and Agid (19) have shown that the ventral tegmental area of the human mesencephalon is rich in tyrosine hydroxylase, which is most likely present in dopaminergic neurons. Enzyme activity in this area was decreased in PD patients. It is possible, therefore, that in human, as in rat, there is a tegmental dopaminergic system which projects to cortical areas (the so-called mesocortical system). Depletion of dopamine in this system may relate to some of the cognitive and affective changes observed in PD.

Lawton and MacDermott (20) have shown that PD patients do not show normal levodopa inhibition of thyrotropin releasing hormone (TRH)-induced prolactin release, suggesting that hypothalamic-hypophyseal dopaminergic pathways may be abnormal.

Clinical Signs. There is now agreement that dementia occurs with increased frequency in PD, but the clinical features and the pathological substrate of the dementia are not precisely known. On the one hand, it has been suggested on clinical grounds that in PD lesions of subcortical nuclear structures may be responsible for a subcortical dementia, as described for progressive supranuclear palsy (21). On the other hand, Alvord and associates (22) have suggested, on the basis of pathology, that the demented PD patient may have coexisting Alzheimer's disease. Recently, Hakim and Mathieson have shown an association between Lewy bodies and Alzheimer changes (23).

Two recent studies are relevant to these issues. In a postmortem analysis, Boller and coworkers (24) selected 36 patients with pathologically verified PD and retrospectively reviewed clinical data for the presence of dementia. The brains were independently reviewed for the presence of Alzheimer changes. Of the 36 patients, 16 had clinical dementia; 9, severe; and 7, mild. All 9 patients with severe dementia had histological changes of Alzheimer's disease, and 3 of the 7 mildly demented patients had such changes. A control population of random autopsies had a prevalence of 5% of dementia and Alzheimer changes, compared to 33% in the PD group. The authors conclude that there may be two forms of PD. One is characterized clinically by typical PD signs and dementia, and pathologically by subcortical parkinsonian changes and cortical Alzheimer changes. The other is characterized clinically by PD signs in the absence of dementia and pathologically by subcortical changes only.

Sroka and coworkers (25) have studied dementia in PD patients in relation to atypical clinical features and computed tomography (CT) scan abnormalities. They classified 93 PD patients as typical or atypical on the basis of pyramidal tract signs, cerebellar or brain stem signs, or an unusual clinical evolution. These 93 patients were evaluated for presence of dementia, and all patients had CT scans, which were reviewed independently of their clinical status. Controls were 72 age-matched patients with normal neurological examinations. Typical PD patients (N = 71) had dementia in 15% of cases and abnormal CT scans in 56% of cases, whereas atypical patients (N = 22) were demented in 68% of cases and had abnormal CT scans in 91% of cases. Disease duration did not correlate with either mental status or scan findings. There was no difference in the age profile of the typical and atypical groups. The authors suggest that there are 2 groups of PD patients. Atypical patients tend to have dementia and abnormal CT scans (usually ventricular enlargement or cortical atrophy), and typical patients tend to have normal intellect and CT scans which are no more frequently abnormal than those of a control population. These latter patients may be the ones originally described by James Parkinson.

The conclusion of these two studies, that there may be two forms of PD, one associated with dementia, atypical signs, abnormal CT scans and Alzheimer changes, and the other a more pure parkinsonian syndrome, is reminiscent of the conclusion drawn by Lieberman and colleagues (26) in their study of dementia in PD. They noted that nondemented patients tended to have a younger age of onset and were more likely to develop clinical fluctuations during levodopa therapy. Similarly, Granerus and associates (27) in a study of patients with on-off phenomenon noted that they tended to be younger and to be less often demented. Sroka and coworkers (25) did not find any age difference between their typical and atypical patients.

It is not possible at this point to reconcile these different conceptions of two types of PD patients, but collectively these studies represent growing evidence that there may be two forms of PD. The evidence is enough at this point that future studies of any aspect of PD must try to recognize the possible existence of different forms of the disease.

A number of studies have suggested that depression frequently occurs in PD (28, 29). Mayeux and coworkers (30) studied the prevalence of depression among PD patients and the relationship between depression and specific aspects of the disease. Fifty-five consecutive PD patients, excluding those with overt dementia, were assessed neurologically, neuropyschologically with a mini-

mental state examination, and psychiatrically with the Beck Depression Inventory. Spouses were used as controls. Depression was present in 47% of patients and in only 13% of controls. There was a small but significant correlation between severity of depression and severity of PD. Degree of intellectual impairment also correlated with severity of depression. The question arises as to whether depression may not be secondary to having a chronic neurological illness, and whether comparison to spouses would control for such a relationship. The authors cite other studies which used other medical illnesses as controls and which also found an increased prevalence of depression in PD. They also point out that 43% of their depressed patients were depressed before the clinical onset of PD.

Nausieda and coworkers (31) have studied dystonia affecting the feet in PD patients. They describe the dystonic foot response of parkinsonism as a tonic extension of the great toe, arching of the sole of the foot with flexion of the toes, inversion of the foot, or extension at the ankle. They observed this response in 24 of 73 (33%) of consecutive PD patients screened for it. Prior to therapy, 6 patients (8%) had dystonic foot response, but the prevalence did increase with longer duration of therapy. Half of the patients treated for 8 years had the response. Walking elicited the response in 33% of patients. Other forms of stimulation (e.g., stroking the plantar surface of the sole) failed to elicit the response, and for this reason, the authors distinguish parkinsonian foot dystonia from the tonic foot response which has been described with frontal lobe disease. The dystonic foot response of parkinsonism was painful in 58% of patients. Interestingly, baclofen lessened the problem in 7 patients.

The phenomenon of sudden, transient "freezing" in PD is not well understood. It can be a most debilitating problem, as it often is not improved by levodopa. Stern and coworkers (32) have examined some of the clinical aspects of this problem. Patients and their families often describe the problem as being suddenly frozen to the spot, until the ability to move returns with equal abruptness. The episodes often are linked with an external trigger such as people or obstacles in the path, surprise or sudden anxiety, or a change in the texture of the walking surface. The episodes tend to occur when the patient is tired, and they can culminate in a fall. Many patients have tricks to try to overcome the periods of immobility, such as walking sideways, sliding a foot back and then throwing it forward, marching to command, or singing a march. Stern and colleagues note the ineffectiveness of levodopa in dealing with these episodes; indeed, Fahn and associates have suggested that freezing may at times be induced by excessive levodopa (33).

Guiloff and coworkers (34) draw attention to an interesting neuro-ophthalmological observation in 2 PD patients. These patients, aged 72 and 75, showed transient supra-nuclear ophthalmoplegia during intercurrent infection which led to an erroneous initial diagnosis of progressive supranuclear palsy. In both, the ophthalmoplegia cleared with treatment of the infection, and the correct diagnosis of PD became apparent.

Klawans has described a new syndrome of hemiparkinsonism as a late complication of hemiatrophy (35). At the ages 31 to 40, 4 men with hemiatrophy, presumably due to hemispheric injury in early life, developed parkinsonism on the atrophied side. Two patients had CT scans which were normal. The parkinsonism has remained unilateral for 5 to 35 years and has been minimally progressive. There was minimal benefit from levodopa. The pathogenesis of this syndrome, which occurs many years after a presumably static cerebral insult, is unknown. This phenomenon resembles the delayed onset of another movement disorder, dystonia, which has recently been described and which occurs years after presumably static insults (see **DYSTONIA**).

Two short reports have described parkinsonism in association with disorders of calcium metabolism and calcification of the basal ganglia. Margolin and coworkers (36) reported 2 women aged 64 and 84 with parkinsonism associated with hyperparathyroidism and bilateral basal ganglia calcification. The occurrence of parkinsonism and basal ganglia calcification with hypoparathyroidism has been described, but this is the first report of their occurrence with hyper-

parathyroidism. Berger and Ross (37) described a woman who underwent thyroidectomy at age 39 and who presented at age 62 with parkinsonism, a serum calcium level of 4.2 mg/100 ml, a parathormone level < 10 μlEq per milliliter (normal 10 to 150), and bilateral basal ganglia calcification. The parkinsonism resolved completely with restoration of normal calcium levels, unlike most previously described cases.

Usually, calcification of the basal ganglia is asymptomatic. Brannan and coworkers (38) reviewed 38 cases of basal ganglia calcification detected by CT scan and found that only 1 had parkinsonism, an 81-year-old woman who responded well to levodopa. Two patients (5%) had hypoparathyroidism with no basal ganglia signs. Koller and coworkers (39) examined 4219 consecutive CT scans and found basal ganglia calcification in 14 (0.33%). PD was present in 1 patient who had a minimal response to levodopa. No patients had abnormal calcium metabolism. Murphy (40) reviewed 7081 CT scans and found 53 (0.75%) with basal ganglia calcification. Of these 75% occurred in patients older than 50 years. One patient had PD. Serum calcium and phosphorus levels were normal in 46 patients who had these tests done. Basal ganglia calcification in younger patients was associated with a history of cranial irradiation in 5. Thus, calcification of the basal ganglia, especially in older patients, is often asymptomatic and infrequently associated with disturbances of calcium metabolism. Nevertheless, such calcification can occur in hypo- or hyperparathyroidism, in pseudohypoparathyroidism, in a levodopa-resistant form of parkinsonism, and in familial calcification of the basal ganglia, which may be associated with chorea or parkinsonism (41). Therefore, basal ganglia calcification has to be interpreted in the clinical context.

Williams and coworkers (42) reported the presence of oligoclonal bands in the cerebrospinal fluid (CSF) of 2 patients who developed parkinsonism 10 and 2 years after probable encephalitis at ages 19 and 49, respectively. Analysis of CSF for oligoclonal bands therefore may be of help in differentiating idiopathic PD from postencephalitic parkinsonism.

Treatment

Levodopa. It has been 13 years since the introduction of high-dosage levodopa to treat PD (43). Controversy continues to exist about its appropriate use, particularly about how soon and how much levodopa should be used early in the management of PD. Fahn and Calne (44) suggested that not all patients with PD should be treated with as much levodopa as possible at the outset of their disease, because levodopa appears to have a limited period of maximum usefulness in most patients (45). Rather, levodopa should be utilized only when it is needed to help preserve important motor functions required for competence at work or for a satisfactory home life. In support of this idea Lesser and coworkers (46) found in a retrospective analysis of levodopa therapy in 146 PD patients that those treated longer with levodopa were more impaired than patients treated for shorter periods, even when matched for duration of disease and clinical stage at the start of levodopa therapy. The authors indicate, however, that prospective study is required to confirm this point.

This conservative approach to the use of levodopa has been challenged by Markham and Diamond (47). They conducted a longitudinal study of 58 PD patients treated with maximum tolerated doses of levodopa (mean daily dose 4.77 g). They grouped patients according to duration of disease prior to initiation of levodopa therapy: group 1—symptoms for 1 to 3 years (N = 19); group 2—symptoms for 4 to 6 years (N = 16); group 3—symptoms for 7 to 9 years (N = 23). They serially evaluated patients in these groups for 6 years of therapy. They found that the determinant of disability was duration of disease and not duration of therapy. For example, group 1 patients who had disease for 8 years, and levodopa therapy for 6 years, had a disability score very similar to group 2 patients during their eighth year of disease who at that point had been on levodopa for only 3 years. They found on a plot of PD disability score (dependent variable) against years since onset of disease (independent variable) that a line connecting pre-levodopa scores of the 3 groups ran precisely parallel to a plot of their progression of disease with levodopa treatment. In other words, disability in a group at any particular year of disease was equal to disability from progression of the disease minus the amount of improvement provided by levodopa therapy, and that amount stayed constant regardless of duration of therapy. The authors also found that incidence of choreoathetosis did not differ among the 3 groups at any time in the 6 treatment years. They did not investigate other types of involuntary movement. Of their 58 patients, only 5 (8%) developed the on-off effect. They fault the Lesser and coworkers' study in its retrospective nature and insensitivity of scales used to assess disability.

The clinician at this point is in the unfortunate position of not having a clear consensus from investigators of PD on this very important and fundamental issue. For the present, the decision about when to start levodopa and how much to use will have to depend on the clinician's personal judgment and assessment of the conflicting data. While it would be unfair for us to take the opportunity provided by this review to unilaterally air our views on this issue, it is appropriate to point out at least two reservations about the Markham and Diamond study. It is troubling that they report only an 8% incidence of on-off fluctuation in their patients. This figure is considerably less than that reported by other investigators: 47% at 5 years (Sweet and McDowell [48]); 60% at 7 to 9 years (Rinne and coworkers [49]). Fluctuation in performance is a major source of disability late in the course of levodopa therapy (50), which has been related to duration of therapy (46, 51). Why Markham and Diamond have encountered this problem so infrequently is not clear. It is also troublesome that they do not note a progressive increase in the incidence of abnormal involuntary movements during treatment. Again, this is a major source of disability late in the treatment of PD which has been noted by most workers to become more frequent with longer duration of therapy (48, 51, 52). Whether or not levodopa efficacy diminishes simply as a result of disease progression as Markham and Diamond suggest, or also because of levodopa therapy itself, as others believe (45, 46), will be best answered by a prospective study of high- and low-dose levodopa in matched PD patients, which has yet to be done. It is noteworthy that in a prospective, long-term study of bromocriptine used as the only therapeutic agent in PD, no patients have yet developed fluctuation of performance (53).

Several investigators have found levodopa drug holidays to be useful in the management of late complications of levodopa therapy. Weiner and coworkers (54) studied 16 patients aged 50 to 81, treated with levodopa for 2 to 9 years. Levodopa was decreased to one-half dosage for 5 days, then discontinued for 5 to 7 days. After the holiday, many patients were improved in functional disability scores and had fewer levodopa adverse effects. Twenty to thirty percent of patients did not benefit from the holiday. This group of investigators found on long-term follow-up that there was a gradual return to a preholiday level over 1 year (55). Six patients had resolution of levodopa-induced hallucinations after the holiday, and four of them remained asymptomatic at 1 year. Direnfeld and coworkers (56) have likewise found a drug holiday to be beneficial. Complications, such as aspiration, from severe parkinsonism could occur during the holiday. Whether a drug holiday is a useful approach to the long-term management of loss of levodopa efficacy and levodopa adverse effects compared to simply reducing the dosage of levodopa remains to be determined. Why a drug holiday works is not known. Weiner and coworkers (54) speculated that dopamine receptor changes induced by long-term levodopa therapy, which may relate to loss of efficacy and increased sensitivity to adverse effects, might be reversed by a holiday. It should be pointed out that if Markham and Diamond's (47) analysis of disability in PD is correct, that is, if it is solely determined by progression of disease and not by prolonged levodopa therapy, then it would be very difficult to understand why a levodopa holiday should lead to an improvement in disability.

Hoehn studied the effect of increased daily dosage of carbidopa in patients receiving less than 750 mg/day levodopa (57). The rationale for her study was that between 75 and 150 mg carbidopa a day are required to inhibit peripheral dopa decarboxylation, and a patient unable to tolerate more than 750 mg/day of levodopa in a fixed 1:10 (carbidopa:levodopa) preparation is therefore not receiving an adequate amount of carbidopa. She studied 21 patients who had PD for a mean of 8.9 years. Their carbidopa dose was increased by about twofold after 15 months treatment, whereas levodopa dose remained about the same. There was a significant improvement in their neurological deficit score with a reduction of gastrointestinal complaints and orthostatic hypotension. Her study suggests that patients who cannot tolerate more than 750 mg levodopa in 1:10 preparations are likely to benefit from higher ratios, such as the recently available 25/100 mg form.

Dopaminergic Agonists. Bromocriptine has proven efficacy in the treatment of PD (58), but its precise role in the practical management of PD patients is still being clarified. Bromocriptine does not appear to be superior to levodopa as a primary drug for PD. Stern and coworkers (53) have treated 40 PD patients with bromocriptine as their initial and only therapy. At 2 years 23 patients had stopped bromocriptine; 19 of these subsequently responded to levodopa. Ten patients were still taking bromocriptine alone and had an overall benefit similar to that experienced with levodopa, but, interestingly, dyskinesias and fluctuations of performance have not been observed. Godwin-Austin (59) studied 24 patients, who had initially responded to levodopa, in a double-blind crossover trial comparing levodopa to bromocriptine. He found no significant difference between the response to levodopa and bromocriptine. He points out that there has been no investigation finding bromocriptine alone superior to levodopa alone. Duvoisin and coworkers (60) compared bromocriptine alone to levodopa (and carbidopa) and found levodopa to be substantially more effective than bromocriptine.

If bromocriptine has not supplanted levodopa as the primary therapy for PD, should it, nevertheless, be tried in patients who are primary levodopa failures—that is, who do not respond to or cannot tolerate levodopa? Experience indicates that bromocriptine usually does not help in this situation (59). For example, Stern and coworkers (53) found that none of their 18 levodopa failures received significant benefit from bromocriptine. There are some reports, however, of response to bromocriptine in primary levodopa failures (61), so a trial of bromocriptine may be worthwhile, depending on the clinical circumstances.

The role of bromocriptine is probably as an adjunct to levodopa therapy when complications arise, although there are disagreements about the benefits provided by bromocriptine even in this setting. Lieberman and coworkers (62, 63) added bromocriptine to a levodopa regimen in patients who were becoming increasingly disabled despite optimal levodopa therapy. They found an improvement in motor performance and a great improvement in fluctuations; time spent in "on" periods increased by 57%, and time in "off" periods decreased by 45% (62). Fahn and coworkers (61) found that 6 of 11 patients with fluctuations improved. Only 3 of these patients maintained sustained benefit. Stern and coworkers (53), however, found that none of their 14 patients with oscillations of performance improved.

From their experience with bromocriptine in 130 PD patients treated during 5 years, Calne and coworkers (17) have the impression that the major indication for bromocriptine is as an adjunct to levodopa in patients with severe levodopa-induced dyskinesia. They give an initial test dose of 1 mg, since some patients initially develop significant hypotension. They gradually increase the dosage to a range of 40 to 90 mg/day over 6 to 10 weeks. Previous dosage of levodopa should be gradually decreased as bromocriptine is increased. Adverse reactions include psychiatric symptoms (confusion, hallucinations, and personality change [64]), nausea, cardiac arrhythmias, abnormal liver function tests, and an erythromelagia-like syndrome.

Lisuride is an ergot derivative which acts as a dopamine agonist at D-2 receptors. Unlike levodopa and bromocriptine, it has motor effects which are independent of the formation or presence of dopamine stores (65). Lisuride also has complex actions on serotonin receptors (66). Intravenous administration of lisuride demonstrated antiparkinsonian efficacy in patients with idiopathic, postencephalitic, and drug-induced parkinsonism (65). A study of oral lisuride likewise demonstrated efficacy (66). Like bromocriptine and levodopa, lisuride induced psychiatric symptoms (66) and involuntary movements (65). In the study by Gopinathan and associates (66), drowsiness occurred in 9 of 20 patients and was a persistent problem in 4. Whether lisuride offers any advantage over levodopa and bromocriptine remains to be studied.

Another dopamine agonist ergot derivative, pergolide, was the subject of an encouraging report by Lieberman and coworkers (67) who studied 13 nonambulatory PD patients no longer responsive to levodopa, bromocriptine, or lergotrile. Pergolide had considerable efficacy in these advanced patients. Nine patients completed the initial trial and remained on pergolide at 10 months. These 9 patients were incapacitated and homebound before treatment; during treatment 8 of them could leave their homes independently. Three patients developed psychiatric symptoms, one requiring discontinuation of pergolide. Pergolide appears to be a promising new drug, and it undoubtedly will be studied carefully to determine the extent of its efficacy and its role in the management of PD.

Other Therapeutic Approaches. Dopamine is catabolized in brain by monoamine oxidase (MAO) and catechol-*O*-methyltransferase (COMT). To try to prolong the action of dopamine in brain, MAO inhibitors were used in treating PD in the early 1960s, but they occasionally caused severe hypertensive crises and significant morbidity. It is now recognized that there are two forms of MAO, MAO A and MAO B, and the latter is more selectively involved in dopamine catabolism. Deprenyl, a selective inhibitor of MAO B, does not cause hypertensive reactions. It also increases cerebral dopamine levels with minimal effect on other transmitters.

Deprenyl has been studied for possible efficacy in treating fluctuations in performance late in the course of levodopa therapy. In a double-blind trial, Schacter and associates (68) found that deprenyl frequently diminished end-of-dose deteriorations in performance. However, in patients with random fluctuations in performance, unrelated to dose, deprenyl seemed to exacerbate the response swings. Eisler and colleagues (69) studied 11 patients and did not find substantial benefit from deprenyl. They do not specify how many of their patients had fluctuations in performance or what type of fluctuation they had—that is, end-of-dose or random—but they report that on-off phenomenon increased in 3 patients. The apparent difference in the results of these two studies may relate to lack of precision and confusion that surrounds use of the term "on-off." Deprenyl will need to be studied in larger groups of patients with careful definition of the types of fluctuation under study.

There have been reports that electroconvulsive therapy (ECT) has a beneficial effect on motor performance in depressed patients with PD (70). Balldin and coworkers (71) studied the effect of ECT on 5 PD patients with on-off fluctuations. All 5 patients improved after ECT, 3 considerably, 2 slightly. Improvement seemed unrelated to coexistent depression. Ward and associates (72), however, studied 5 patients, without depression or dementia, who had random fluctuations in motor performance. None of them showed any improvement in parkinson disability, mental state, or fluctuations. They suggest that prior reports of benefit were probably related to relief of depression by ECT.

Summary
We do not have much further insight into the cause of PD, except that there are a growing number of negative studies that have sought evidence for an underlying viral infection. A study of HLA antigens in patients with postencephalitic parkinsonism has found an increased frequency of HLA-B14, indicating that there may be a genetic susceptibility to that disease. There may also be a genetic factor in the development of idiopathic PD,

as suggested by the low incidence of PD in Mediterranean people. A preliminary study of PD in identical twins, however, has not found evidence for a genetic factor. Several studies indicate that the incidence of smoking is less in PD patients, but the significance of the finding is not clear.

EMG techniques used to study simple motor paradigms have been very useful in elucidating the pathophysiological mechanisms underlying the signs of PD. Bradykinesia appears to be related to an inability of the PD patient to increase the amount of muscle activity during a single triphasic agonist-antagonist-agonist cycle which occurs with ballistic movements. The patient consequently must repeat cycles to perform long ballistic movements, which results in slower movement. Anticipatory postural reflexes are often absent in PD, and this may be one factor in postural instability. Spectral analysis of accelerometer tracings has identified three tremor frequencies in PD, two of which (4-5.3 Hz and 6 Hz) may cause tremor at rest, and two of which (6 Hz and 8-9 Hz) are associated with cogwheeling and action tremor.

There is evidence that dopa may be decarboxylated to dopamine in striatal neurons in PD. It is decarboxylated there rather than in remaining dopaminergic terminals or other monaminergic terminals.

There is growing evidence that there may be two forms of idiopatic PD. One is more often associated with dementia, CT scan abnormalities, atypical clinical features, and probably with Alzheimer changes at autopsy. The other is less often associated with dementia and CT abnormalities and may be the group of patients originally described by James Parkinson.

Levodopa is the primary therapy of clinically significant PD, but there is disagreement about when in the course of the disease to start it, and how much to use. Some investigators believe that levodopa has a limited period of optimum usefulness, which is best reserved for treatment of significant disability and that chronic levodopa therapy results in complications, which are difficult to treat, such as fluctuations in response and dyskinesias. Others question the concept of a limited period of usefulness of levodopa and encourage its use in maximum tolerated doses early in the course of the disease. The issue needs to be studied in a long-term prospective trial.

Bromocriptine has some usefulness as an adjunct to levodopa therapy, when fluctuations in response and dyskinesias due to levodopa become problematic. Pergolide and lisuride are promising new ergot derivatives for the treatment of PD.

Shy-Drager Syndrome

Studies of neurological autonomic failure syndromes (not associated with peripheral neuropathy) suffer at present from a lack of agreement on their classification. For example, Polinsky and coworkers (73) distinguish between idiopathic orthostatic hypotension (IOH), which is not associated with other neurological signs (74), and Shy-Drager syndrome (75) [or multiple system atrophy] which is. They present pharmacological data that distinguish the two. Others lump IOH and Shy-Drager syndrome (76) and instead recognize a classification based on clinical and pathological features (77). This latter approach proposes that there are two types of autonomic failure syndrome. One either occurs in isolation or with signs of parkinsonism, and at autopsy shows Lewy-type inclusion bodies in pigmented nuclei. The second type occurs with multiple neurological signs (e.g., cerebellar) with or without parkinsonism. At autopsy this type shows cell loss at a variety of sites (striatum, substantia nigra, pons, cerebellum), but no Lewy-type inclusions. These differences in classification stem from our ignorance of the etiology and fundamental pathophysiology of these syndromes, and at present the best one can do is to keep both classifications in mind until a better understanding resolves the differences.

Polinsky and associates (73) have studied 21 patients with orthostatic hypotension by norepinephrine, tyramine, and angiotensin infusion. They found different responses to these infusions between IOH and Shy-Drager syndrome patients. IOH patients had lower resting levels of serum norepinephrine and a greater blood pressure response to infused norepinephrine, compatible with norepinephrine denervation supersensitivity. In response to tyramine infusion, which releases endogenous norepinephrine, IOH patients had lower increases in plasma norepinephrine levels than Shy-Drager patients. These results suggest that IOH is associated with degeneration of post-ganglionic norepinephrine-containing neurons, whereas Shy-Drager syndrome is associated with degeneration of central neurons. These results are consistent with those obtained by Kontos and coworkers (78) and Ziegler and coworkers (79). Kontos's group has strengthened the argument by showing that catecholamine specifie fluroescence is absent in sympathetic nerves of patients with IOH. One possible conceptual problem with this seemingly valid approach to classification of autonomic failure syndromes is that not infrequently patients will clinically have IOH for up to 10 years (80) before they develop other neurological signs that make a diagnosis of Shy-Drager syndrome more appropriate. As Polinsky and associates state, longitudinal study of these patients is needed.

Oppenheimer (81) measured cell loss in the intermediolateral columns of the thoracic cord in patients with progressive autonomic failure. Using cell-counting techniques he showed that all cases of autonomic failure showed severe loss. Interestingly, three cases of multiple system atrophy without autonomic failure had lost an intermediate number of cells. He reaffirms the belief that there are two types of autonomic failure, as described above (77). He points out that the average age at death is different for the two groups: 72 years for the autonomic failure with parkinsonism group; 58 years for the autonomic failure with multiple-neurological-signs group.

Khurana and associates (76) have emphasized that cholinergic autonomic dysfunction may be a major source of disability in Shy-Drager syndrome patients, causing constipation, urinary symptoms, and impotence. They documented such dysfunction in 2 patients. They had some success in managing bowel and bladder symptoms in their patients with use of oral bethanechol chloride, a muscarinic agonist, which does not cross the blood-brain barrier.

CHOREIC SYNDROMES

Huntington's Disease

Huntington's disease (HD) is a tragic degenerative neurological disease which usually presents in the fourth or fifth decade of life. It may present with chorea, dementia, or psychiatric symptoms, but in its course it often causes all of these signs. It is inherited as an autosomal dominant trait with complete penetrance, such that each offspring of an affected individual has a 50% chance of developing the disease. The main thrust of current research is aimed at identifying the primary biochemical defect in this disease, so that antenatal detection and perhaps definitive treatment will become possible. We will review significant recent investigations related to possible generalized cell membrane abnormalities in HD patients. Since knowledge of neurochemical alterations will provide the rationale for future therapeutic trials in HD, we will review important new data in this area. There have been many therapeutic trials in HD, many of the latest intended to augment cerebral γ-aminobutyric acid (GABA) content, with disappointing results. These unsuccessful trials underscore the need for a more fundamental understanding of HD and the importance of basic research.

Etiology

There are reports suggesting a generalized cell membrane defect in HD. Butterfield and his associates have found evidence on electron-spin resonance studies of HD erythrocytes that there is an alteration of membrane proteins (82). Additionally, they have reported abnormalities of HD erythrocyte morphology (83), deformability (84), and sodium-potassium adenosine triphosphatase activity (85), each of which is suggestive of a membrane abnormality. More recently, they have found that treatment of HD erythrocytes with proteolytic enzymes abolishes the abnormalities observed in electron-spin resonance studies (86). This suggests that the membrane protein abnormality resides on the external surface of the erythrocyte. In addition, Bialas and coworkers have found slightly increased Cl transport in HD red cells (87). Since Cl transport is regulated at the

external aspect of a red cell membrane protein (87), this result also suggests an external membrane protein abnormality.

Pettegrew and colleagues have used fluorescence spectroscopy to study intact HD erythrocytes. With this technique, fluorescent probes with affinities for different membrane components can be used to study membrane dynamics in different regions. Fluorescamine, for example, binds to amines on the cell surface. They have found abnormalities of fluorescamine spectroscopy in HD erythrocytes, which indicate an abnormality of the cell surface (88). They had previously also found abnormalities in HD fibroblast and lymphocyte membranes. Membrane surface abnormalities as reported by these two groups are compatible with early reports of abnormal growth patterns of HD fibroblasts (89).

Possibly also related to a membrane abnormality is the recent finding of L-glutamate toxicity in HD fibroblasts. Gray and coworkers (90) have found that HD fibroblasts have a specific, dose-related diminution of viability in media containing L-glutamate. This susceptibility was quite specific. For example, D-glutamate did not have the effect. This toxicity was prevented by simultaneous incubation with glutamine, but not GABA. This interesting finding potentially relates the observed membrane abnormalities in HD to the observation that intrastriatal injection of the glutamate analog kainic acid causes lesions histologically and biochemically comparable to those of HD (91, 92). Confirmation of these results will be most important.

Another type of fundamental defect in HD cells has been suggested by an abnormal sensitivity of HD lymphocytes to x-rays (93). This sensitivity implies that HD cells may be deficient in their capacity to repair deoxyribonucleic acid (DNA). Cultured lymphocytes from 4 patients with HD and 2 of 5 patients at risk for HD showed this sensitivity. Specificity of this finding is supported by the lack of sensitivity of control cells to x-rays and the lack of sensitivity of the cells to ultraviolet radiation. This report is compatible with a prior study which showed increased sensitivity of HD fibroblasts to ionizing radiation (94). Study of additional patients will be of great interest.

Neurochemistry

Spokes has performed extensive neurochemical studies of postmortem HD brain tissue (95). Various brain regions of 56 HD patients were analyzed and compared to 53 controls (without neurological or psychiatric disease) and 59 schizophrenic patients. Dopamine content was elevated in striatum, pallidum, nucleus accumbens, and substantia nigra of HD brains. Prior treatment with neuroleptics did not affect these differences. There was a trend for rigid HD patients to have lower brain dopamine content, but the difference did not achieve significance.

There are several ways of interpreting these findings. It is possible that destruction of nondopaminergic neurons in a structure, such as straitum, could lead to an increased concentration of dopamine. In fact, if one takes into account the loss of striatal volume in HD (about 60%), one would expect a 150% increase in dopamine concentration. Spokes suggests that his finding of only a 70% increase may actually be indicative of dopamine loss, in absolute terms, in HD striatum. In accumbens, however, the elevation in dopamine content is out of proportion to tissue shrinkage and may therefore represent an absolute increase in dopamine content (95).

The functional significance of elevated brain dopamine levels is not clear because such levels do not necessarily reflect dopaminergic activity. Spokes cites several studies which have looked at CSF homovanillic acid (HVA) levels as an index of dopamine turnover and found them reduced in HD. Another study lately has confirmed this finding (96). If there is not an absolute dopaminergic overactivity in HD, how might we explain the clinical observation that chorea is improved by drugs which block or deplete dopamine? Spokes discounts the idea that postsynaptic dopamine receptor supersensitivity may be responsible for a relative overactivity of dopaminergic transmission, because measurements of dopamine receptor binding have actually shown decreases in HD striatum (97). Spokes proposes that a relative dopaminergic overactivity may occur in HD because of loss of neurotransmitters or neuromodulators, which normally oppose dopamine activity.

In Spokes's study, glutamic acid decarboxylase (GAD), the synthetic enzyme for GABA, was decreased in all HD brain areas. However, a protracted terminal illness of any kind tends to lower brain GAD levels, and when HD brains were compared to brains of controls dying of such illnesses, only GAD decreases in striatum and globus pallidus were significant. This finding is consistent with prior studies of GAD and reports of reduced GABA concentrations in the basal ganglia of HD brains. Spokes and colleagues (98) have also shown that GABA is reduced by about 25% in the substantia nigra of HD brains, confirming previous studies by Perry. It is not known what role reduced GABA has in the symptoms of HD.

Another important synthetic enzyme, choline acetyltransferase (CAT), which synthesizes acetylcholine, was also decreased in the striatum, accumbens, and hippocampus of HD brains (95). Spokes comments that the rather inconsistent clinical results with drugs intended to enhance cholinergic transmission could relate to extensive loss of cholinergic neurons or to loss of cholinergic receptors, which has been reported by Enna and coworkers (99).

Much remains to be learned about the role of neuropeptides in control of cerebral function, but it is becoming clear that many of these peptides are altered in HD. Substance P, which may act as an excitatory neurotransmitter in a striatonigral pathway, is depleted in HD globus pallidus and substantia nigra (100). Angiotensin II may also be a neurotransmitter in brain, and angiotensin converting enzyme, which converts angiotensin to its active form, is depleted in HD striatum (101). Emson and colleagues lately have shown depletion of methionine (Met)-enkephalin (102) and cholecystokinin (103) in the globus pallidus and substantia nigra of HD brains.

Thus, it appears that a wide spectrum of neurochemical alterations take place in association with degeneration of striatal neurons in HD, but we do not know how to translate these findings into specific symptoms.

Clinical Features

The rigid, akinetic variant of HD (the

Westphal variant) is less well known than the choreic form, and it occurs in approximately 10% of all cases. This form can cause diagnostic confusion, being mistaken for idiopathic torsion dystonia, juvenile Parkinson's disease, or other neurological disorders. It more commonly occurs in childhood (in one-third of those presenting before age 20), which is an unusual age of presentation for HD. Juvenile HD also has the unusual features of mental retardation and seizures (104). This mode of presentation can be especially confusing if the parent, usually the father, does not show signs of the disease until some years after the child becomes symptomatic. Rigidity is associated with a graver prognosis. Bruyn (104) has suggested that juvenile HD patients are more frequently female and more often receive the gene from the father. Brackenridge (105) has studied parental factors associated with the occurrence of rigidity in HD. Relationships among offspring, parental sex, age at onset, and rigidity were investigated. Rigidity in the offspring was associated with rigidity in the parent and with paternal transmission of the gene. No relationship between rigidity and the sex of the patient was found. However, Brackenridge had previously shown that girls are more susceptible to rigidity at an earlier age than boys (106). The proportion of rigid males almost doubles as the age of onset extends from childhood to middle age.

Management

The issue of whether or not we should develop and use tests which would allow presymptomatic detection of HD has been a controversial one. Many equally well-informed and well-intended neurologists and investigators of HD have taken opposed positions in this debate. At the center of the debate is the fact that we have no treatment for HD. Therefore, any benefit provided by a presymptomatic test to individuals at risk, in terms of ability to plan their lives in accordance with the test result (107), must be weighed against the suffering of a protracted death sentence (108) imposed on the asymptomatic patient with a positive result. An analysis of the suffering relieved and caused by the availability of a presymptomatic test is very much a personal assessment, and it is understandable that

some oppose (109) but others favor it (110). At present no presymptomatic test has been demonstrated to be valid (i.e., no false positives or false negatives), and none are recommended for general use, including the levodopa provocation test (111). It is quite possible, though, as research continues, that a presymptomatic detection test will become available, and then it will become a matter of judgment for the individual clinician as to how and when to use it. Although many patients at risk for HD have expressed a positive attitude towards a presymptomatic test (112), the preference is undoubtedly a personal one, and the patient's wishes will need to be taken into account.

Klawans and colleagues (111) and Propert (110) have reviewed proposed tests for presymptomatic detection of HD. Eye movement abnormalities occur in HD, and they have been noted in asymptomatic relatives of HD patients. However, such abnormalities are not specific, and they could be genetically linked but unrelated to HD (111). Electroencephalograms (EEG) have not proven useful in presymptomatic detection of HD patients. Use of CT scans to measure degree of caudate atrophy has likewise not been useful. Patients with HD have sometimes claimed that by observing personality traits within the family, they could predict who would develop the disease. Thus far, however, no battery of neuropsychological tests has been effective as a presymptomatic test (111). Various biochemical tests, such as CSF GABA determinations and platelet type B monoamine oxidase activity, have not been able to clearly delineate at-risk subjects into those with and without the abnormal gene.

Fundamental abnormalities in HD cells, such as those of fibroblast, erythrocyte, and lymphocyte membranes, have not been sought in at-risk patients (110, 111). Increased sensitivity of lymphocytes to x-rays has been noted in 2 of 5 patients at risk for HD (93), but, of course, more patients and follow-up are required. Unfortunately, studies of linkage of the HD trait with red cell markers or HLA types have not had positive results, nor have searches for an identifiable protein abnormality.

The levodopa provocation test was

performed by Klawans and colleagues (113) on 30 patients at risk for HD in 1972. The idea behind the test is that levodopa might produce choreic movements in presymptomatic individuals with HD, but not in those without it. At the time of the test, 10 of the 30 patients developed chorea. At most recent follow-up (111), 5 of the 10 who had developed chorea currently have been diagnosed to have HD, and the other 5 are under continued observation. One patient who did not have chorea now has HD. To determine the validity of this test will require years of continued observation, and the authors are no longer enrolling patients in this study. We do not recommend use of this test in clinical practice. Its validity has not been established, and yet the results are apparent to the patient, who would undoubtedly take the results seriously, perhaps with tragic results.

In view of the marked depletion of GABA and GAD in HD basal ganglia, several therapeutic trials have aimed to increase brain GABA content in HD patients. Perry and associates (114) reported an improvement in HD patients treated with isoniazid, an inhibitor of GABA transaminase, a GABA degradative enzyme. Manyam and colleagues treated 8 patients with isoniazid and studied CSF GABA levels (115). Two patients developed anorexia associated with abnormal liver function tests. Of the remaining 6 patients, only 2 showed a mild decrease in choreic symptoms, in spite of a threefold increase in average CSF GABA levels. In a similar study, treatment of 14 HD patients with γ-acetylenic GABA, an irreversible inhibitor of GABA transaminase, did not result in clinical improvement in spite of increases in CSF GABA and homocarnosine (a GABA-containing dipeptide [116]). Perry and colleagues treated 7 HD patients with aminooxyacetic acid, another inhibitor of GABA transaminase, and found no benefit (117). Rather, the drug had a high degree of toxicity, inducing drowsiness, ataxia, seizures, and psychosis.

These discouraging results have several possible explanations. As we have seen, many neurochemical alterations occur in HD, and increasing brain GABA may affect only a small part of the problem. It is also possible that the increases in brain GABA achieved with these drugs has no functional significance. For example, the GABA increase may occur in intracellular GABA pools that do not participate in neurotransmission. It is also possible that decreased basal ganglia GABA is not related to choreic movements, the symptom that most investigators analyze.

At present, it is possible to suppress choreic movements with dopamine receptor blocking drugs or catecholamine-depleting drugs, such as reserpine and tetrabenazine The former class of drugs may also be helpful in treating psychiatric manifestations of the disease.

In the absence of an effective treatment of this disease, a major role of the physician is to be supportive and understanding, not only of the patient, but also of the spouse. A paper by Hans and Koeppen (118) lucidly describes the tragic consequences of HD experienced by the spouse. The spouse suffers years of financial, social, and personal hardship as the patient deteriorates, often only to find that the suffering must be recapitulated as a child becomes symptomatic with the disease. As Hans and Koeppen express it: "The impact of the disease on the spouse is permanent; the trauma never terminates." A reading of their paper is recommended for physicians who treat HD patients.

Summary

Several investigators have found evidence for a cell membrane abnormality in HD erythrocytes, lymphocytes, and fibroblasts. The abnormality seems to be in the external protein component of the cell membrane. Perhaps related to a membrane abnormality is the recent demonstration that L-glutamate is toxic to HD fibroblasts. Another type of fundamental abnormality, that of deficient DNA repair, is proposed to affect HD lymphocytes on the basis of their increased sensitivity to x-rays.

Neurochemical studies have shown depletion in HD brain of GABA and its synthetic enzyme GAD, choline acetyltransferase, substance P, met-enkephalin and cholecystokinen. Although dopamine concentration is increased in HD striatum, the increase is less than what would be expected from the degree of tissue shrinkage, suggesting that dopamine levels, in absolute terms, may actually be decreased. The rigid, akinetic variant of HD must be considered in the differential diagnosis of dystonia, mental retardation, and seizures in childhood. The rigid form is more likely to occur in patients who have a parent with the rigid form and who receive the gene from the father. Controversy exists over the benefits of presymptomatic tests for HD. At present, no valid, clinically applicable test exists. Trials of drugs which augment brain GABA levels have been uniformly disappointing in the treatment of HD.

Other Choreas

The incidence of Sydenham's chorea has diminished greatly in recent years, but its importance as a diagnostic consideration for chorea in childhood remains. Nausieda and coworkers (119) reviewed 240 cases of Sydenham's chorea diagnosed at their institution between 1951 and 1976. Of these cases, 92% were diagnosed before 1968. The average age at onset was 9.3 years. The overall incidence was higher in girls (57.5%) than in boys (42.5%), but this was primarily due to a higher incidence in girls older than 10 years. Chorea was generalized in 80% of patients and unilateral in the remainder. The duration ranged from 1 to 22 weeks, with a median duration of 12 weeks. Associated signs were dysarthria in 40%, weakness in 5%, encephalopathy (including personality change) in 10%. Most patients (80%) did not have recurrences, but those who did usually had only 1, on the average about 2 years after the first attack. Recurrences many years after the first episode were unusual, and this suggests that late recurrences may be due to reactivation by other mechanisms, such as pregnancy (chorea gravidarum) or drugs (oral contraceptives, phenytoin). CSF HVA levels were increased acutely in a 10-year-old girl with Sydenham's chorea (120). She was not improved by haloperidol but was by reserpine. This case suggests that dopamine turnover may be increased in this condition.

Two cases of bilateral chorea in patients with bilateral subdural hematomas have been reported (121, 122). Both patients had resolution of their chorea following evacuation of their hematomas. The pathophysiological basis for this occurrence is obscure.

Glutaric acidemia can cause progressive choreoathetosis in children. This disorder is caused by a defect in the oxidation of glutamyl-CoA, an intermediate in the catabolism of lysine and tryptophan. A case described by Leibel and associates (123) exemplifies the clinical and pathological features. The child presented with developmental delay and metabolic acidosis. He then developed progressive choreoathetosis, pseudobulbar signs, extensor plantar responses, and died at 3½ years of age. Glutaric acid concentrations were elevated in the plasma and urine. Postmortem examination showed neuron loss in the striatum, and glutaric acid was present in increased amounts in the brain. Glutaric acidemia therefore must be considered in the differential diagnosis of chorea and dystonia in childhood, along with Wilson's disease, Hallervorden-Spatz disease, Leigh's disease, Lesch-Nyhan syndrome, juvenile HD, idiopathic torsion dystonia, and some lipid storage diseases.

Several drugs are well known to induce chorea, including levodopa, phenytoin, birth control pills, antipsychotics (after prolonged use), and amphetamines. Two other drugs have recently been added to the list. Nausieda and associates have reported a child who developed chorea following accidental ingestion of pemoline, a central stimulant used to treat minimal brain dysfunction (124). Wasserman and Yahr have reported an interesting case of chorea induced by chronic methadone use (125). There is some suggestion that their patient may have had pre-existing cerebral injury. The authors point out that in some cases of drug-induced chorea asymptomatic lesions, which presumably preceded drug use, have been found in the basal ganglia at autopsy.

TARDIVE DYSKINESIA

Tardive dyskinesia (TD) is usually a choreic movement disorder which affects the oromandibular region. It also can be associated with other involuntary movements, such as dystonia and myoclonus and can affect any body region. The variable nature and severity of its manifestations have led to a wide range of diagnostic criteria and assessment scales with resulting confusion about its prevalence, predisposing factors, prognosis, and treatment.

It is now universally agreed that TD is an iatrogenic disease induced by chronic antipsychotic drug treatment. The evidence for this consists of epidemiological studies which have shown antipsychotic use to be associated with an increased prevalence of TD (126, 127). In addition, there is a temporal relationship between use of antipsychotics and the appearance of TD historically and in individual cases. Lastly, pharmacological and biochemical investigations of antipsychotic treatment and TD make plausible a causal role for antipsychotics in the occurrence of TD.

The clinical pharmacology of TD, like other choreic movement disorders, is in many ways opposite to that of PD. TD is improved by dopamine blocking or depleting drugs; it is aggravated by levodopa; it is improved by drugs which enhance acetylcholine transmission; it is aggravated by anticholinergic drugs. This clinical pharmacology of dopaminergic overactivity in TD can be understood as a consequence of antipsychotic drug treatment. Prolonged treatment with antipsychotic drugs has been shown to increase animal behavioral responses to dopamine agonists, the sensitivity of striatal dopamine-sensitive adenylate cyclase, and striatal electrophysiological responses to dopamine (128, 129). These phenomena, in turn, can be understood in terms of increased dopamine receptor binding following prolonged antipsychotic drug treatment, which has been demonstrated by several investigations (130-132).

In spite of the appeal of the dopamine receptor supersensitivity hypothesis of TD, it does have some weaknesses which should not be overlooked. Baldessarini and Tarsy (128, 129) point out that the duration of behavioral supersensitivity in laboratory animals is brief, whereas TD clinically can persist indefinitely in some cases. In one primate model of TD, however, behavioral supersensitivity to apomorphine has lasted for months (133). In addition, Muller and Seeman have argued that the duration of behavioral supersensitiv-ity in laboratory animals correlates with duration of antipsychotic drug treatment, which does correspond to clinical experience (134).

Baldessarini and Tarsy also note that the biochemical and behavioral changes indicative of dopaminergic supersensitivity have generally been small and rapidly reversible (128, 129). They suggest that an antipsychotic-induced anatomical lesion is more likely to underlie TD, given its persistence clinically. However, no definite pathological lesions have been demonstrated. It has been suggested that perhaps chronic neuroleptic treatment, by blocking dopamine receptors, induces cerebral dopaminergic neuron sprouting, thus providing an anatomical basis for persistent dopaminergic supersensitivity (135). This hypothesis is interesting but has no data to support it at the present time.

Many fundamental epidemiological facts about TD, such as its prevalence, incidence, prognosis, and predisposing factors, remain either unknown or controversial because of widely different findings among investigators. Some methodological difficulties in epidemiological studies of TD include: (1) varying clinical definitions of TD; (2) questionable reliability of rating scales; (3) inability to generalize findings from one patient population to another; (4) the confounding effect of antipsychotic treatment, which can influence the severity and prevalence of TD observed (136). For example, estimates of the prevalence of TD have ranged from 0.5% to 56% (126). A likely prevalence range is from 10% to 20% (136). Whether or not the prevalence of TD is increasing is not known. Gardos and Cole have pointed out that prevalence estimates up until 1972 averaged about 15%, whereas more recent estimates have been closer to 50% in both in- and outpatient populations (137). However, it seems possible that some of this difference may be accounted for by an increased awareness of the syndrome and its milder forms.

There is little data available on the incidence of TD. Gardos and Cole estimated the risk of developing TD for a schizophrenic inpatient to be 4%-5% for 1 year of observation in their institution.

Epidemiological data about the natural history of TD also varies greatly. Estimates of the rate of spontaneous remission range from 5% to 92% (136). More recent estimates, which take into account more brief and mild forms of the disease, are probably more accurate, and they suggest that one-fourth to one-half of patients may improve within a year (136). The likelihood of spontaneous remission may be greater in patients treated for a shorter period of time (137). Increasing age, however, may be associated with a decreased likelihood of spontaneous remission.

There is growing evidence that age increases the prevalence, severity, and likelihood of irreversibility of TD. Smith and Baldessarini studied the relationship between these variables and age by reviewing data from their own patient population and from the literature (138). They found that the prevalence of TD had a very close linear correlation with age. Prevalence in a younger than 40-year group was 10%, whereas it was 40% in an older than 60-year group. Likewise, severity increased linearly with age. Degree of recovery in TD was inversely related to age. In a younger than 60-year group, 83% improved or recovered; whereas only 36% did so in an older than 60-year group. Crane also found increased age to be associated with more severe TD (139). The female sex is also associated with more severe cases of TD (136).

It seems intuitive that duration and dosage of antipsychotic drug therapy should correlate with prevalence and severity of TD, but the evidence on this point is not definite. In an analysis of 669 chronically hospitalized patients, Crane diagnosed TD in 300 (45%), and he found duration and dose of antipsychotic drug treatment to be correlated with severity of TD (139). Gardos and associates (127) studied several drug variables and found duration of therapy (i.e., time since initial therapy began) to correlate with the occurrence of TD, but total amount of neuroleptics and maximum dose did not. A review of other studies does not support a relationship between drug variables and severity of TD (138), and the American Psychiatric Association Task Force Report

on TD summarizes the studies on this issue as inconclusive (136). The methodological difficulties previously mentioned could account for the conflicting results of these epidemiological studies. Klawans observed that the TD of an individual patient can become more severe as antipsychotic drugs are continued (140). Therefore, it seems reasonable, even with the lack of confirmatory epidemiological data, to try to discontinue antipsychotics when TD occurs and, as a preventive measure, to minimize the dose and duration of therapy in treating schizophrenia.

Fundamental questions about the clinical presentation of TD also remain unanswered. For example, Gardos and Cole have remarked that there is little information available on how often TD is severe and disabling (137). In an informal survey of investigators of TD, they found that only an estimated 10% of patients with TD were functionally impaired. In a survey of 89 patients with TD in their institution, none were disabled because of it. These figures are, of course, derived only from casual surveys, and the true incidence of functional impairment in TD is unknown. It is of interest in this regard that none of the commonly used scales for TD include an assessment of functional disability (141).

It has been mentioned that the clinical variability of the nature and severity of involuntary movements in TD has led to differing diagnostic criteria and assessment scales. The extent of this variability has suggested to some investigators that TD may actually consist of separate sub-syndromes. Barnes and coworkers (142) and Kidger and colleagues (143) used multivariate statistical methods to analyze involuntary movements in TD. Patients under treatment with antipsychotics (N = 182) and normal volunteers (N = 85) were studied by behavioral rating and videotape analysis; patients and videotape raters were unaware of the design and intent of the study. All movements that had no obvious purpose were recorded. They found that three separate, identifiable groups of movements were present. One group consisted of hand and lip tremor and it corresponded to a parkinsonian syndrome. Another group consisted of movements of the lips, tongue, jaw, and neck. This constellation of movements best corresponded to the classical description of the oral-buccal-lingual masticatory movements of TD. A third group consisted of trunk, arm, hand, and leg movements. These movements appeared to be restless or fidgety movements such as occur in akathisia. However, many of the patients with these movements did not complain of restlessness. The authors suggest that these movements correspond to late onset akathisia, which has been described by Simpson (144), which is frequently associated with oral choreic TD, and which may less often have a subjective component as in acute akathisia. It is interesting to note in view of these findings a report by Bobruff and associates (145) that orofacial movements have a different pharmacological response than axial and extremity movements. The former responded better to clonazepam, whereas the latter responded better to phenobarbital. These authors suggest that future treatment studies should consider selective effects on different body regions.

Polizos and Engelhardt (146) have studied movement disorders induced by antipsychotic drug treatment of children. They have treated 95 children, most diagnosed as childhood schizophrenics with autistic features. TD is rare in children, as the authors observed only two instances during 11 years of treatment of this patient population. A common problem in children is withdrawal emergence syndrome, which occurred in 51% of 184 instances of neuroleptic withdrawal. Withdrawal emergence syndrome usually occurs within 2 weeks of drug withdrawal. It consists primarily of choreic movements, but there may be myoclonus, and all body regions may be involved. Oral choreic movements in this syndrome were infrequent (less than 20% of cases) and mild. Ataxia was observed in 86% of cases. The mean duration of these movements was 15 days. These authors have not been able to completely study the natural history of this syndrome because often antipsychotic therapy needed to be reinstituted. However, the movements seem usually to remit spontaneously.

There is no universally effective therapy for TD, so efforts must be made to prevent it. The American Psychiatric Association Task Force Report on TD provides an excellent review of considerations in the use of antipsychotic drugs (136), and it is recommended reading. Choice of psychiatric therapy rests primarily on a careful psychiatric diagnosis. There has been a tendency for the term schizophrenia to be used too broadly, to refer to any severe psychiatric disorder, including affective disorders and personality disorders. Long-term maintenance treatment with antipsychotics is of demonstrated value only in the management of schizophrenia. Commitment of a patient to long-term treatment with antipsychotics requires: (1) more than one acute psychotic episode; (2) objective evidence of continuing psychosis; (3) a likelihood of further psychotic episodes; (4) evidence of responsiveness to antipsychotic treatment (136). Once a commitment has been made to long-term antipsychotic drugs, the dose should be kept to a minimum, and the need for their continued use should be periodically re-evaluated.

If TD occurs, it is desirable to stop antipsychotic drugs. A significant number of patients will improve partially or completely within a few months. Most patients will transiently worsen following withdrawal of antipsychotics, but this does not imply a decreased likelihood of spontaneous recovery. If antipsychotic drugs cannot be withdrawn because of debilitating psychiatric symptoms, the family, patient, and physician must discuss the therapeutic dilemma and weigh the risk of severe or irreversible TD against the risk of uncontrolled psychiatric symptoms. If antipsychotic drugs must be continued, and TD becomes a debilitating problem, then therapeutic approaches to TD as outlined below can be administered concomitantly with antipsychotic drugs.

If antipsychotic drugs are withdrawn, it is desirable to follow the patient without therapy, because they may recover spontaneously. However, if the TD is so severe that the patient cannot tolerate watchful waiting, or if months of waiting have not shown improvement, then any of the therapeutic approaches discussed below should be considered.

The major approaches to treating TD involve manipulation of dopaminergic, cholinergic, or GABAergic neurotransmission. There are other approaches which will be touched upon briefly. In his review, Klawans (140) states that agents which deplete cerebral dopaminergic stores, such as reserpine or tetrabenazine, are the mainstays of current therapy for TD, and we agree with this. These drugs often ameliorate TD signs, they both have some efficacy as antipsychotics, and the risk of causing or exacerbating TD with their chronic use appears to be low. They can, however, cause parkinsonism, depression, and orthostatic hypotension, which can limit their use.

A D-2 receptor antagonist, oxiperomide, has been reported to suppress levodopainduced dyskinesias without exacerbating parkinsonism. Casey and Gerlach found that oxiperomide suppressed dyskinesia in TD without inducing parkinsonism (147). However, it is possible that oxiperomide, like other dopamine receptor blocking agents, may, with chronic use, aggravate TD. Its apparent selective ability to suppress levodopa and TD dyskinesias without inducing parkinsonism is of theoretical interest.

Albert and Friedhoff (148) have taken another approach to modifying dopaminergic activity in TD. The idea is that if chronic dopamine receptor blockade can induce dopamine receptor supersensitivity (and therefore, hypothetically, cause TD), then perhaps sustained treatment with levodopa might reverse this supersensitivity. They treated 3 patients with levodopa (2-6 g/day) for 10 to 60 days and then evaluated TD following discontinuation of levodopa. Two patients had an excellent response, and one patient a good response. Bjorndal and associates tried this approach in 7 patients (149). In 4 patients who remained on neuroleptics, it produced no benefit. In 3 patients who were not on neuroleptic treatment, it produced complete remission in 1 and 25% improvement in 2 others. Study of this approach with blind trials in more patients is needed.

Another therapeutic approach to TD is to attempt to augment cholinergic neurotransmission. Deanol, as a possible choline precursor, has been used for this purpose. In a review of clinical trials using deanol to treat TD, Domino and Kovacic (150) note that 161 patients have been treated and 37% reported improved. If only blind trials of deanol are considered, only 16% of patients are reported improved. Cole and his colleagues (151) found deanol to be of no benefit. The conflicting results with deanol may be related to the fact that although deanol elevates serum choline levels, it also competes with choline to cross the blood-brain barrier (152).

Zeisel and associates (152) have used oral choline and lecithin to augment cerebral acetylcholine. In a double-blind crossover trial of choline in treating 20 patients with TD, 9 improved. Choline, however, has unpleasant side effects; it causes diarrhea and an unpleasant fishy body odor. They, therefore, have studied lecithin as choline precursor. They have treated 7 patients with lecithin and all 7 improved, with minimal side effects. This is a promising approach, and additional patients need to be studied.

Agents that enhance cerebral GABA transmission have been used to treat TD. One possible rationale is that a striatonigral GABA pathway seems to exist, and it may inhibit dopaminergic activity. Although some benefit has been reported with these drugs, they have unacceptable side effects and are more of theoretical interest than practical use. Casey and associates studied γ-acetylenic GABA, which is an irreversible inhibitor of GABA-transaminase, and found improvement in 9 out of 10 patients (153). The drug has side effects of sedation and confusion, which the authors believe will preclude it from clinical use. Chase and Tamminga studied muscimol in treating TD, and although it suppressed dyskinesia, it aggravated psychiatric symptoms and induced myoclonic twitching (154). Nair and colleagues studied sodium valproate and baclofen (155). In high doses, valproate inhibits GABA-transaminase. Baclofen, although it is a GABA analog, has an uncertain relationship to GABA transmission. They found that neither sodium valproate nor baclofen alone suppressed TD in 10 patients.

Klawans and his associates (156) and others

have shown that lithium given concurrently with a neuroleptic such as haloperidol will prevent the occurrence of dopaminergic supersensitivity. This observation has provided a rationale for treatment of TD patients with lithium. Mackay and coworkers treated 11 TD patients with lithium and noted no benefit (157).

GILLES DE LA TOURETTE SYNDROME

Gilles de la Tourette syndrome (GTS) is characterized by chronic, multiple motor and vocal tics which wax and wane in their severity and evolve in their nature. Motor tics are rapid movements, which may be simple, such as eye blinking, or complex, such as clapping. Likewise, vocal tics may be simple sounds, such as grunts, or complex, such as coprolalia. GTS almost always begins in childhood; the age of onset, in the series of Shapiro and coworkers, ranged from 2 to 15 years (158). In addition to tics, GTS patients may have a variety of other neurological and psychiatric manifestations. There seems to be an increased prevalence of learning disabilities (158), sleep disorders (159), and possibly obsessive-compulsive and self-destructive behaviors (160). These associated problems can be prominent, as pointed out by O'Quinn and Thompson (161), who noted that 4 of their 5 patients were referred for academic difficulties due to distractibility and disruptive behavior.

GTS is likely to be an organic illness rather than a functional, psychiatric one, although as we learn more about brain function this classic distinction becomes less meaningful. The arguments in favor of an organic basis for this disease include its frequent association with signs of preceding cerebral injury (158); its amelioration by dopamine blocking agents (158) and induction by dopamine agonists (162); reports that it can occur as an acquired disorder following antipsychotic therapy (163); its familial occurrence (160); and reports of abnormalities of CSF monoamines (164).

There is increasing evidence that GTS can be genetically transmitted. Nee and associates examined 50 patients with GTS and carefully ascertained family histories for the presence of the syndrome or tics alone (160). Sixteen families contained a member other than the proband who had GTS. Another 16 families reported at least 1 member who had motor tics. These investigators observed parent to child transmission in several instances and noted the occurrence of TDS and tics in several generations. These observations make an autosomal recessive mode of transmission unlikely. The authors declined to suggest a specific possible mode of transmission because of potential inaccuracies in their ascertainment of data. They noted that patients with a positive family history of GTS were more likely than patients with a negative history to have sleep disturbances, obsessive-compulsive behaviors, and a favorable response to haloperidol therapy. This observation suggests that there may be subtypes of GTS with different underlying pathophysiological processes and responses to therapy.

The study by Nee and associates (160) also indicates that GTS and simple motor tics may occur within families, suggesting that the two are probably related. A similar finding was reported by Kidd and coworkers (165). Abe and Oda have found that simple tics also have a familial occurrence which probably has a genetic basis (166).

Klawans and associates have reported the occurrence of GTS in a 28-year-old schizophrenic woman treated for 6 years with neuroleptics (163). Following discontinuation of chlorpromazine, she developed barking noises and tics of the face, neck, and arms, which fluctuated in their severity and location. There are several recent additional reports of this occurrence. A 65-year-old man developed grunting and tic-like movements of the mouth after discontinuation of neuroleptics (167). A 28-year-old man developed facial tics, grunting, and involuntary limb movements when neuroleptics were discontinued after 13 years of treatment (168). Fog and Pakkenburg (169) reported 3 similar cases in patients aged 20 to 54 years. These cases seem compatible with the concept of dopaminergic overactivity in GTS, because they can be explained on the basis of neuroleptic-induced dopamine supersensitivity, as postulated for tardive dyskinesia.

Although these cases are of interest, they must be viewed with caution, because some of them do not conform to criteria for GTS. It is reasonable to set aside the criterion of childhood onset for these cases, given that they are acquired, but it is not reasonable to set aside the criteria of waxing and waning of tics and evolution of the character of tics. Few of these reports document these aspects. Furthermore, late onset akathisia associated with TD can present with grunting, even shouting, and complex movements such as face rubbing or scratching, which may resemble tics. The oral movements of TD can be rapid and repetitive and can resemble tics. Future reports of antipsychotic-induced GTS will need to carefully specify the nature of vocal and motor tics, document a waxing and waning course, and the evolution of tics.

Reports of antipsychotic-induced GTS do raise concern about treating GTS with haloperidol, which is said to be effective in 80% of cases (158). These reports raise the theoretical concern that antipsychotic drugs, by inducing dopaminergic supersensitivity, might ultimately exacerbate the disease. In addition, it is possible that chronic haloperidol therapy might induce typical TD, as recently reported in 1 case (170). It would be desirable to know the consequences of long-term haloperidol treatment in GTS patients and to develop alternate medical therapy. Cohen and associates have reported that clonidine, in doses up to 0.30 mg/day improved 70% of 25 GTS patients who had not responded to haloperidol therapy (171). No serious side effects occurred. This promising result needs to be confirmed with double-blind trials. Stahl and Berger using double-blind format have shown that intravenous physostigmine improves tics in GTS (172). A central cholinergic effect of physostigmine is suggested by their demonstration that proprantheline (a peripherally-acting anticholinergic) did not block the beneficial response. They suggest that treatment with lecithin, to augment acetylcholine transmission, might be a plausible chronic therapy.

DYSTONIA

Dystonia refers to sustained or twisting involuntary movements which may be slow or rapid. They are influenced by posture and may be induced by voluntary motor activity (action dystonia). Dystonia may occur without apparent cause, or it may occur with a large number of degenerative or metabolic neurological diseases or following a variety of cerebral insults. In the latter instance, it is referred to as secondary or symptomatic dystonia.

Since Eldridge's comprehensive survey of dystonic patients in the United States in 1970, it has been believed that primary dystonia shows two patterns of inheritance: autosomal recessive in patients of Ashkenazic Jewish descent, and autosomal dominant in non-Jews (173). Recently, Korczyn and coworkers (174) questioned the pattern of inheritance in Jewish patients. They conducted a country-wide search for cases of dystonia in Israel diagnosed between 1969 and 1975. Of 137 patients tentatively diagnosed to have primary dystonia, 42 were confirmed to have that diagnosis and were available for study. European Jews had the highest prevalence of dystonia. Family data were available for 40 Jewish patients: 25 had a negative family history; 1 had parents who were first cousins; 14 were in family aggregates. These 14 patients occurred among 4 families. In 2 of the families, a parent and 3 children were affected; in the other 2 families, dystonia occurred in more than 1 generation. These authors conclude that the pattern of inheritance in European Jews is likely to be autosomal dominant with incomplete penetrance.

Eldridge (175) has questioned this interpretation of their data, because only 2 of their 29 families had parent and child affected. This is a small number for an autosomal dominant trait, unless the mutation rate is extraordinarily high. He interprets their parent-to-child transmission cases as possible examples of pseudodominance in which 1 parent is homozygous for a recessive trait, and the other parent is heterozygous, resulting in an average of 50% homozygous children. Korczyn and associates (176) have replied that to invoke pseudodominance to explain these occurrences postulates a higher frequency of the dystonia trait in the population than probably exists. Until this controversy is resolved, one must keep an open mind about the pattern of inheritance in Jews.

One form of primary dystonia is idiopathic dystonia affecting predominantly the face, which has been called blepharospasm-oromandibular syndrome, Meige's syndrome (177), and Brueghel's syndrome (178). Tolosa has reviewed the clinical features of the condition in 17 of his patients (179). In general, the facial muscle spasms tend to be bilateral, symmetric, tonic, nonrhythmic contractions. A partial list of the spasms (in order of decreasing frequency) seen among his patients includes spasms of eye closure, mouth retraction, eyebrow elevation and frowning, neck spasms, jaw opening, lip pursing, and abdominal and truncal spasms. In the majority of patients, certain actions triggered the spasms, such as walking, talking, opening the eyes, or reading. The clinical course was very variable. The time from onset of symptoms to their maximum severity ranged from 2 months to 18 years. Tolosa noted tremor in 8 of his patients. He also noted a high prevalence of depression (7 of 17). In 5 patients, depression preceded dystonia. He noted that the sister of 1 patient also had the disease. Nutt also recently reported the occurrence of blepharospasm-oromandibular dystonia in sisters (180).

Tolosa previously concluded from pharmacological studies that blepharospasm-oromandibular syndrome is associated with cerebral dopaminergic overactivity (181). Casey supports this view with his finding that 2 patients were improved by perphenazine, but made worse by levodopa (182). He also found that benztropine made both patients worse, and deanol improved them. The clinical pharmacology of this condition, however, is likely to be complex and to require further study. We have noted, for example, that although dopamine-depleting agents may in some cases provide significant benefit, they often do not.

The pathophysiological basis of blepharospasm-oromandibular dystonia syndrome is unknown. Postmortem analysis of 1 case, with careful examination of the basal ganglia, was normal (183). Thus, as with other idiopathic dystonias, blepharospasm-oromandibular dystonia is believed to be a disorder of the basal ganglia, but pathological evidence is lacking.

We have recently drawn attention to a phenomenon of prolonged delay between the occurrence of static cerebral lesions and the appearance of dystonia due to the lesion (184). We described 1 patient with head trauma, 2 with cerebral infarctions, and 5 children with perinatal insults who developed dystonia 1 or more years after the injury. The children are of particular interest because they were often diagnosed early in their course to have idiopathic dystonia. Our first case provides an example. This girl was the full term product of a normal pregnancy. Delivery was difficult; forceps were used; and the Apgar score was 3. She thereafter appeared to develop normally, except for clumsiness and dysarthria, for which she received speech therapy. At 7 years she developed left hemidystonia, and a CT scan showed right cerebral hemiatrophy. Similar cases have previously been described by others (185). Since our report, we have encountered a number of additional cases due to perinatal injury. Descriptions of more cases are needed to have a better concept of the clinical spectrum of this problem, as well as its prognosis and response to treatment.

Goldman and associates (186) have described a child with GM_1 gangliosidosis whose clinical course was marked by progressive, generalized dystonia. At age 2 years, this boy developed unsteady gait and was thought to have cerebral palsy. By 6 years dysarthria became apparent, and at 10 years dystonic posturing of the legs and back appeared. Intellectual impairment was mild. Dystonia progressed, and the patient died at 27 years. Postmortem examination showed findings relatively localized to the basal ganglia. The caudate, putamen, and globus pallidus were shrunken. Neurons of the caudate were swollen with numerous intracytoplasmic inclusions. β-Galactosidase activity was deficient in several tissues, and GM_1 ganglioside was increased in brain (187). Thus GM_1 gangliosidosis must be considered in the differential diagnosis of symptomatic dystonia in childhood, which includes cerebral palsy and delayed onset dystonia, HD, PD, Wilson's disease, Hallervorden-Spatz syndrome, and other cerebral lipidoses. Ataxia-telangiectasia must also be added to the list, because a recent case report described dystonia as the predominant presenting feature (188).

CT scan may be helpful in an evaluation for Hallervorden-Spatz syndrome. This disease usually presents in childhood and is often familial (189). Dystonia is generally a prominent clinical feature, as are intellectual deterioration, dysarthria, and pyramidal tract signs. Dooling and associates (190) reported that a CT scan in a patient showed diffuse cerebral atrophy and ventricular dilatation.

Very little is known about the biochemical or physiological basis of chronic dystonias, either primary or secondary. Perhaps by studying acute dystonia induced by antipsychotic drugs we might gain some insight into the mechanisms of the chronic dystonias. Kolbe and associates have studied the dynamics of dopamine metabolism alterations following a single dose in rats of butaperazine (191). They observed that a single dose causes increased dopamine turnover, as measured by HVA and DOPAC concentrations, for about 48 hours. At about 24 hours, dopaminergic supersensitivity, as measured by apomorphine-induced stereotypy, begins to appear. Thus, there is a period of overlap of these two events between 24 and 48 hours, during which time dopamine turnover is heightened in the presence of dopaminergic supersensitivity. This time interval corresponds to the time of peak occurrence of acute dystonic reactions in patients following butaperazine ingestion, and the authors suggest that these dynamics of dopamine metabolism may be responsible for dystonic reactions. Their hypothesis is a good starting point for trying to understand acute dystonia, and it merits further study.

TREMOR

The classification, diagnosis, pathophysiology, and management of tremors was recently reviewed by Jankovic and Fahn (192). Tremor is an involuntary oscillatory movement which can be classified according to clinical appearance or etiology. Classification by appearance is most useful for the clinician, and it categorizes tremors according to presence at rest, during action (either on posture-holding against gravity or during an isometric contraction), or during intention (i.e., during a goal-directed act such as finger-to-nose testing).

Tremor at rest is usually associated with PD, and the reader is referred to our section on that subject for review of recent research. It will suffice to mention here two clinical points brought out by Jankovic and Fahn (192). First, the typical 3 to 7 Hz rest tremor of PD usually begins in the fingers and thumb; the lips and jaw may become involved, but tremor of the head is rare. Head tremor, in the absence of rigidity, bradykinesia, or postural instability, should suggest a diagnosis of essential tremor or spasmodic torticollis. Second, tremor may be resistant to levodopa therapy, and addition of an anticholinergic drug can be beneficial.

Physiological tremor and essential tremor are both action tremors. Physiological tremor is present in normal individuals and is usually asymptomatic. It has a frequency of 6 to 12 Hz and is most readily observed on posture holding (e.g., hands outstretched). Physiological tremor can become symptomatic if it is accentuated, as it can be by a variety of factors, including fatigue, emotional stress, metabolic derangements (e.g., thyrotoxicosis, and hypoglycemia), and drugs (e.g., isoproterenol, caffeine, and lithium). Young and Hagbarth (193) have shown that physiological tremor can be enhanced by maneuvers which augment the segmental stretch reflex. During tonic muscle contraction, for example, physiological tremor becomes more apparent as EMG bursts become more grouped. Each of the EMG bursts follows a primary spindle afferent burst, suggesting that the segmental stretch reflex is involved in maintaining the enhanced tremor. This effect is actually observed before the subject becomes aware of fatigue. Performance of the Jendrassik maneuver and application of a vibration stimulus to the muscle, both of which enhance the segmental stretch reflex, also augment physiological tremor (193).

It has been shown that intra-arterial

infusion of isoproterenol can enhance the amplitude of physiological tremor, and intra-arterial propranolol can block this effect (194). Thus, physiological tremor can be modified by pharmacological effects of peripheral β-adrenergic receptors, whereas this is not the case with essential tremor. The precise peripheral localization of β-adrenergic receptors, and their physiological role in modification of tremor is not known. Nevertheless, β-adrenergic receptor blocking drugs, such as propranolol, can be useful in the treatment of physiological tremor, which becomes symptomatic under stress (195). Small doses of benzodiazepines taken on an as-needed basis can also be helpful.

Essential tremor, like physiological tremor, is rapid (7-11 Hz) and is most prominent with action. It may be hereditary, sporadic, or associated with other neurological diseases such as torsion dystonia or Charcot-Marie-Tooth disease. Sporadic cases in the elderly are referred to as senile tremor, but sporadic cases can occur at any age. Essential tremor often begins in the hands, but it can affect the head, causing horizontal (negation) or vertical (affirmation) movements. It can also affect the voice. Essential tremor is exacerbated by stress and by coordinated, voluntary acts such as handwriting or bringing a cup to the lips. It is alleviated by alcohol and oral propranolol (196). Unlike physiological tremor, essential tremor is not relieved by intra-arterial propranolol, so the beneficial effect of propranolol is thought to be on a central basis. Essential tremor may be relieved by low doses of propranolol, but sometimes doses up to 320 mg/day are required (192). In a study of 5 patients with essential tremor, Sorensen and associates found no relation between plasma propranolol levels and clinical effect (197). Some patients noted benefit before plasma levels were measurable; thus measurement of such levels is unlikely to be useful in clinical management. Patients with a history of congestive heart failure or obstructive pulmonary disease cannot be treated with propranolol. There are reports that metoprolol, which has selective B_1 blocking properties, is beneficial in essential tremor (198, 199), and it may be a suitable alternative to propranolol in patients with obstructive lung disease.

Intention tremor is commonly caused by cerebellar disease. It is a 3-5 Hz coarse tremor which is accentuated by target directed movements. Intention tremor is not well understood, and there is currently no effective pharmacotherapy for it. It has been said that weighting the affected limbs decreases the amplitude of the tremor (200). There is a recent report of intention tremor suppressed in 2 patients by contralateral electrical stimulation of the midbrain-thalamic junction (201). The physiological implications of this observation and its ultimate role, if any, in clinical management are uncertain.

PAROXYSMAL DYSKINESIAS

The paroxysmal dyskinesias are intriguing disorders which bridge the realms of epilepsy and movement disorders. They are uncommon diseases with peculiar features, which often lead to an initial diagnosis of hysteria. Lance (202) has proposed that the paroxysmal dyskinesias be classified into two groups: paroxysmal dystonic choreoathetosis (PDC) and paroxysmal kinesogenic choreoathetosis (PKC).

The age of onset of PDC is usually in early infancy, but it may be as late as 22 years (202). The disorder consists of attacks of abnormal involuntary movements which may be dystonic or choreoathetotic. The movements can be unilateral, sometimes alternating sides in the same patient during different attacks, or bilateral. Although the patient may be anarthric during an attack, consciousness is preserved. The attacks may last from minutes to hours. The maximum frequency of attacks has been about three per day. Alcohol, fatigue, coffee, tea, and stress are frequently precipitating factors. Four reported families with this disorder, reviewed by Lance (202), have shown an autosomal dominant pattern of inheritance. PDC does not generally respond to phenytoin or carbamazepine. Lance (202) and more recently Tibbles and Barnes (203) have reported improvement with clonazepam.

PKC is also characterized by attacks of abnormal involuntary movements, either dystonic or choreoathetotic. Unlike PDC, the age of onset in familial cases is usually 5 to 15 years, although it can be quite variable in acquired cases. The attacks are brief in PKC, lasting no more than 5 minutes. They can be as frequent as 100 a day. The most common precipitating factor is sudden movement after rest. In Lance's review (202), 72% of PKC cases were familial, 28% were sporadic. Most familial cases appear to follow an autosomal dominant pattern of transmission but some may be autosomal recessive. The causes of sporadic cases include cerebral palsy, hypocalcemia, multiple sclerosis, and structural lesions (202). Unlike PDC, PKC often responds to phenytoin and carbamazepine. Homan and coworkers (204) have shown in 5 cases that minimal effective phenytoin levels in children are about equal to those required to control epileptic seizures. In adults, however, the minimum levels appeared to be less than those required for seizure control, suggesting that age-related changes in brain alter the expression of the disease.

The pathophysiology of these disorders is not known, and there has been discussion about whether they should be classified as epilepsy (205) or movement disorder (206). In favor of the former is that the episodes are paroxysmal, and they respond to anticonvulsants. In favor of the latter is that the movements resemble those of movement disorders (dystonia, choreoathetosis), the movements can occur bilaterally without alteration of consciousness, evolution of attacks to focal or generalized seizures has not been described, EEG is unchanged during attacks in the majority of cases, and interictal chorea has been described (204). In 2 autopsied cases, slight asymmetry of the substantia nigra was described in 1 (207), and abnormalities of the locus ceruleus were reported in another (208). Classification of these disorders depends a great deal on how one chooses to define epilepsy and movement disorders and ultimately will be resolved by a better understanding of their pathophysiology.

REFERENCES

1. Calne DB, Kebabian JK: Parkinson's disease; unanswered questions. *J Neural Transm* [Suppl] 16:1-5, 1980

2. Marttila R, Rinne UK, Halonen P, et al: Herpes viruses and parkinsonism. Herpes simplex viruses types 1 and 2, and cytomegalovirus antibodies in serum and CSF. *Arch Neurol* 38:19-21, 1981

3. Elizan TS, Madden DL, Noble GR, et al: Viral antibodies in serum and CSF of parkinsonian patients and controls. *Arch Neurol* 36:529-534, 1979

4. Elizan TS, Terasaki PI, Yahr MD: HLA-B14 antigen and postencephalitic Parkinson's disease. *Arch Neurol* 37:542-544, 1980

5. Rosati G, Granieri E, Pinna L, et al: The risk of Parkinson disease in Mediterranean people. *Neurology* 30:250-255, 1980

6. Duvoisin RC, Eldridge R, Williams A, et al: Twin study of Parkinson disease. *Neurology* 31:77-80, 1981

7. Baumann RJ, Jameson HD, McKean HE, et al: Cigarette smoking and Parkinson disease. I. A comparison of cases with matched neighbors. *Neurology* 30:839-843, 1980

8. Hallett M, Khoshbin S: A physiological mechanism of bradykinesia. *Brain* 103:301-314, 1980

9. Flowers KA: Ballistic and corrective movements on an aiming task: intention tremor and parkinsonian movement disorders compared. *Neurology* 25:413-421, 1975

10. Evarts EV, Teravainen H, Calne DB: Reaction time in Parkinson's disease. *Brain* 104:167-186, 1981

11. Traub MM, Rothwell JC, Marsden CD: Anticipatory postural reflexes in Parkinson's disease and other akinetic-rigid syndromes and in cerebellar ataxia. *Brain* 103:393-412, 1980

12. Lance JW, Schwab RS, Peterson EA: Action tremor and the cogwheel phenomenon in Parkinson's disease. *Brain* 86:95-110, 1963

13. Findley LJ, Gresty MA, Halmagyi GM: Tremor, the cogwheel phenomenon and clonus in Parkinson's disease. *J Neurol Neurosurg Psychiatry* 44:534-546, 1981

14. Melamed E, Hefti F, Liebman J, et al: Serotonergic neurons are not involved in action of L-DOPA in Parkinson's disease. *Nature* 293:772-774, 1980

15. Melamed E, Hefti F, Wurtman RJ: Nonaminergic striatal neurons convert exogenous L-DOPA to

dopamine in parkinsonism. *Ann Neurol* 8:558-563, 1980

16. Melamed E, Hefti F, Pettibone DJ, et al: Aromatic L-amino acid decarboxylase in rat corpus striatum: implications for action of L-DOPA in parkinsonism. *Neurology* 31:651-655, 1981

17. Calne DB, Eisler T, Gopinathan G, et al: Progress in the pharmacotherapy of parkinsonism. In *Ergot Compounds and Brain Function: Neuroendrocrine and Neuropsychiatric Aspects.* Edited by Goldstein M, et al. New York, Raven Press, 1980, pp 237-243

18. Schacter M, Bedard P, Debono AG, et al: The role of D-1 and D-2 receptors. *Nature* 286:157-159, 1980

19. Javoy-Agid F, Agid Y: Is the mesocortical dopaminergic system involved in Parkinson's disease. *Neurology* 30:1326-1330, 1980

20. Lawton NF, MacDermott J: Abnormal regulation of prolactin release in idiopathic Parkinson's disease. *J Neurol Neurosurg Psychiatry* 43:1012-1015, 1980

21. Albert ML, Feldman RG, Willis AL: The 'subcortical dementia' of progressive supranuclear palsy. *J Neurol Neurosurg Psychiatry* 37:121-130, 1974

22. Alvord EC, Forno LS, Kusske JA, et al: The pathology of parkinsonism: a comparison of degenerations in cerebral cortex and brain stem. *Adv Neurol* 5:175-193, 1974

23. Hakim AM, Mathieson G: Dementia in Parkinson's disease: a neuropathologic study. *Neurology* 29:1209-1214, 1979

24. Boller F, Mizutani T, Roessman U, et al: Parkinson disease, dementia, and Alzheimer disease: clinicopathological correlations. *Ann Neurol* 7:329-335, 1980

25. Sroka H, Elizan TS, Yahr MD, et al: Organic mental syndrome and confusional states in Parkinson's disease. *Arch Neurol* 38:339-342, 1981

26. Lieberman A, Dziatolowski M, Kupersmith M, et al: Dementia in Parkinson's disease. *Ann Neurol* 6:355-359, 1979

27. Granerus AK, Carlsson A, Svanborg A: The aging neuron: influence on symptomatology and therapeutic response in Parkinson's syndrome. *Adv Neurol* 24:327-334, 1979

28. Mindham RHS: Psychiatric symptoms in parkinsonism. *J Neurol Neurosurg Psychiatry* 33:188-191, 1970

29. Celesia GC, Wanamaker WM: Psychiatric disturbances in Parkinson's disease. *Dis Nerv Syst* 33:577-583, 1972

30. Mayeux R, Stern Y, Rosen J, et al: Depression, intellectual impairment, and Parkinson's disease. *Neurology* 31:645-650, 1981

31. Nausieda PA, Weiner WJ, Klawans HL: Dystonic foot response of parkinsonism. *Arch Neurol* 37:132-136, 1980

32. Stern GM, Lander CM, Lees AJ: Akinetic freezing and trick movements in Parkinson's disease. *J Neural Transm* [Suppl] 16:137-141, 1980

33. Fahn S, Cote LJ, Snider SR, et al: The role of bromocriptine in the treatment of parkinsonism. *Neurology* 29:1077-1083, 1979

34. Guiloff RJ, George RJ, Marsden CD: Reversible supranuclear ophthalmoplegia associated with parkinsonism. *J Neurol Neurosurg Psychiatry* 43:552-554, 1980

35. Klawans HL: Hemiparkinsonism as a late complication of hemiatrophy: a new syndrome. *Neurology* 31:625-627, 1981

36. Margolin D, Hammerstad J, Orwell E, et al: Intracranial calcification in hyperparathyroidism associated with gait apraxia and parkinsonism. *Neurology* 30:1005-1007, 1980

37. Berger JR, Ross DB: Reversible Parkinson syndrome complicating postoperative hypoparathyroidism. *Neurology* 31:881-882, 1981

38. Brannan TS, Burger AA, Chandary MY: Bilateral basal ganglia calcifications visualized on CT scan. *J Neurol Neurosurg Psychiatry* 43:403-406, 1980

39. Koller WC, Cochran JW, Klawans HL: Calcification of the basal ganglia: computerized tomography and clinical correlation. *Neurology* 29:328-333, 1979

40. Murphy MJ: Clinical correlations of CT scan-detected calcifications of the basal ganglia. *Ann Neurol* 6:507-511, 1979

41. Moskowitz MA, Winickoff RN, Heinz ER: Familial calcification of the basal ganglions. *N Engl J Med* 285:72-77, 1971

42. Williams A, Houff S, Lees A, et al: Oligoclonal banding in the cerebrospinal fluid of patients with postencephalitic parkinsonism. *J Neurol Neurosurg Psychiatry* 42:790-792, 1979

43. Cotzias GC, Papavasiliou PS, Gellene R: Modification of parkinsonism. Chronic treatment with L-dopa. *N Engl J Med* 280:337-345, 1969

44. Fahn S, Calne DB: Considerations in the management of parkinsonism. *Neurology* 28:5-7, 1978

45. Yahr MD: Long-term levodopa in Parkinson's disease. *Lancet* 1:706-707, 1977

46. Lesser RP, Fahn S, Snider SR, et al: Analysis of clinical problems in parkinsonism and the complications of long-term therapy. *Neurology* 29:1253-1260, 1979

47. Markham CH, Diamond SG: Evidence to support early levodopa therapy in Parkinson's disease. *Neurology* 31:125-131, 1981

48. Sweet RD, McDowell FH: Five year's treatment of Parkinson's disease with levodopa. *Ann Intern Med* 83:456-463, 1975

49. Rinne UK, Sonninen V, Siirtola T, et al: Long-term responses of Parkinson's disease to levodopa therapy. *J Neural Transm* [Suppl] 16:149-156, 1980

50. Marsden CD, Parkes JD: 'On-off' effects in

patients with Parkinson's disease on chronic levodopa therapy. *Lancet* 1:292-296, 1976

51. Barbeau A: Six years of high-level levodopa therapy in severely akinetic patients. *Arch Neurol* 33:333-338, 1976

52. Yahr MD: Overview of present day treatment of Parkinson's disease. *J Neural Transm* 43:227-238, 1978

53. Stern GM, Lees AJ, Shaw KM, et al: The role of bromocriptine in the treatment of Parkinson's disease. In *Ergot Compounds and Brain Function: Neuroendrocrine and Neuropsychiatric Aspects.* Edited by Goldstein M, et al. New York, Raven Press, 1980, pp 267-270

54. Weiner WJ, Koller WC, Perlik S, et al: Drug holiday and management of Parkinson disease. *Neurology* 30:1257-1261, 1980

55. Koller WC, Weiner WJ, Perlik S, et al: Complications of chronic levodopa therapy: long-term efficacy of drug holiday. *Neurology* 31:473-475, 1981.

56. Direnfeld LK, Feldman RG, Alexander MP, et al: Is L-dopa drug holiday useful? *Neurology* 30:785-787, 1980

57. Hoehn MM: Increased dosage of carbidopa in patients with Parkinson's disease receiving low doses of levodopa. A pilot study. *Arch Neurol* 37:146-149, 1980

58. Calne DB, Teychenne PF, Leigh PN, et al: Treatment of parkinsonism with bromocriptine. *Lancet* 2:1355-1356, 1974

59. Godwin-Austen RB: Levodopa compared with bromocriptine in the treatment of Parkinson's disease. In *Ergot Compounds and Brain Function: Neuroendocrine and Neuropsychiatric Aspects.* Edited by Goldstein M, et al. New York, Raven Press, 1980, pp 261-265

60. Duvoisin RC, Mendoza MM, Yahr MD: A comparative study of bromocriptine and levodopa in Parkinson's disease. In *Ergot Compounds and Brain Function: Neuroendocrine and Neuropsychiatric Aspects..* Edited by Goldstein M, et al. New York, Raven Press, 1980, pp 271-275

61. Fahn S, Cote L, Barrett RE, Further experiences with low doses of bromocriptine in Parkinson's disease. In *Ergot Compounds and Brain Function: Neuroendocrine and Neuropsychiatric Aspects.* Edited by Goldstein M, et al. New York, Raven Press, 1980, pp 271-275

62. Lieberman A, Kupersmith M, Neophytides A, et al: Long-term efficacy of bromocriptine in Parkinson disease. *Neurology* 30:518-523, 1980

63. Lieberman AN, Kupersmith M, Neophytides A, et al: Bromocriptine in Parkinson's disease. Report on 106 patients treated for up to five years. In *Ergot Compounds and Brain Function: Neuroendocrine and Neuropsychiatric Aspects.* Edited by Goldstein, M, et al. New York, Raven Press, 1980, pp 245-253

64. Serby M, Angrist B, Lieberman A: Psychiatric effects of bromocriptine and lergotrile in parkinsonian patients. In *Ergot Compounds and Brain Function: Neuroendocrine and Neuropsychiatric Aspects.* Edited by Goldstein M, et al. New York, Raven Press, 1980, pp 245-253

65. Parkes JD, Schacter M, Marsden CD, et al: Lisuride in parkinsonism. *Ann Neurol* 9:48-52, 1981

66. Gopinathan G, Teravainen H, Dambrosia JM, et al: Lisuride in parkinsonism. *Neurology* 31:371-376, 1981

67. Lieberman A, Goldstein M, Leibowitz M, et al: Treatment of advanced Parkinson disease with pergolide. *Neurology* 31:675-682, 1981

68. Schacter M, Marsden CD, Parkes JD, et al: Deprenyl in the management of response fluctuations in patients with Parkinson's disease on levodopa. *J Neurol Neurosurg Psychiatry* 3:1016-1021, 1980

69. Eisler T, Teravainen H, Nelson R, et al: Deprenyl in Parkinson disease. *Neurology* 31:19-23, 1981

70. Asnis G: Parkinson's disease, depression and ECT: a review and case study. *Am J Psychiatry* 134:191-195, 1977

71. Balldin J, Eden S, Granerus A-K, et al: Electroconvulsive therapy in Parkinson's syndrome with 'on-off' phenomenon. *J Neural Transm* 47:11-21, 1980

72. Ward C, Stern GM, Pratt RTC, et al: Electroconvulsive therapy in parkinsonian patients with the 'on-off' syndrome. *J Neural Transm* 49:133-135, 1980

73. Polinsky RJ, Kopin IJ, Ebert MH, et al: Pharmacologic distinction of different orthostatic hypotension syndromes. *Neurology* 31:1-7, 1981

74. Bradbury S, Eggleston C: Postural hypotension: a report of three cases. *Am Heart J* 1:73-86, 1925

75. Shy GM, Drager GA: A neurological syndrome associated with orthostatic hypotension; a clinico-pathologic study. *Arch Neurol* 2:511-527, 1960

76. Khurana RK, Nelson E, Azzarelli B, et al: Shy-Drager syndrome: diagnosis and treatment of cholinergic dysfunction. *Neurology* 30:805-809, 1980

77. Bannister R, Oppenheimer DR: Degenerative diseases of the nervous system associated with autonomic failure. *Brain* 95:457-474, 1972

78. Kontos HA, Richardson DW, Norvell JE: Norepinephrine depletion in idiopathic orthostatic hypotension. *Ann Intern Med* 82:336-341, 1975

79. Ziegler M, Lake C, Kopin I: The sympathetic nervous system defect in primary orthostatic hypotension. *N Engl J Med* 296:293-297, 1977

80. Thomas JE, Schirger A: Idiopathic orthostatic hypotension: a study of its natural history in 57 neurologically affected patients. *Arch Neurol* 22:289-293, 1970

81. Oppenheimer DR: Lateral horn cells in progressive autonomic failure. *J Neurol Sci* 46:393-404, 1980

82. Butterfield DA, Oewswin JQ, Markesberry WR: Electron spin resonance study of membrane protein alterations in erythrocyte in Huntington's disease. *Nature* 267:453-455, 1977

83. Markesberry WR, Butterfield DA: Scanning electron microscopy studies of erythrocytes in Huntington's disease. *Biochem Biophys Res Commun* 78:560-564, 1977

84. Butterfield DA, Purdy MJ, Markesberry WR: Electron spin resonance, hematological and deformability studies of erythrocytes from patients with Huntington's disease. *Biochem Biophys Acta* 551:452-458, 1979

85. Butterfield DA, Oeswein JQ, Punty ME, et al: Increased sodium plus potassium adenosine triphosphatase activity in erythrocyte membranes in Huntington's disease. *Ann Neurol* 4:60-62, 1978

86. Butterfield DA, Doorley PF, Markesberry WR: Evidence for a membrane surface defect in erythrocytes in Huntington's disease. *Life Sci* 27:609-615, 1980

87. Bialas WA, Markesberry WR, Butterfield DA: Increased chloride transport in erythrocytes in Huntington's disease. *Biochem Biophys Res Commun* 95:1895-1900, 1980

88. Pettegrew JW, Nichols JS, Stewart RM: Membrane studies in Huntington's disease. Steady-state fluorescence studies of intact erythrocytes. *Ann Neurol* 8:381-386, 1980

89. Goetz I, Roberts E, Comings DE: Fibroblasts in Huntington's disease. *N Engl J Med* 293:1225-1227, 1975

90. Gray PN, May PC, Mundy L, et al: L-glutamate toxicity in Huntington's disease fibroblasts. *Biochem Biophys Res Commun* 95:707-714, 1980

91. Coyle JT, Schwarcz R: Lesions of striatal neurons with kainic acid provides a model for Huntington's chorea. *Nature* 263:244-246, 1976

92. McGeer EG, McGeer PL: Duplication of biochemical changes of Huntington's chorea by intrastriatal injections of glutamic and kainic acids. *Nature* 263:517-519, 1976

93. Moshell AN, Tarone RE, Barrett SF, et al: Radiosensitivity in Huntington's disease: implications for pathogenesis and presymptomatic diagnosis. *Lancet* 1:9-11, 1980

94. Arlett CF, Muriel WJ: Radiosensitivity in Huntington's chorea cell strains: a possible preclinical diagnosis. *Heredity* 42:276, 1979

95. Spokes EGS: Neurochemical alterations in Huntington's chorea. A study of postmortem brain tissue. *Brain* 103:179-210, 1980

96. Cunha L, Oliveira CR, Diniz M, et al: Homovanillic acid in Huntington's disease and Sydenham's chorea. *J Neurol Neurosurg Psychiatry* 44:258-261, 1981

97. Reisine TD, Fields JZ, Bird ED, et al: Characterization of brain dopaminergic receptors in Huntington's disease. *Commun Psychopharmacol* 2:79-84, 1978

98. Spokes EGS, Garrett NJ, Rossor MN, et al: Distribution of GABA in postmortem brain tissue from control, psychotic and Huntington's chorea subjects. *J Neurol Sci* 48:303-313, 1980

99. Enna SJ, Bennett JP, Bylund DB, et al: Alterations of brain neurotransmitter receptor binding in Huntington's chorea. *Brain Res* 116:531-537, 1976

100. Gale JS, Bird ED, Spokes EGS, et al: Human brain substance P: distribution in controls and Huntington's chorea. *J Neurochem* 30:633-634, 1978

101. Arregui A, Bennett JP, Bird ED, et al: Huntington's chorea: selective depletion of angiotensin converting enzyme in the corpus striatum. *Ann Neurol* 2:294-298, 1977

102. Emson PC, Arregui A, Clement-Jones V, et al: Regional distribution of methionine-enkephalin and substance P-like immunoreactivity in normal human brain and in Huntington's disease. *Brain Res* 199:147-160, 1980

103. Emson PC, Rehfeld JF, Langerin H, et al: Reduction in cholecystokinin-like immunoreactivity in the basal ganglia in Huntington's disease. *Brain Res* 198:497-500, 1980

104. Bruyn GW: Huntington's chorea. Historical, clinical and laboratory synopsis. In *Handbook of Clinical Neurology*. Edited by Vinken PJ, Bruyn GW. Amsterdam, North-Holland, 1968, pp 298-378

105. Brackenridge CJ: Parental factors associated with rigidity in Huntington's disease. *J Med Genet* 17:112-114, 1980

106. Brackenridge LJ, Chamberlin M: The relation of sex of choreic and rigid subjects to the age at onset of Huntington's disease. *Clin Genet* 5:248-255, 1974

107. Goetz CG, Klawans HL: Letter. *Ann Neurol* 10:203, 1981

108. Marsden CD: Prediction of Huntington's disease (letter). *Ann Neurol* 10:202-203, 1981

109. Emory AEH: Whether or not predictive tests. *Neurology* 30:345-346, 1980

110. Propert DN: Presymptomatic detection of Huntington's disease. *Med J Aust* 1:609-612, 1980

111. Klawans HL, Goetz CG, Perlik S: Presymptomatic and early detection in Huntington's disease. *Ann Neurol* 8:343-347, 1980

112. Barette J, Marsden CD: Attitudes of families to some aspects of Huntington's chorea. *Psychol Med* 1:327-336, 1979

113. Klawans HL, Paulson GW, Ringel SP, et al: Use of levodopa in detection of presymptomatic Huntington's chorea. *N Engl J Med* 286:1332-1334, 1972

114. Perry TL, Wright JM, Hansen S, et al: Isoniazid therapy of Huntington's disease. *Neurology* 29:270-275, 1979

115. Manyam BV, Katz L, Hare TA, et al: Isoniazid-induced elevation of CSF GABA levels and effects on chorea in Huntington's disease. *Ann Neurol* 10:35-37, 1981

116. Tell G, Bohlen P, Schechter PJ, et al: Treatment of Huntington disease with γ-acetylenic GABA, an irreversible inhibitor of GABA-transaminase: increased CSF GABA and homocarnosine without clinical amelioration. *Neurology* 31:207-211, 1981

117. Perry TL, Wright JM, Hansen S, et al: Failure of aminooxyacetic acid therapy in Huntington's disease. *Neurology* 30:772-775, 1981

118. Hans MB, Koeppen AH: Huntington's chorea. Its impact on the spouse. *J Nerv Ment Dis* 168:209-214, 1980

119. Nausieda PA, Grossman BJ, Koller WC, et al: Sydenham chorea: an update. *Neurology* 30:331-334, 1980

120. Nardu S, Narasimhachari N: Sydenham's chorea. A possible presynaptic dopaminergic dysfunction initially. *Ann Neurol* 8:445-447, 1980

121. Bal SH, Vates TS, Kenton EJ: Generalized chorea associated with chronic subdural hematomas. *Ann Neurol* 8:449-450, 1980

122. Kotagal S, Shuter E, Horenstein S: Chorea as a manifestation of bilateral subdural hematoma in an elderly man. *Arch Neurol* 38:195, 1981

123. Leibel RL, Shih VE, Goodman SI, et al: Glutaric acidemia: a metabolic disorder causing progressive choreoathetosis. *Neurology* 30:1163-1168, 1980

124. Nausieda PA, Koller WC, Weiner WJ, et al: Pemoline-induced chorea *Neurology* 31:356-360, 1981

125. Wasserman S, Yahr M: Choreic movements induced by the use of methadone. *Arch Neurol* 37:727-728, 1980

126. Crane G, Smith RC: The prevalence of tardive dyskinesia. In *Tardive Dyskinesia.* Edited by Fann, WE, et al. New York, Spectrum Publications, 1980, pp 269-279

127. Gardos G, Cole JO, LaBrie RA: Drug variables in the etiology of tardive dyskinesia: application of discriminant function analysis. In *Tardive Dyskinesia.* Edited by Fann WE, et al. New York, Spectrum Publications, 1980, pp 291-296

128. Baldessarini RJ: Dopamine and pathophysiology of dyskinesia induced by antipsychotic drugs. *Annu Rev Neurosci* 3:23-41, 1980

129. Baldessarini RJ, Tarsy D: The pathophysiologic basis of tardive dyskinesia. In *Tardive Dyskinesia.* Edited by Fann WE, et al. New York, Spectrum Publications, 1980, pp 181-186

130. Burt DR, Creese I, Snyder SH: Antischizophrenic drugs: chronic treatment elevates dopamine receptor binding in brain. *Science* 196:326-328, 1977

131. Friedhoff AJ, Bonnet K, Rosengarten H: Reversal of two manifestations of dopamine receptor supersensitivity by administration of L-dopa. *Res Commun Chem Pathol Pharmacol* 16:411-423, 1977

132. Muller P, Seeman P: Brain neurotransmitter receptors after long-term haloperidol. *Life Sci* 21:1751-1758, 1977

133. Gunne L, Barany S: A primate model for tardive dyskinesia. In *Tardive Dyskinesia.* Edited by Fann WE, et al. New York, Spectrum Publications, 1980, pp 1-12

134. Muller P, Seeman P: Effect of long-term neuroleptic treatment on neurotransmitter receptors: relation to tardive dyskinesia. In *Tardive Dyskinesia.* Edited by Fann WE, et al. New York, Spectrum Publication, 1980, pp 115-125

135. Staton RD, Brumback RA: Neuroleptic-induced reinnervative sprouting in the central nervous system. *J Clin Psychiatry* 41:427-428, 1980

136. Baldessarini RJ, Cole JO, Davis JM, et al: Tardive dyskinesia: summary of a task force report of the American Psychiatric Association. *Am J Psychiatry* 137:1163-1172, 1980

137. Gardas G, Cole JO: Overview: public health issues in tardive dyskinesia. *Am J Psychiatry* 137:776-781, 1980

138. Smith JM, Baldessarini RJ: Changes in prevalence, severity, and recovery in tardive dyskinesia with age. *Arch Gen Psychiatry* 37:1368-1373, 1980

139. Crane GE: Neuroleptic drugs and other factors predisposing to tardive dyskinesia. In *Tardive Dyskinesia.* Edited by Fann WE, et al. New York, Spectrum Publications, 1980, pp 281-290

140. Klawans HL, Coetz CG, Perlik S: Tardive dyskinesia: review and update. *Am J Psychiatry* 137:900-908, 1980

141. Tardive dyskinesia scales in current use. In *Tardive Dyskinesia.* Edited by Fann WE, et al. New York, Spectrum Publications, 1980, pp 243-267

142. Barnes TRE, Kidger T, Traver T, et al: Re-classification of the tardive dyskinesia syndrome. *Adv Biochem Psychopharmacol* 24:565-568, 1980

143. Kidger T, Barnes TRE, Traver T, et al: Subsyndromes of tardive dyskinesia. *Psychol Med* 10:513-520, 1980

144. Simpson GM: Neurotoxicity of major tranquilizers. In *Neurotoxicology.* Edited by Roizin L, Shiraki H, Grcevic N. New York, Raven Press, 1977, pp 1-7

145. Bobruff A, Gardos G, Tarsy D, et al: Clonazepam and phenobarbital in tardive dyskinesia. *Am J Psychiatry* 138:189-193, 1981

146. Polizos P, Engelhardt DM: Dyskinetic and neurological complications in children treated with psychotropic medications. In *Tardive Dyskinesia.* Edited by Fann WE, et al. New York, Spectrum Publications, 1980, pp 193-199

147. Casey De, Gerlack H: Oxiperomide in tardive dyskinesia. *J Neurol Neurosurg Psychiatry* 43:264-267, 1980

148. Alpert M, Friedhoff AJ: Clinical application of receptor modification treatment. In *Tardive Dyskinesia.* Edited by Fann WE, et al. New York, Spectrum Publications, 1980, pp 471-473

149. Bjorndal N, Casey D, Gelach J: Dopamine antagonist and agonist treatment in tardive

dyskinesia. *Adv Biochem Psychopharmacol* 24:541-545, 1980

150. Domino EF, Kovacic B: Status of deanol as a cholinergic precursor-experimental evidence and clinical uses in tardive dyskinesia. In *Tardive Dyskinesia.* Edited by Fann WE, et al. New York, Spectrum Publications, 1980, pp 379-393

151. Cole JO, Gardas G, Tarsy D, et al: Drug trials in persistent dyskinesia. In *Tardive Dyskinesia.* Edited by Fann WE, et al. New York, Spectrum Publications, 1980, pp 419-427

152. Zeisel SH, Geleberg AJ, Growdon JH, et al: Use of choline and lecithin in the treatment of tardive dyskinesia. *Adv Biochem Psychopharmacol* 24:463-470, 1980

153. Casey DE, Gerlach J, Magelund G, et al: γ-Acetylenic GABA in tardive dyskinesia. *Arch Gen Psychiatry* 37:1376-1379, 1980

154. Chase, TN, Tamminga CA: Pharmacologic studies of tardive dyskinesia. *Adv Biochem Psychopharmacol* 24:457-461, 1980

155. Nair NPV, Lal S, Schwartz G, et al: Effect of sodium valproate and baclofen in tardive dyskinesia; clinical and neuroendocrine studies. *Adv Biochem Psychopharmacol* 24:437-441, 1980

156. Klawans HL, Nausieda PA, Weiner WJ: The effect of lithium on haloperidol-induced supersensitivity to D-amphetamine and apomorphine. In *Tardive Dyskinesia.* Edited by Fann WE, et al. New York, Spectrum Publications, 1980, pp 165-170

157. Mackay AVP, Sheppard GP, Saha BK, et al: Failure of lithium treatment in established tardive dyskinesia. *Psychol Med* 10:583-587, 1980

158. Shapiro AK, Shapiro ES, Brunn RD, et al: *Gilles de la Tourette Syndrome.* New York, Raven Press, 1978

159. Mendelsohn WB, Caine ED, Goyer P, et al: Sleep in Gilles de la Tourette syndrome. *Biol Psychiatry* 15:339-343, 1980

160. Nee LE, Caine ED, Polinsky RJ, et al: Gilles de la Tourette syndrome: clinical and family study of 50 cases. *Ann Neurol* 7:41-49, 1980

161. O'Quinn AN, Thompson RJ: Tourette's syndrome: an expanded view. *Pediatrics* 66:420-424, 1980

162. Golden GS: Gilles de la Tourette's syndrome following methylphenidate administration. *Dev Med Child Neurol* 16:76-78, 1974

163. Klawans HL, Falk DK, Nausieda PA, et al: Gilles de la Tourette syndrome after long-term chlorpromazine therapy. *Neurology* 28:1064-1066, 1978

164. Butler I, Koslow SH, Seifert WE, et al: Biogenic amine metabolism in Tourette syndrome. *Ann Neurol* 6:37-39, 1979

165. Kidd KK, Prusoff BA, Cohen DJ: Familial pattern of Gilles de la Tourette syndrome. *Arch Gen Psychiatry* 37:1336-1339, 1980

166. Abe K, Oda N: Incidence of tics in the offspring of childhood tiquers: a controlled follow-up study. *Dev Med Child Neurol* 22:649-653, 1980

167. DeVeough-Geiss J: Tardive Tourette syndrome. *Neurology* 30:562, 1980

168. Stahl SM: Tardive Tourette syndrome in an autistic patient after long-term neuroleptic administration. *Am J Psychiatry* 137:1267-1269, 1980

169. Fog R, Pakkenberg H: Theoretical and clinical aspects of the Tourette syndrome. *J Neural Transm* [Suppl] 16:211-215, 1980

170. Mizrahi EM, Holtzman D, Tharp B: Haloperidol-induced tardive dyskinesia in a child with Gilles de la Tourette syndrome. *Arch Neurol* 37:780, 1980

171. Cohen DJ, Detlor J, Young G, et al: Clonidine ameliorates Gilles de la Tourette syndrome. *Arch Gen Psychiatry* 37:1350-1357, 1980

172. Stahl SM, Berger PA: Physostigmine in Tourette syndrome: evidence for cholinergic underactivity. *Am J Psychiatry* 138:240-242, 1981

173. Eldridge R: The torsion dystonias: literature review and genetic and clinical studies. *Neurology* 20:1-78, 1970

174. Korczyn AD, Kahana E, Zilber N, et al: Torsion dystonia in Israel. *Ann Neurol* 8:387-391, 1980

175. Eldridge R: Inheritance of torsion dystonia in Jews. *Ann Neurol* 10:203, 1981

176. Korczyn A, et al: Letter. *Ann Neurol* 10:204, 1981

177. Meige H: Les convulsions de la face, une forme clinique de convulsion facial, bilaterale et mediane. *Revue Neurol (Paris)* 20:437-443, 1910

178. Marsden CD: Blepharospasm-oromandibular dystonia syndrome (Brueghel's syndrome). *J Neurol Neurosurg Psychiatry* 39:1204-1209, 1976

179. Tolosa E: Clinical features of Meige's disease (idiopathic orofacial dystonia). *Arch Neurol* 38:147-151, 1981

180. Nutt JG, Hammerstad JP: Blepharospasm and oromandibular dystonia (Meige's syndrome) in sisters. *Ann Neurol* 9:189-191, 1981

181. Tolsoa ES, Lai C: Meige's disease: striatal dopaminergic preponderance. *Neurology* 29:1126-1130, 1979

182. Casey DE: Pharmacology of blepharospasm-oromandibular dystonia syndrome. *Neurology* 30:690-695, 1980

183. Garcia-Albea E, Frande O, Munoz D, et al: Brueghel's syndrome, report of a case with postmortem studies. *J Neurol Neurosurg Psychiatry* 44:437-440, 1981

184. Burke RE, Fahn S, Gold AP: Delayed onset dystonia in patients with 'static' encephalopathy. *J Neurol Neurosurg Psychiatry* 43:789-707, 1980

185. Hansen RA, Berenberg W, Byers RK: Changing motor patterns in cerebral palsy. *Dev Med Child Neurol* 12:309-314, 1970

186. Goldman JE, Katz D, Rapin I, et al: Chronic GM_1 gangliosidosis presenting as dystonia: I. Clinical and pathological features. *Ann Neurol* 9:465-475, 1981

187. Kobayashi T, Suzuki K: Chronic GM_1 ganglio-

sidosis presenting as dystonia: II. Biochemical studies. *Ann Neurol* 9:476-483, 1981

188. Bodensteiner JB, Goldblum RM, Goldman AS: Progressive dystonia masking ataxia in ataxia-telangiectasia. *Arch Neurol* 37:464-465, 1980

189. Dooling EC, Schoene WC, Richardson EP: Hallervorden-Spatz syndrome. *Arch Neurol* 30:70-83, 1974

190. Dooling EC, Richardson EP, Davis KR: Computed tomography in Hallervorden-Spatz disease. *Neurology* 30:1128-1130, 1980

191. Kolbe H, Clow A, Jenner P, et al: Neuroleptic-induced acute dystonic reactions may be due to enhanced dopamine release or to supersensitive postsynaptic receptors. *Neurology* 31:434-439, 1981

192. Jankovic J, Fahn S: Physiologic and pathologic tremors. *Ann Int Med* 93:460-465, 1980

193. Young RR, Hagbarth K: Physiological tremor enhanced by maneuvers affecting the segmental stretch reflex. *J Neurol Neurosurg Psychiatry* 43:248-256, 1980

194. Marsden CD, Meadows JC, Lowe RD: The influence of noradrenaline, tyramine, and activation of sympathetic nerves on physiological tremor in man. *Clin Sci* 37:243-252, 1969

195. James IM, Pearson RM, Griffith DNW, et al: Effect of oxprenolol on stage-fright in musicians. *Lancet* 2:952-954, 1977

196. Winkler GF, Young RR: Efficacy of chronic propranolol therapy in action tremors of the familial, senile or essential varieties. *N Engl J Med* 290:984-988, 1974

197. Sorensen PS, Paulson OB, Steiness E, et al: Essential tremor treated with propranolol: lack of correlation between clinical effect and plasma propranolol levels. *Ann Neurol* 9:53-57, 1981

198. Britt CW, Peters BH: Metoprolol for essential tremor. *N Engl J Med* 301:331, 1979

199. Newman RP, Jacobs L: Metoprolol in essential tremor. *Arch Neurol* 37:596-597, 1980

200. Hewer RL, Coopre R, Morgan MH: An investigation into the value of treating intention tremor by weighting the affected limb. *Brain* 95:579-590, 1972

201. Brice J, McLellan L: Suppression of intention tremor by contingent deep-brain stimulation. *Lancet* 1:1221-1222, 1980

202. Lance JW: Familial paroxysmal dystonic choreo-athetosis and its differentiation from related syndromes. *Ann Neurol* 2:285-293, 1977

203. Tibbles JAR, Barnes SE: Paroxysmal dystonic choreoathetosis of Mount and Reback. *Pediatrics* 65:149-151, 1980

204. Homan RW, Vasko MR, Blaw M: Phenytoin plasma concentrations in paroxysmal kinesigenic choreoathetosis. *Neurology* 30:673-676, 1980

205. Hudgins RL, Corbin KB: An uncommon seizure disorder: familial paroxysmal choreoathetosis. *Brain* 89:199-204, 1966

206. Goodenough DJ, Farrello RG, Annis BL, et al: Familial and acquired paroxysmal dyskinesias. *Arch Neurol* 35:827-831, 1978

207. Stevens H: Paroxysmal choreoathetosis: a form of reflex epilepsy. *Arch Neurol* 14:415-420, 1966

208. Kertesz A: Paroxysmal kinesigenic choreo-athetosis. *Neurology* 17:680-690, 1967

5

Metabolic Disorders

Thomas K. Koch and Ivan Diamond

This chapter reviews the recent literature of several metabolic encephalopathies related to liver function. The reviews of Reye's syndrome and hepatic encephalopathy supplement information presented in *Current Neurology*, vol. 3, and include new sections on therapy. The reviews of Wilson's disease and bilirubin encephalopathy present recent information about the pathogenesis and management of these conditions.

REYE'S SYNDROME

In 1963 Reye and coworkers (1) reported 21 children ranging from 5 months to 8 1/2 years of age with an acute noninflammatory encephalopathy accompanied by fatty degeneration of the liver. The authors recognized that the onset of the disease usually began with a mild viral illness with upper respiratory or gastrointestinal tract symptoms which progressed to recurrent vomiting, disturbed consciousness, convulsions, and altered muscle tone and reflexes. Seven of the original twenty-one patients had liver function studies, and all had increased transaminase activities. Hypoglycemia frequently complicated the management of these patients. Seventeen of the twenty-one children died, and at autopsy all had striking cerebral swelling and enlarged firm fatty livers often associated with fatty infiltration of the kidneys. Although an acute noninflammatory encephalopathy of childhood had

been recognized before, it was not until this report that an association was made with fatty degeneration of the liver. Since then, Reye's syndrome has become recognized as a major cause of death in childhood from a potentially reversible central nervous system disease.

Epidemiology

The epidemiology of Reye's syndrome is not well understood. It has been recognized since the initial report of Reye and coworkers (1) that the disease often follows a mild illness. Epidemics of influenza B virus in 1974 were shown to correspond temporally and geographically to outbreaks of Reye's syndrome (2). However, other infectious diseases were also shown to be associated with Reye's syndrome. These include: varicella (3); influenza A (4); parainfluenza (4); echovirus (4): reovirus (4); rubella (4); rubeola (4): polio virus type 1 (4); respiratory syncytial virus (5); Epstein-Barr virus (6); herpes simplex type 1 (7); coxsackievirus A, A_1, B_1, and B_4 (4); live virus vaccines (5); *Hemophilus influenzae* (8); and *Yersinia pestis* (5). Some reports have implicated varicella in 10% to 20% of cases of Reye's syndrome (9). Approximately 77% of patients with uncomplicated chickenpox have an elevated serum glutamic-oxaloacetic transaminase (SGOT) as a subclinical hepatic change to the varicella (9). This elevation does not suggest that such patients have Reye's syndrome or that there is a relationship

---

Preparation of this manuscript was supported in part by grants from the National Institutes of Health.

between varicella hepatitis and Reye's syndrome.

In addition to infectious agents, toxins have also been reported to cause a Reye-like illness. Aflatoxin B_1 (10) and hypoglycin A (11) cause an encephalopathy with fatty visceral changes. Recently there have been several reports of a Reye-like syndrome in patients receiving valproic acid therapy (12, 13). Perhaps this is related to the similarities between valproic acid (2-propylpentanoic acid) and the known potent inhibitors of fatty acid oxidation, 4-pentonic acid (12) and hypoglycin (12). High-dose long-term salicylate therapy may also lead to a metabolic disturbance characterized by hepatic failure, hyperammonemia, and toxic metabolic encephalopathy (14). Recently a 4-year-old child on long-term salicylates for rheumatoid arthritis developed a fatal Reye's syndrome after symptoms of a trivial infection (15). Previous reports did suggest a relationship between Reye's syndrome and aspirin taken during an associated antecedent illness. The Center for Disease Control (CDC) reported the results of two controlled studies, indicating that patients with Reye's syndrome are more than 11 times as likely to have taken salicylates than controls (16). They concluded that during certain viral illnesses the use of salicylates—even before the onset of vomiting—may be a factor in the pathogenesis of Reye's syndrome (16). A third study recently reported similar findings supporting the CDC's conclusions (17). In addition, a correlation was found between salicylate consumption and the severity of the encephalopathy (17).

Although Reye's syndrome is usually considered to be a disease of childhood and adolescence, there are now several reports of Reye's syndrome in adults (18, 19). Moreover, Reye's syndrome in infants has been reported with increasing frequency, and it appears that there are several distinguishing features to the clinical presentation in the infantile age group. Huttenlocher and Trauner (20) reported the clinical findings of 8 infants less than 6 months of age and noted that the patients tend to develop a sudden onset of respiratory distress with tachypnea and apneic episodes. Although vomiting usually occurs, it is not a prominent feature. Seizures tend to occur with high frequency early in the course of the disease. Increased intracranial pressure is often present, but the fontanelle is rarely so tense that the intracranial pressure becomes life-threatening. This is in contrast to the older child who has severe and often fatal cerebral edema (20, 21). Despite the decreased severity of the cerebral edema in infancy, infants appear to be more susceptible to the metabolic derangements that occur in Reye's syndrome; they also have a higher morbidity and mortality rate (20). In addition to these clinical findings, Huttenlocher and Trauner (20) also reported that infants with Reye's syndrome come from predominantly urban and low socioeconomic groups. This socioeconomic bias was confirmed recently by reviewing epidemiologic information about 54 children less than 1 year of age who were reported to the CDC from 1974 through 1978. This study found that 48% of the children less than 1 year of age with Reye's syndrome were black, while only 8% of all children affected were black (23).

The appearance of Reye's syndrome in siblings has been reported and has been shown to exceed that of the general population (22). HLA typing has been performed on the siblings in an attempt to identify a common genetic marker, but none has been found (23).

Clinical Features

The diagnosis of Reye's syndrome should be suspected in patients—particularly patients less than 20 years of age—who develop an acute alteration in mental status after a mild viral-like illness. The diagnostic criteria have been reviewed in detail (5, 19). In 1972 Huttenlocher (24) described four clinical stages of the disease, and in 1974 Lovejoy and coworkers (25) described five stages (Table 1). Recently, some clinicians have become very aggressive in the management of mild to moderate Reye's syndrome, while others reserve this approach for moderate to severe Reye's syndrome. Therefore, the diagnostic criteria used to establish the stage of the illness and the indications for aggressive management are controversial (26). Some authors advocate vigorous management with intra-

Table 1: Clinical Stages in Reye's Syndrome

Stage	Huttenlocher*	Lovejoy et al†
I	Stupor or delirium	Vomiting, lethargy, abnormal liver function tests (LFTs), and slow electroencephalogram (EEG) predominant theta
II	Coma with withdrawal to pain or flexion posturing (decorticate)	Disorientation, delirium, combativeness, hyperventilation, hyperactive reflexes, withdrawal to pain, abnormal LFTs, and slow EEG predominantly delta
III	Coma with extensor posturing (decerebrate) of upper limbs, preserved pupillary responses, and spontaneous respirations	Obtundent, coma, hyperventilation, decorticate rigidity, intact pupillary and oculovestibular responses, and slow EEG predominantly delta
IV	Flaccid paralysis without response to pain, absent respirations and pupillary reflexes	Deepening coma with decerebrate rigidity, large fixed pupils, abnormal oculovestibular response, other evidence of brain stem dysfunction, and low voltage EEG with burst suppression or isoelectric intervals
V	. . .	Seizures, loss of reflexes, respiratory arrest, flaccidity, and isoelectric EEG

* Huttenlocher PR: Reye's syndrome: relation of outcome to therapy. *J Pediatr* 80:845-850,1972.

† Lovejoy FH, Smith AL, Bresnan MJ, et al: Clinical staging in Reye syndrome. *Am J Dis Child* 128:36-41, 1974.

cranial monitoring, mechanical ventilation, and the induction of barbiturate coma when the patient reaches Lovejoy-stage II (27). Others reserve this management for Lovejoy-stage III (28, 29). At the University of California, San Francisco, we begin aggressive management for children who are either at or rapidly approaching Lovejoy-stage III. Trauner (28) proposed the use of the Glasgow coma scale (30) and recommended aggressive management for children who are either at or rapidly approaching Lovejoy-stage III. Trauner (28) proposed the use of the Glasgow coma scale (30) and recommended aggressive management with a score of 7 or less.

There have been two reports of computer assisted tomography in Reye's syndrome (31, 32), and noncontrast scans show acute and residual changes. The acute changes indicate diffuse cerebral edema with low density deep in white matter, increased gray-white matter differentiation, and evidence of secondary ventricular compression (32). The residual changes after severe disease are nonspecific and atrophic in nature, reflecting cytotoxic damage and anoxia with resultant cerebral degeneration (32). There is a frontal predominance for these findings (32).

In addition to hepatic dysfunction and a severe metabolic encephalopathy, Reye's syndrome can be complicated by other organ system involvement. A frequent complication is acute pancreatitis associated with hypotension, hypocalcemia, and labile blood glucose levels (33, 34). Acute renal failure is a life-threatening complication in a patient who is receiving osmotic diuretics for increased intracranial pressure since it may lead to hypervolemia, cardiac failure, and worsening of the cerebral edema (5, 35). The occurrence of neurologic pulmonary edema is not a surprising complication in a disease characterized by intracranial hypertension (36). This may begin as progressive pulmonary insufficiency after cerebral and hepatic function have become normal (36). Retinal hemorrhages have been reported as a manifestation of central retinal vein occlusion in Reye's syndrome (37).

Pathology

Morphologic abnormalities have been detected in brain, liver, kidney, heart, pancreas, lungs, gastrointestinal tract, spleen, thymus, and lymph nodes of patients with Reye's syndrome (4, 5). The brain characteristically weighs 10%-15% more than normal and is diffusely edematous with flattened cortical surfaces and gyral enlargement. There is often evidence of uncal and cerebellar herniation (4). Microscopically there is necrosis of cortical neurons, loss of Purkinje cells, astrocytic swelling, reactive astrocytosis, and myelin bleb formation (4, 5). Alzheimer type II glia cells seen in hepatic encephalopathy are absent in Reye's syndrome (4). Examination of the mitochondria reveals pleomorphism and matrix expansion limited to neurons (5, 21). Liver pathology consists of diffuse microvesicular fatty change and occasional mild periportal hepatic necrosis (38). In a recent review of the liver pathology in Reye's syndrome, Bentz and Cohen (38) described a case with hemorrhagic periportal necrosis. They support the hypothesis that fatty acids are the toxins that cause mitochondrial injury, especially in periportal hepatocytes (39). These cells are the first to be exposed to high levels of fatty acids and are less capable of metabolizing the fatty acids. Aflatoxin B causes a similar periportal necrosis in rats (38). Ultrastructural studies of hepatocytes, heart, and pancreas in Reye's syndrome reveal the same mitochondrial changes as in neurons (38, 39). Occasionally, the encephalopathy in Reye's syndrome develops before there is biochemical or histological evidence of liver dysfunction (38, 40). This suggests that brain involvement may not be dependent upon hepatic dysfunction and that there may be a common mitochondrial insult. A more complete discussion about mitochondrial involvement was presented in *Current Neurology*, vol. 3 (5).

Pathophysiology

Pathological and biochemical studies con-tinue to support the idea that the mitochondria is the primary site of injury in Reye's syndrome (5). There are many reports about abnormal mitochondrial enzyme activity in liver, brain, and muscle (41-46). Elevated plasma and urinary tyramine levels (41, 42) have suggested a disruptive effect upon hepatic monoamine oxidase (41-43). This enzyme activity was reported to be about 60% reduced in stage V Reye's syndrome patients (42). Mitchell and coworkers (43) studied nine enzymes in liver specimens obtained from four children who died with Reye's syndrome; activities were compared to activities of control children who died from unrelated causes. They found that the ratio of cytosolic:mitochondrial enzyme activity was significantly greater in Reye's syndrome than in the control group (43). This study confirmed previous work which proposed that depressed liver enzymes were related to mitochondrial disease. The investigators speculated that the decrease in activity of monoamine oxidase, an outer mitochondrial membrane enzyme, may be related to elevated tyramine and octopamine (43). Severe hepatic dysfunction has been correlated with elevated levels of octopamine in the hypothalamus in both Reye's and non-Reye's encephalopathies (47). In *Current Neurology*, vol. 3, we cited a report of elevated levels of monoamine metabolites in ventricular fluid from patients with Reye's syndrome. Interestingly, this increased rate of monoamine metabolism by the brain occurs at the same time that liver monoamine oxidase activity is impaired. Mitchell and coworkers (42, 43) commented on possible dys-synchronous mitochondrial involvement. Shaywitz and coworkers (48) postulated that the increased homovanillic acid (HVA) levels in the cerebrospinal fluid (CSF) may be due to cerebral ischemia and release of vasoactive amines from the brain and not directly related to increased monoamine oxidase activity.

Serum from patients with Reye's syndrome has been shown to cause mitochondrial swelling (48) and to stimulate oxygen utilization in preparations of isolated rat liver mitochondria. Aprille and coworkers (49) attempted to identify the "serum factor" responsible for the swelling and stimulation.

They employed three different methods of isolation, and all three approaches yielded uric acid as a common factor. Moreover, uric acid was capable of stimulating oxygen utilization, but it did not produce mitochondrial swelling. Thus, these investigators postulated the presence of another "swelling factor." Further studies by Ansevin (44) disclosed that serum from patients with Reye's syndrome when added to rat brain mitochondria stimulated the resting respiratory rate, decreased respiratory control, stimulated ATPase activity, and decreased the rate of phosphorylation. These changes were most marked when serum from deeply comatose patients was used, but the effects could be blocked by the addition of fatty acid-free albumin (43). One explanation is that short- and medium-chain fatty acids, which have high affinity for albumin, may be the factors in serum responsible for the mitochondrial injury (43). It is known that short-chain fatty acids have a disruptive effect on normal mitochondrial energy production (5) and increased concentrations of short-chain fatty acids may play a crucial role in coma production in Reye's syndrome (5). Trauner (50) has shown that infusions of sodium octanoate in rabbits produces increased intracranial pressure with pressure plateau waves and electroencephalographic (EEG) abnormalities with generalized slowing of the background activity. Further studies of lipid homeostasis in Reye's syndrome have shown markedly increased hepatic triglyceride concentrations which correlate well with severe panlobular fatty changes (51). These changes were not found in non-Reye's hyperammonemic encephalopathies.

Many inborn errors of metabolism are known to produce hyperammonemic hepatic encephalopathy (5). At least three of these disorders may present as a recurrent Reye-like syndrome. The first is systemic carnitine deficiency (52, 53). In a report by Chapoy and coworkers (52) treatment was attempted with oral carnitine supplementation; substantial clinical and chemical responses were produced. Unfortunately, studies of carnitine levels in patients with Reye's syndrome have not been helpful. One study reported increased serum levels during the acute phase of the illness (54), while a second study reported reduced liver and muscle carnitine concentrations during the acute phase of the disease (55). Patients with glutaric acidemia type II can develop repeated episodes of hypoglycemia, elevated serum levels of free fatty acids, and fatty infiltration of the liver, precipitated by infection (56). Hydroxymethylglutaryl CoA lyase deficiency can also cause a clinical syndrome similar to that of Reye's syndrome when the patient is stressed by an acute viral infection (57). The common link between these inborn errors of metabolism and hypoglycin toxicity—a known inhibitor of isovalenyl CoA dehydrogenase and fatty acyl CoA transport—is the ability to interrrupt normal acyl CoA metabolism (57). It has been postulated that if hepatic mitochondrial integrity is compromised early in Reye's syndrome then a block in acyl CoA metabolism occurs which may be responsible for the majority of the observed clinical features (57).

At present we do not understand the role these metabolic pathways play in the development of Reye's syndrome. It seems likely that mitochondrial injury is of primary importance in the pathophysiology of this condition, but it is not certin whether elevations of medium- and short-chain fatty acids are cause or effect.

Treatment

In Reye's original report in 1963 (1) the mortality rate for acute encephalopathy with fatty infiltration of the viscera was 80%. In 1969 Huttenlocher and coworkers (58) associated hyperammonemia with Reye's syndrome and suggested treatment with exchange transfusions. Despite this intervention, the mortality rate still loomed near 60%. It was not until the mid-1970s that the morbidity and mortality rates began to decline. This is probably due to the development of effective intracranial pressure monitoring, controlled ventilation, cardiovascular monitoring, vigorous management of increased intracranial pressure, and the early identification of the patients. Shaywitz and coworkers (29) reported the outcome of 29 children with Reye's syndrome admitted to Yale-New Haven Hospital since initiating a regimen of intracranial pressure monitoring, controlled respiration, and administration of mannitol and barbiturates to patients whose clinical status deteriorated to Lovejoy-stage III coma. Since 1975 they have had 2 deaths in a group of 29 children (6.9%), and significant neurologic residua developed in only 3 patients (10.3%).

An outline for the management of patients with Reye's syndrome as proposed by Trauner (59) is presented in Table 2. As discussed earlier, aggressive management with controlled ventilation, intracranial and cardiovascular monitoring, and vigorous management of intracranial pressure is most commonly instituted at or near Lovejoy-stage III coma (28, 29). Once the decision is made that aggressive management is warranted, the patient should be intubated immediately and placed on a mechanical respirator. This usually requires the administration of pancuronium bromide (Pavulon) in a dose of 0.1 to 0.2 mg/kg of body weight to produce muscle paralysis so that the patient will not resist the respirator. The tidal volume and respirator rate should be adjusted to maintain a P_{CO_2} at about 25 mm Hg (27, 59). This P_{CO_2} level produces enough vasoconstriction to help reduce intracranial pressure but not enough to compromise perfusion (60). If the P_{CO_2} is too low, ischemic damage to the brain may result from severe vascoconstriction (60).

Table 2. Outline of Management for Patients with Reye's Syndrome

1. Temperature should be maintained below 37°C with a cooling blanket.
2. Nasotracheal intubation is performed.
3. Controlled hyperventilation via a mechanical respirator should be used to maintain carbon dioxide tension at 25 mm Hg.
4. Hypertonic glucose (15% to 20% solution) should be given intravenously to keep blood glucose levels between 150 and 200 mg/100 ml.
5. Insulin is administered intravenously, 1 unit per 10 g of glucose every 4 hours initially, increasing the dose according to blood glucose concentration. Alternatively, insulin can be given as a continuous intravenous infusion if albumin is added to the intravenous solution. Dextrostix should be used to check blood glucose immediately before and ½ hour after insulin is given. Quantitative serum glucose determination should be performed every 4 hours.
6. Fluid and electrolyte balance should be carefully maintained. A bladder catheter and nasogastric tube should be inserted so that accurate intake and output can be calculated.
7. Neomycin enemas may be given to help reduce serum ammonia levels.
8. Central venous and arterial pressures should be monitored.
9. A ventricular or subdural monitoring device should be inserted for continuous recording of intracranial pressure. If prothrombin time is prolonged, fresh-frozen plasma can be given or a partial exchange transfusion performed to correct it so the monitor can be inserted safely.
10. If intracranial pressure is elevated or if the patient is fighting the respirator, pancuronium bromide (Pavulon) in a dose of 0.1 to 0.2 mg/k of body weight should be given for muscle paralysis *after* a careful neurological assessment has been completed. Pavulon can be discontinued briefly if neurological reassessment is required, but intracranial pressure should be watched closely, as it may rise.
11. Mannitol, 0.25 g/k per dose, should be given intravenously if intracranial pressure rises above 20 mm Hg.
12. Serum osmolality should be measured every 4 hours and kept below 320 mOsm/L.
13. Careful chest physiotherapy and suctioning should be performed every 2 hours. The patient should not be turned but should be positioned on the back with the head elevated 30 degrees.
14. If these measures fail to control intracranial pressure, barbiturate coma should be instituted.

Note.—Reprinted with permission from Trauner DA: Treatment of Reye's syndrome, *Ann Neurol* 7:2-4, 1980.

General Management

Strict attention needs to be given to the patient's blood chemistries and gases and serum and urine osmolalities. Fluids should be carefully maintained to keep the patient's pulmonary capillary wedge pressure at 4-6 mm Hg (27). The serum glucose should be maintained between 150-200 mg/100 ml (59). Administration of intravenous insulin has been proposed (59), but this is not universally accepted. Lactulose or neomycin enema may be given to help reduce the amount of ammonia in the gastrointestinal tract. Vitamin K should be administered and fresh frozen plasma may be necessary if bleeding becomes excessive. Patients must be monitored for complications of Reye's syndrome, including pancreatitis (33, 34), acute renal failure (5, 35), and neurogenic pulmonary edema (36).

Management of Increased Intracranial Pressure

Severe intracranial hypertension is the most life-threatening problem in patients with Reye's syndrome. Continuous intracranial monitoring is essential in the management of this complication. The patient's cerebral perfusion pressure can be calculated as the difference between the mean arterial pressure and intracranial pressure. This perfusion pressure should be maintained at greater than 50 mm Hg at all times to insure adequate perfusion and to prevent cerebral ischemia. Intracranial pressure levels above 20 mm Hg should should be reduced. Manual hyperventilation for several minutes can be very effective in reducing moderately elevated intracranial pressure. The effect of such a maneuver is almost immediate, and a beneficial response can be produced despite low P_{CO_2} levels (27).

Administration of osmotic diuretics such as mannitol has been very helpful. Trauner (59) reported that doses as low as 0.25 g/kg of body weight were quite effective in the treatment of acute increases in intracranial pressure. It has been Trauner's experience that most patients with Reye's syndrome can be managed with hyperventilation and osmotic agents. However, with continued use of mannitol therapy, it is imperative that the serum osmolality be monitored every 4 to 6 hours. A serum osmolality above 320 mOsm/L should be avoided because of the deleterious effects of the hyperosmolar state (61) and because mannitol is not as effective when the serum osmolality is high.

Botterell and coworkers (62) first reported that intracranial pressure was markedly reduced during hypothermia. Hypothermia is now used widely in the management of increased intracranial pressure (27, 59, 60) with recommendations that the patient's temperature be reduced to 31°C (27, 60). This requires paralysis of the patient to prevent shivering. Care should be taken to avoid temperatures below 31°C since there is an increased risk for cardiac arrhythmias at such low temperatures. Rewarming should not be done actively with heating blankets, particularly if hypothermia was used in conjunction with barbiturates. Sudden rewarming may cause barbiturates to be released into the circulation from fatty tissues, and this large bolus delivered to the heart can cause a cardiac arrest, which may not respond to electroshock therapy (60).

Barbiturate therapy was first reported in advanced Reye's syndrome by Marshall and coworkers (63) with good results. Now, many clinicians use barbiturates in the treatment of increased intracranial pressure (19, 27, 29, 59, 60). Unfortunately, the efficacy of barbiturate therapy and its mechanism of action are still unknown, although patients receiving barbiturates may require less mannitol. The most commonly employed barbiturate is pentobarbital. The dosage schedule at the University of California, San Francisco, includes induction with 5 mg/kg of pentobarbital every hour for 4 hours and then maintenance with 1-2 mg/kg every hour. The maintenance dosage is guided by the cerebral perfusion pressure (maintain above 50 mm Hg), the EEG (burst-suppression or flat line), and blood barbiturate levels (25-40 mcg/ml). The major complications of pentobarbital treatment are depression of the cardiac output and a fall in arterial blood pressure. This problem increases as the barbiturate levels rise. We reserve the use of barbiturates for those patients who cannot be controlled with mannitol and hyperventilation alone or for those patients who require constant infusions of mannitol. Small doses of thiopental at 1 - 2 mg/ kg have been reported to be helpful in reducing mild elevations of intracranial pressure (27).

Craniotomy has been advocated as a final effort for refractory intracranial hypertension in Reye's syndrome (27). This drastic procedure has had life-saving results but commonly with neurologic sequelae.

Experimental Studies

Pettegrew and coworkers (64) reported the rapid recovery of a patient with Lovejoy-stage III Reye's syndrome following administration of a single intravenous dose of physostigmine (64). This was tried unsuccessfully in a second patient as reported by Dobyns and colleagues (65). Further studies using this form of therapy have yet to be reported.

Dimethyl sulfoxide (DMSO) is a strong organic solvent which has attained popular recognition as a possible therapy for arthritis (66). In addition, there have been scattered reports about protective and therapeutic effects of DMSO on cerebral ischemia (66- 68). In one study of experimental head injury DMSO has been shown to result in a higher blood pressure, improved cerebral perfusion, improved cerebral blood flow, and higher cerebral oxidative metabolism (69). Several studies that investigate the use of DMSO in the treatment of other causes of increased intracranial pressure are under way. At our institution we have witnessed the use of DMSO in 1 patient with Reye's syndrome and refractory intracranial hypertension. There was no beneficial effect in this patient.

Outcome

The mortality rate for Reye's syndrome has dramatically decreased because of aggressive management and early recognition. Morbidity, including mild neuropsychological disturbances, has not been studied extensively. Brunner and colleagues (70) reported the evaluation of 40 children 1 or more years after their recovery from Reye's syndrome. They studied intelligence, school achievement, visual-motor coordination, social maturity, and Halstead-Reiton Neuropsychological Batteries. They reported a strong correlation between the degree of impaired neuropsychological function, the clinical stage at admission, the duration of impaired consciousness, and the number of exchange transfusions given. Some of these deficits such as language and perceptual-motor disturbances were transient, while disturbances of higher cognitive functions appeared to be subtle but lasting. This important study indicates that some patients with Reye's syndrome may experience permanent neuropsychological sequelae after recovery.

HEPATIC ENCEPHALOPATHY

Nervous system dysfunction associated with hepatic failure was recognized during the time of Hippocrates. Subsequently, hepatic encephalopathy was documented by Johannes Baptista Morgagni, a teacher at the Padua Medical School in the 18th century.

Clinical Features

Hepatic encephalopathy is a syndrome characterized by abnormal behavior, failure of memory and attention, tremor, extrapyramidal signs, and progressive impairment of consciousness which leads to deep coma (70). This syndrome occurs in association with metabolic alterations which result from hepatic failure (71, 72). Hepatic encephalopathy may be divided into two major categories: encephalopathy with acute hepatic failure and encephalopathy with subacute or chronic hepatic failure (73). With acute hepatic failure, the patient rapidly develops mental confusion, loss of contact with the environment, agitation, and emotional lability followed by obtundation. With chronic hepatic failure, the patient experiences fluctuating confusional states, disorientation, memory impairment, and asterixis. Frequently, the two clinical groups merge with one another (74). Hepatic failure may be endogenous or exogenous in origin. It may be induced by such precipitating factors as: gastrointestinal bleeding, excess ingestion of protein or ammonia-producing substances, shock and hypoxia, infections, toxins, electrolyte depletion, renal failure, and sedatives (71, 72). Recently it has been reported following open heart surgery (75).

The earliest indication of hepatic encephalopathy may be subtle psychomotor disturbances on psychometric testing (76, 77). Marchesini and coworkers (76) found that approximately 33% of clinically normal patients with cirrhosis have neuropsychological deficits and that there was a significant correlation between the scores on testing and levels of plasma amino acids, particularly tryptophan. Gilberstadt and coworkers (77) found that 50% of alcoholic patients with cirrhosis had abnormalities on psychometric testing as compared to alcoholic patients without cirrhosis. With progression of hepatic dysfunction a spectrum of mental and neuromuscular signs precede the development of coma and death. Examination of a comatose patient with hepatic encephalopathy reveals signs of multilevel incomplete brain stem involvement. Recognized findings include: decorticate and decerebrate posturing (78), absent oculovestibular reflexes (79), ocular bobbing (80), and dysconjugate gaze on caloric stimulation (81). EEG alterations have been divided into several steps ranging from a slight slowness of rhythm, to the appearance of the typical "triphasic waves," and finally the complete absence of electrical activity in deep coma (82). However, these EEG abnormalities may not have prognostic value. Tanaka and coworkers (83) reported a patient who made a complete recovery from fulminant hepatic failure in which the EEG was flat for 62 hours. This experience is unusual since fulminant hepatic failure is usually associated with an 80% mortality rate (84). Unlike other forms of hepatic encephalopathy, patients with sudden and severe hepatic failure usually develop cerebral edema. Silk and coworkers (85) reported the presence of cerebral edema at necropsy in over 80% of patients who died as a result of fulminant hepatic failure. Hanid and coworkers (86) reported the value of recording the intracranial pressure in such patients. They commented on the efficacy of mannitol therapy for increases in intracranial

pressure. The association of cerebral edema with hepatic dysfunction and the pattern of intracranial pressure increases are similar to those described in Reye's syndrome (86).

Pathogenesis

The pathogenesis of hepatic encephalopathy still remains a subject of speculation and investigation. Proposed mechanisms are thought to be related to such changes as: hyperammonemia, increased free fatty acids, altered amino acid concentrations, and the appearance of false neurotransmitters and mercaptans (71-73).

Although hyperammonemia is frequently thought to account for hepatic encephalopathy, it has been recognized both clinically and experimentally that there is poor correlation between blood ammonia levels and the degree of encephalopathy (71). However, glutamine in the CSF, which results from the reaction of α-ketoglutaric acid with excess brain ammonia, appears to be elevated during hepatic coma and may reflect the patient's neurological status (70). Oei and coworkers (87) demonstrated a significant correlation between the natural logarithm of CSF glutamine levels and the EEG stage of hepatic encephalopathy. They proposed that CSF glutamine levels and EEG changes together can provide useful diagnostic and prognostic information for patients with hepatic encephalopathy.

As discussed above in the section on Reye's syndrome, free fatty acids disrupt normal mitochondrial function. They are also capable of interfering with the disposition of ammonia in the body, and they appear to increase the potential for ammonia and mercaptans to produce coma (88). Teychenne and coworkers (89) described the relationship between slow-wave activity on the EEG and the concentration of five carbon fatty acids in the CSF of rabbits. An accumulation of short-, medium-, and long-chain fatty acids can be found in chronic hepatic failure, but this has not been a consistent finding in fulminant hepatic failure (71). It appears that fatty acids may augment the toxic effect of ammonia, aromatic amino acids, and mercaptans, but the precise mechanism of action is not clear.

Since the liver regulates amino acid metabolism, it is not surprising that a grossly altered pattern of amino acid levels in the circulation occurs with advanced liver disease. The most striking change is a decrease in the level of branched-chain amino acids (valine, leucine, and isoleucine) and an increase in the levels of aromatic amino acids (phenylalanine, tyrosine, and tryptophan) and methionine (73, 90, 91). The reason for this altered pattern may be related to the selective catabolism of amino acids by different organs. The aromatic amino acids are catabolized mainly in liver, while the branched-chain amino acids are catabolized mostly in muscle (73). Changes in the blood level of different amino acids affect the uptake and utilization of amino acids by the brain. For example, both the branched-chain and aromatic amino acids share the same carrier system for transport across the blood-brain barrier (92). Thus, in the blood, an elevation of aromatic amino acids and a decrease of branched-chain amino acids, which compete for the same carrier, tend to increase the amount of aromatic amino acids that enter the brain. This could lead to the synthesis of unusual neurotransmitters from these precursors or have a direct effect on other amino acid pathways in brain. In fact, the increase of aromatic amino acids in the brain even exceeds their rise in the plasma (73). Perhaps this is related to an alteration of the blood-brain barrier itself in hepatic failure (93). Methionine is also increased in the circulation in liver disease and methionine levels above 300 μmol have been reported to be diagnostic of acute liver failure (94). Moreover, early in the development of hepatic encephalopathy methionine levels may correlate with the presence and severity of the encephalopathy (94). Because of the changes in amino acid patterns, several investigators have attempted to normalize blood amino acid levels by active intervention. Infusions of branched-chain amino acids in cirrhotic patients has been shown to depress the elevated levels of aromatic amino acids and methionine (90). These same mixtures have also been used successfully to reverse

hepatic encephalopathy produced in dogs by portacaval shunts and that observed in patients with cirrhosis of the liver (71).

Intravenous administration of the branched-chain amino acid L-valine to patients with hepatic coma has resulted in a significant fall in the brain concentration of tryptophan, serotonin, and 5-hydroxyindoleacetic acid (95). Clinical improvement was associated with this change, and ammonia metabolism became normal. It was suggested that L-valine may play a crucial role in intermediary metabolism and is able to restore an anabolic state (95).

It is not clear how elevated aromatic amino acids are involved in the pathogenesis of hepatic encephalopathy. These amino acids are precursors for neurotransmitter synthesis. Therefore, it has been proposed that hepatic encephalopathy may be secondary to a disturbance in cerebral catecholamines with a decline in dopamine and noradrenaline and a rise in "false neurotransmitters," especially octopamine (71, 74, 91, 96-98). Cuilleret and coworkers (96) studied this possibility directly and found that brain levels of dopamine and noradrenaline were identical in cirrhotic patients with and without encephalopathy and in patients without liver disease. In addition, they found that brain octopamine levels were higher in control subjects than in patients with cirrhosis or hepatic encephalopathy. Moreover, Bucci and Chiaverelli (74) studied 30 patients with and without hepatic encephalopathy and found no relationship between brain octopamine levels and the presence or degree of hepatic encephalopathy.

Other trace amines such as tryptamine have also been implicated in the pathogenesis of hepatic coma. Young and Lal (97) reported significantly higher levels of CSF indoleacetic acid (IAA) in patients with hepatic coma than in cirrhotic patients not in coma. Additionally there appears to be a close relationship between CSF levels of IAA and the grade of coma (97). Phenylethylamine has also been shown to be elevated in CSF and to correlate with the grade of hepatic coma (98). Despite these correlations, however, cause and effect are not clear.

Wardle and Williams (99) have shown that tyramine and phenylethylamine can decrease serotonin uptake in platelets. Since serotonin uptake by platelets may be similar to that in neurons (26), Wardle and Williams (99) proposed that in hepatic coma neurons may not be able to reaccumulate all the serotonin that is released. They suggested that this may predispose to a depressed level of consciousness, especially when there is concurrent ammonia intoxication. Perhaps this is related to Jouvet's (100) observation that serotonin plays a role in sleep.

Increased blood glucagon levels (400%) have been documented in liver cirrhosis. Despite mild elevations of insulin levels (50%) the insulin:glucagon ratio is depressed (71, 101). This hormonal alteration has been proposed to account for the plasma amino acid imbalance which may underlie the pathogenesis of hepatic encephalopathy. Marchesini and coworkers (101) found that increased glucagon secretion occurs in cirrhotic patients and correlates with their mental status. Additionally they found no alteration in the insulin: glucagon ratio until neurological symptoms appeared. In a second report (102) they proposed and demonstrated that oral glucose is capable of suppressing hyperglucagonemia and increasing the insulin:glucagon ratio; this change appears to lower elevated tryptophan levels.

James and coworkers (103) presented a hypothesis that attempts to encompass many of the above-mentioned factors. They proposed that the hyperammonemia in liver cirrhosis or after portacaval shunt contributes to plasma amino acid imbalance and increases aromatic amino acid transport across the blood-brain barrier. The abnormal pattern of plasma amino acids is thought to be due in part to ammonia stimulation of glucagon secretion and a resulting high rate of gluconeogenesis. In addition, ammonia is utilized for glutamine synthesis from glutamate in brain, which then results in a rapid exchange of brain glutamine for plasma aromatic amino acids. Therefore, hyperammonemia may indirectly contribute to hepatic encephalopathy by raising the concentration of aromatic amino acids in brain, which then may disrupt catecholamine metabolism.

Mercaptans are extremely toxic sulfur-containing compounds that appear to be derived largely from methionine metabolism by bacteria in the gastrointestinal tract. Similar to ammonia, mercaptans normally are detoxified and removed from the circulation by the liver. Methylmercaptan (methanethiol) was first isolated in 1955 from the urine of a woman in deep hepatic coma (104). Subsequently, small amounts of mercaptans have been shown to produce a reversible coma in animals and to act synergistically with ammonia and fatty acids (71). McClain and coworkers (105) studied blood methanethiol levels in patients with possible hepatic encephalopathy. They found good correlation between the direction of change in methanethiol levels and change in mental status. Chang and Lister (106) have shown that hemoperfusion over albumin-collodion-coated activated charcoal effectively removes mercaptans and helps to restore consciousness in the comatose patient. They postulated that the recovery of consciousness in patients with hepatic coma is secondary to removing toxic molecules from the circulation. These include mercaptan and other molecules loosely bound to protein.

Treatment

The standard therapy for hepatic encephalopathy is to eliminate gastrointestinal bacteria and the nitrogenous substances they utilize and to carefully monitor fluids, electrolytes, and acid-base balance. Extracorporeal liver hemoperfusion has become accepted as treatment for acute hepatic failure. Albumin-collodion-coated activated charcoal hemoperfusion is an effective means of promoting recovery to consciousness within 1 to 2 hours. Patients in hepatic coma who are improved by hemoperfusion and who survive develop a sustained rise in the blood level of α-fetoprotein, while those who die do not (107).

Infusions of special amino acid mixtures produced improvement in hepatic encephalopathy (71, 90, 95, 108, 109). Herlog and coworkers (110) demonstrated marked clinical and EEG improvement in 8 patients with chronic portal-systemic encephalopathy who were given ornithine salts of branched-chain ketoacids. This treatment was much more effective than either branched-chain amino acids, branched-chain ketoacids, or ornithine alone. The investigators proposed that the synergism between ornithine and branched-chain ketoacids in improving the encephalopathy may be due to a stimulatory effect of ornithine on the urea cycle and the promotion of an anabolic state by the branched-chain ketoacids.

The use of catecholamine agonists and precursors has been suggested because hepatic encephalopathy might be due to an abnormal competitive displacement of normal neurotransmitters by false neuro-transmitters. Michel and coworkers (111) reported the results of a controlled study in which there was no significant difference in the clinical status of 75 cirrhotic patients with hepatic encephalopathy who were treated with either L-dopa, L-dopa with dopa-decarboxylase inhibitor, or a placebo. Uribe and coworkers (112) reported a double-blind controlled clinical trial of the dopamine agonist, bromocriptine, in 7 cirrhotic patients with chronic portal-systemic encephalopathy. They found that bromocriptine was not significantly superior to placebo and was always inferior to standard treatment. In contrast, Morgan and coworkers (113) reported that treatment with bromocriptine produced significant improvement clinically and electroencephalographically in 6 patients with cirrhosis and severe chronic hepatic encephalopathy. As a result of these contradictory observations several letters and editorials (116, 117) appeared in an attempt to explain the paradoxical results. Schenker and coworkers (117) concluded that although bromocriptine may be of benefit to some selected patients with portal-systemic enceph-alopathy, a beneficial response to bromocrip-tine does not necessarily confirm the impaired neurotransmitter hypothesis. Perhaps bromo-criptine influences a different physiological mechanism. This could be analagous to the effect of L-dopa enhancing ammonia output in the urine (118).

Okita and coworkers (119) reported marked improvement of hepatic coma in patients with fulminant hepatic failure when treated with a combination of glucagon and insulin. As mentioned earlier, Marchesini and coworkers (102) proposed that administra-tion of oral glucose is helpful in the management of cirrhotic patients with hepatic encephalopathy. Their data suggest that oral glucose is capable of correcting the abnormal amino acid pattern in the circula-tion.

The role of corticosteroid therapy in acute liver dysfunction with encephalopathy has been studied in acute alcoholic hepatitis. Depew and coworkers (120) investigated 28 patients. They were unable to show any beneficial effect of prednisolone treatment on patient morbidity or mortality. The adverse clinical course of their patients was directly related to the development of specific lethal complications of acute alcoholic hepatitis.

WILSON'S DISEASE

Wilson's disease is an inherited inborn error of copper metabolism believed to be due to an autosomal recessive genetic defect. Wilson (121) presented the first definitive description of this disease in a 1912 monograph entitled "Progressive Lenticular Degeneration: A Familial Nervous Disease Associated with Cirrhosis of the Liver ." Prominent hepatic involvement in the pathogenesis of the disease was emphasized by Hall (122) in 1921; he suggested the name hepatolenticular degen-eration. Disturbed copper metabolism was first recognized in 1913, but this information lay dormant for 3 decades before it was rediscovered. In 1952 several groups working simultaneously found low ceruloplasmin levels in patients with Wilson's disease. Prior to the 1950s a diagnosis of Wilson's disease implied an inevitable progression to death. With the advent of chelating agents this grim outlook has improved substantially.

Clinical Features

The age of onset of symptomatic disease is "variable." In a group of 151 patients none had symptoms prior to 6 years of age, while 50% were recognized by 15 years (123). Dobyns and coworkers (124) reviewed the clinical spectrum of Wilson's disease in 53 symptomatic patients. For those patients who developed liver disease first, the age of onset ranged from 6 to 55 years with a mode of 15 years. For patients who developed neurologic symptoms initially, the age of onset ranged from 9 to 40 years with a mode of 19 years. Of the symptomatic patients, 53% experienced brain disease first, while 47% experienced liver disease first (4). Combined disease was eventually present in 53%. Neurologic involvement included mental or emotional disturbances as well as extrapyramidal, cerebellar, and pseudobulbar findings (124). Clinical evidence of extrapyramidal disease included dysarthria, dysphonia, rigidity, dystonia, and choreoathetosis. Hepatic involvement was heralded by portal hypertension, esophageal varices, hepatosplenomegaly, and hematemesis. Kayser-Fleischer rings were reported in 96% of symptomatic patients (124). Kayser-Fleischer rings are considered the most common nonhepatic non-neurologic manifestation of Wilson's disease. Since 1921 they have been thought to be the only pathognomonic sign of the disease (122), although they may not be present early in the illness. Recent evidence has shown that this is not true. Kayser-Fleischer rings have been reported in chronic progressive hepatitis (125), primary biliary cirrhosis (126), and in a familial cholestatic syndrome (127). In Wilson's disease, Kayser-Fleischer rings may disappear with appropriate chelation therapy (124). Schoenberger and Ellis (128) reported the disappearance of Kayser-Fleischer rings following liver transplantation in a 14-year-old boy with Wilson's disease. Another ophthalmologic manifestation of Wilson's disease is sunflower cataracts. These were present in 12% of patients in the study by Dobyns and coworkers (124). Ocular motility abnormalities are distinctly unique in Wilson's disease. Gadoth and Liel (129) reported a case of transient external ophthalmoplegia precipitated by discontinuation of chelation therapy; this resolved after reinstitution of penicillamine.

Wilson's disease may begin with involvement at other less common sites. Bone and joint disease occurs with mild scoliosis, mild arthralgias, or severe degenerative arthritis and osteochondritis dissecans (124). Renal complications of Wilson's disease include renal tubular abnormalities (Fanconi's syndrome) and renal stones (130). Hematologic disturbances include anemia, leuko-

penia, and thrombocytopenia (123, 124). Endocrinologic dysfunction occurs, presumably on the basis of disrupted hepatic function (123). Disordered esophageal motility has been reported in a patient after 21 years of penicillamine therapy (131).

The clinical manifestations and progression of Wilson's disease have been divided into five stages by Werlin and coworkers (132). During stage 1, which begins at birth, the patient is in positive copper balance but is completely asymptomatic. There is moderate cupriuria, but the Kayser-Fleischer rings may be absent and liver function studies may be normal. Stage 2 begins when the liver becomes saturated with copper. Liver dysfunction and a hemolytic anemia may appear. Cupriuria is increased, but the ceruloplasmin may still be normal and Kayser-Fleischer rings absent. Approximately 60% to 70% of patients pass through this stage without overt liver disease. In stage 3 copper accumulates in the extrahepatic tissues, especially eye, brain, and kidney. Kayser-Fleischer rings almost always appear, and renal manifestations may develop. In stage 4 the neurologic features appear. Stage 5 occurs when therapy is initiated, a negative copper balance is produced, and symptoms begin to resolve.

Diagnosis

The diagnosis of Wilson's disease can be made with ease when the classical triad of Kayser-Fleischer rings, neurologic dysfunction, and hypoceruloplasminemia is present. Unfortunately, not only may the Kayser-Fleischer rings be absent early in the disease, but the serum ceruloplasmin may be normal in about 5% of patients with Wilson's disease (122, 134, 136). Additionally, patients with other forms of hepatic disease may also have very low ceruloplasmin levels (133-135). Edwards and coworkers (137) reported a pedigree with nonwilsonian asymptomatic hypoceruloplasminemia.

A total serum copper concentration below 80 mg/100 ml is typical of Wilson's disease, but as many as 10% of patients may have normal levels (135). In addition, serum copper levels tend to correlate with serum ceruloplasmin levels. Therefore, if the ceruloplasmin is low for any reason, a low serum copper is of little diagnostic value. The 24-hour urinary excretion of copper in Wilson's disease is rarely less than 100 mg, but occasional normal values (less than 60 mg/24 hours) have been reported (135). Elevated urinary copper excretion has also been reported in other hepatic diseases such as chronic active hepatitis (134, 135). Thus, it can be extremely difficult to distinguish wilsonian from nonwilsonian hepatic disease on the basis of serum ceruloplasmin, serum copper, or urinary copper excretion. For this reason, it has been proposed that all patients deserve a liver biopsy for evaluation of hepatic copper content (132, 134, 135) if the diagnosis of Wilson's disease is entertained but cannot be firmly established by ordinary clinical or laboratory studies. Hepatic copper concentrations are always elevated in Wilson's disease, usually in excess of 250 mg/g dry weight (132-134). Although other hepatic diseases may have an elevated hepatic copper concentration, this is rarely in the range seen with Wilson's disease (135). Perman and coworkers (134) studied 20 untreated patients with chronic active hepatitis and 25 patients with Wilson's disease and found that the most reliable test for differentiating the two was the hepatic copper concentration. All of the patients with Wilson's disease had copper levels greater than 400 mg/g dry weight, whereas patients with chronic active hepatitis had levels less than 300 mg/g dry weight. Hepatic copper concentration may also be helpful in distinguishing the heterozygote with low ceruloplasmin from the homozygote with Wilson's disease. The heterozygote may have an increased hepatic copper concentration, but this level does not exceed 250 mg/g dry weight (135). Unfortunately, homozygotes, heterozygotes, and patients with nonwilsonian chronic liver disease may be indistinguishable, even on the basis of the hepatic copper concentrations. In these cases radiocopper uptake has been found to be useful. Also, liver biopsy may be contraindicated, and then radiocopper uptake can usually resolve the diagnostic dilemma. After oral administration of radiocopper, the serum concentration is monitored for 48 hours (135). In normal subjects oral administration results in an early rise in plasma radioactivity reflecting radiocopper bound to albumin and amino acids. This early plasma phase then disappears as the metal is incorporated into liver copper proteins, including ceruloplasmin. A secondary rise follows as these proteins are released back into the circulation (135). Patients with Wilson's disease may have abnormal kinetics because of delayed hepatic uptake, decreased hepatic incorporation, or abnormal excretion and prolonged turnover (135). Sternlieb and Scheinberg (136) propose that radiocopper uptake is most useful in distinguishing the uncommon Wilson's disease patient with a normal ceruloplasmin level from the patient with nonwilsonian liver disease. The test appears less discriminatory when individuals have low ceruloplasmin values.

Other diagnostic studies that are useful in the diagnosis of Wilson's disease include computerized cranial tomography [CT] (138, 139), brain stem auditory evoked responses [BAER] (140), and cultured skin fibroblast copper content (141). Published CT studies in Wilson's disease show low-density abnormalities involving the basal ganglia in all patients with the "cerebral form" of Wilson's disease [Fig. 1] (138, 139). Occasionally low-density lesions may be seen in the cerebellar nuclei and surrounding white matter (139). Ventricular dilatation is not uncommonly seen. None of these abnormalities have been found with the hepatic form of the disease.

Fujita and coworkers (140) have used BAER to study patients with Wilson's disease. They found prolongation of wave latencies in every case of Wilson's disease with neurologic symptoms (Fig. 2). In patients without neurologic involvement, the BAER pattern was normal, as it was in patients with spinocerebellar degenerations.

Cultured skin fibroblasts from patients with Wilson's disease have an elevated intracellular copper content when compared to cultured normal cells (141). The elevation is approximately threefold higher than control cells. This observation indicates that the genetic abnormality of Wilson's disease is

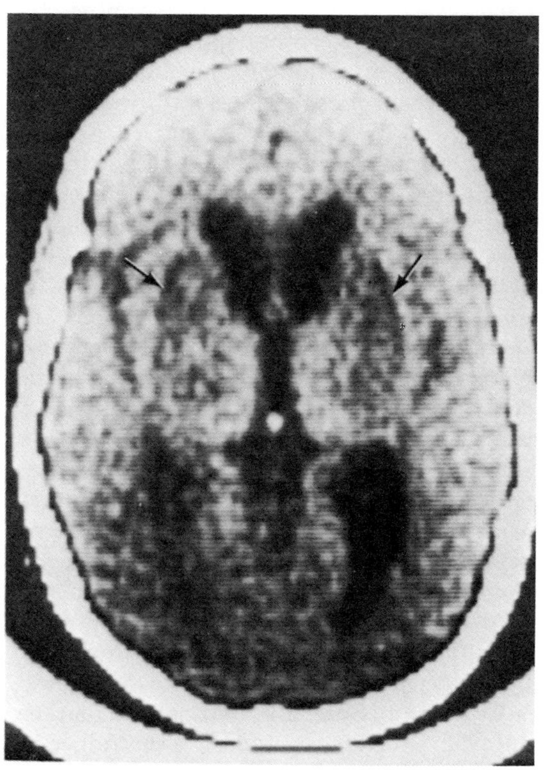

Figure 1. Computed tomography showing large areas of low density (13 EMI units) in the lenticular nuclei (*arrows*) and ventricular dilation. (Reprinted with permission from Harik SI, Post MJ: Computed tomography in Wilson's disease. *Neurology* 31:107-110, 1981.)

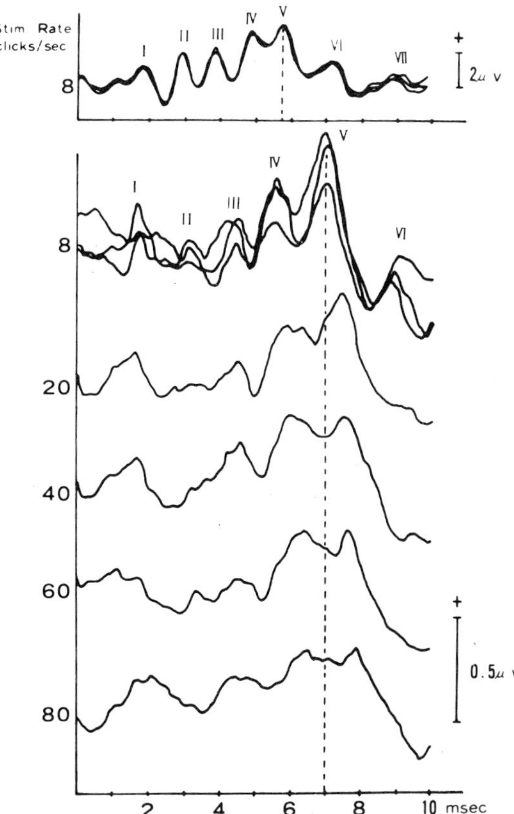

Figure 2. Brain stem auditory evoked responses in Wilson's disease. Each wave from II to VI is markedly prolonged. Normal latency pattern seen at *top* of figure. (Reprinted with permission from Fujita M, Hosoki M, Miyazaki M: Brainstem auditory evoked responses in spinocerebellar degeneration and Wilson's disease. *Ann Neurol* 9:42-47, 1981.)

expressed in cultured fibroblasts. This is an important finding since it provides an in vitro model for studying the pathogenesis of the disease, and it also provides a potential noninvasive method for early diagnosis. At present the fibroblasts studied have been derived from patients ranging from 9-20 years of age, and it is unknown whether this abnormality will be demonstrable earlier in childhood or in prenatal life (141).

Pathology

Wilson's disease is considered to be primarily a hepatic disorder which produces secondary effects in other organs following the release of

copper from the damaged liver (142). Although there are no specific morphological changes unique to Wilson's disease, there are a number of findings that should suggest or confirm the diagnosis. Stromeyer and Ishak (142) were able to separate hepatic specimens from 34 cases of Wilson's disease into three histological groups. The first group consisted of precirrhotic patients characterized by early changes ranging from slight pleomorphism of hepatocytes to fatty metamorphosis, periportal atypical lipofuscin, and vacuolated nuclei. The second group, which consisted of patients with precirrhotic-chronic active hepatitis, had findings similar to those of the first group in addition to obvious periportal degeneration and necrosis. Periportal copper accumulation was found in 43% of these specimens. The last group consisted of cirrhotic specimens which showed either macronodular or mixed micronodular-macronodular cirrhosis. Copper accumulation was found in 87% of these specimens; Mallory bodies were found in 40%. The authors suggested that although many of these findings can be regarded as nonspecific, their combination, particularly in a child or young adult, suggested the possibility of Wilson's disease.

In the central nervous system there are both focal areas of spongy necrosis and diffuse proliferation of abnormal astrocytes (143). Areas involved in spongy necrosis include the lenticular region, thalamus, lower layers of the cerebral cortex, dentate nucleus, and brain stem. The astrocytic proliferation includes sparsely scattered Alzheimer type I glia and more numerous Alzheimer type II cells. In addition, there are occasional large astrocytes with small eccentric pynotic nuclei called Opalski cells. Vallat (144) performed ultrastructural examination of peripheral nerves in Wilson's disease and found no characteristic pathologic changes.

Pathophysiology

Although it is clear that Wilson's disease is a disorder of copper metabolism, the precise underlying pathophysiological mechanism of action is not understood. Normal copper metabolism involves absorption from the gastrointestinal tract into the blood where most of it is loosely bound to albumin. Copper is then cleared promptly by the liver and incorporated into hepatic copper proteins. The copper can then be mobilized by two major routes. The first is by incorporation into the protein ceruloplasmin which is released into the blood; the second is by biliary excretion (123). Studies suggest that the intracellular pools of copper for these two routes of mobilization appear to be separate. The lysosome serves as the major source for biliary copper, and the microsome serves as the site of incorporation of copper into apoceruloplasmin (123). Untreated patients with Wilson's disease are in a positive copper

balance. This could be explained either by increased absorption of copper from the gut or decreased excretion of copper into the bile. The latter proposal is generally accepted. Gibbs and Walshe (145) studied biliary radiocopper excretion in 2 patients and found striking differences between patients and controls. Very little of the injected radio-copper was recovered in the bile of the patients, and there was no evidence of the well-marked secondary rise in the rate of excretion as seen in the controls. The pattern of excretion of copper in the bile found in the controls suggested that an energy-mediated process may participate in copper excretion some hours after its arrival in the hepatocytes. Gibbs and Walshe (145) postulated that Wilson's disease results from the absence or severe deficiency of an energy-mediated secretory mechanism for copper in the hepatocyte. A lysosomal defect was proposed since this appears to be the major source for the biliary pool.

Epstein and Sherlock (146) claimed that the autosomal recessive mode of inheritance in Wilson's disease strongly suggests that a single gene defect is responsible for the disease. A proposed pathogenic mechanism must account for both a reduced ceruloplasmin as well as impaired biliary copper excretion. A structural gene mutation resulting in a single abnormal carrier protein cannot explain depressed ceruloplasmin synthesis and decreased biliary copper excretion, since they are independent pathways with separate copper pools. Alternatively, a lysosomal defect resulting in impaired biliary copper excretion does not explain a decreased ceruloplasmin. Epstein and Sherlock (146) proposed that Wilson's disease results from a controller gene mutation which fails to change the positive copper balance of the fetus to the normal copper balance of the child and adult. In support of this hypothesis is the observation that estrogen administration may increase ceruloplasmin levels in Wilson's disease, indicating that the structural gene responsible for ceruloplasmin synthesis is intact and may be stimulated by hormonal manipulation (146). In addition, the fact that cultured skin fibroblasts from patients with Wilson's disease have elevated copper levels (141) tends to support a controller gene theory with a positive copper balance.

The mechanism by which copper is transported and deposited in the brain, cornea, kidney, and other organ systems affected in Wilson's disease is not known. Brown and Antholine (147) proposed that carnosine and anserine are capable of removing a small fraction of the bound copper from serum albumin in the circulation and then play a role in transporting copper to the kidneys and specific regions of the brain.

Treatment

In 1951 2,3-dimercaptopropanol (BAL) was first introduced as a possible therapeutic agent for Wilson's disease. In 1956 it was replaced by penicillamine which proved to be more effective and easier to administer. Since that time, D-penicillamine has remained the accepted therapeutic agent for inducing cupriuresis in patients with Wilson's disease. Haggstrom and coworkers (148) reported a patient who received continuous penicillamine therapy for 21 years with significant neurological recovery and with no toxic side effects. Unfortunately, however, D-penicillamine therapy can be associated with a variety of toxic and hypersensitivity reactions, including nephrotic syndrome, a lupus-like disease, aplastic anemia, thrombocytopenia, and leukopenia. Approximately 10% of patients with Wilson's disease may develop an absolute intolerance to this drug (149). Triethylene tetramine dihydrochloride (Trien) has been proven a safe and effective alternative to penicillamine (149, 150). Haslam and coworkers (150) reported a case of a 14½-year-old girl who was unable to tolerate D-penicillamine despite steroid coverage. She has tolerated Trien well for 2½ years with good results. A group of tetramines have been surveyed for cupriuretic activity and compared to D-penicillamine in rats (149). 2,3,2-Tetramine proved to be more effective than either Trien or D-penicillamine and thus may become a valuable adjunct for chelation therapy in Wilson's disease.

Hoogenraad and coworkers (151) reported the use of oral zinc sulfate as a long-term treatment for Wilson's disease. It was first described by Schouwink in 1961 (152). Oral zinc sulfate antagonizes copper resorption across the gut mucosa (151). Schouwink proposed that zinc sulfate should be used with penicillamine for several weeks to induce a state of negative copper balance. The negative copper balance could then be maintained by zinc sulfate alone. Hoogenraad and co-workers (151) described a patient who had 6 weeks of penicillamine therapy initially and then zinc sulfate for the next 14 years. On this regimen clinical symptoms were ameliorated, the Kayser-Fleischer rings cleared, and the ceruloplasmin level rose.

Liver transplantation has been successfully performed with Wilson's disease (128). The patient's Kayser-Fleischer rings disappeared gradually over 6 years.

BILIRUBIN ENCEPHALOPATHY (KERNICTERUS)

Bilirubin encephalopathy is a complication of unconjugated hyperbilirubinemia which occurs almost exclusively in the neonatal period. The characteristic neuropathological changes of the disease with yellow staining of the basal ganglia, brain stem, and cerebellum were first reported by Orth in 1875 (153). The term "kernicterus" (nuclear jaundice) was introduced in 1903 by Schmorl (154). Initially, the disease was most commonly seen in term infants with hemolysis resulting from ABO or Rh incompatibility. More recently, it has become a major problem for the ill premature infant.

Clinical Features

Clinically affected infants develop an apathetic and drowsy mental status after several days of life. They may refuse to feed. The Moro reflex is depressed, and there is often downward rotation of the eyes (155). The mental status continues to deteriorate with obtundation and stupor. Intermittent opisthotonic attacks may occur with rigid back arching and hyperextension of the head and neck. These intense spasms associated with a high-pitched cry are frequently precipitated by mild handling. Temperature instability and convulsions may then ensue. Terminally the patients develop pulmonary hemorrhage with frothy red sputum.

If the infant survives after the development of the encephalopathy, then enduring neurologic abnormalities invariably follow (155, 156). With resolution of the jaundice the acute symptoms subside, and the infant may appear normal. By the third month of life, however, hypotonia begins to develop. Over the next 2 years the hypotonia is gradually replaced by choreoathetosis. Before 6 months of age over 90% of patients exhibit impairments in vertical gaze (156). This tends to improve as the child grows older. Hearing abnormalities are a characteristic finding. As many as 75% of children exhibit nerve deafness or a central defect in auditory processing, and 80% of children have enamel dysplasia of the decidous teeth (155, 156).

As a result of studies with infants who had erythroblastosis fetalis, Hsia and coworkers (157) in 1952 reported: "Kernicterus is likely to occur in babies with serum bilirubin levels above 30 mg/100 ml and unlikely to occur when serum bilirubin remains below 20 mg/100 ml." This has been supported by others and has become the basis for the standard practice to perform one or more exchange transfusions to keep the bilirubin concentration below the "danger" level. In 1965 Stern and Denton (158) reported the occurrence of kernicterus in low-birth weight infants at relatively low serum bilirubin concentrations. Further reports have confirmed that small distressed premature infants may develop kernicterus at bilirubin levels of 6 to 9 mg/100 ml (159, 160). These developments have led to the common practice of early exchange transfusion in these infants. Some clinicians perform exchange transfusions when the serum bilirubin (mg/100 ml) exceeds 1% of the infant's weight [g] (160).

Factors that are thought to identify infants susceptible to kernicterus at relatively low bilirubin concentrations include: low birth weight ($<$ 1500g), hypothermia, asphyxia, acidosis, hypoalbuminemia, sepsis, hemolysis, and drug therapy (158-162). Pearlman and coworkers (162) reported the occurrence of kernicterus in 4 of 6 near-term infants who died as a direct result of sepsis. Over a 5-year period there were no other cases of kernicterus. Recently, Turkel and coworkers (163) reported a retrospective matched control study in which it was not possible to identify risk factors for the development of kernicterus. Factors studied included: peak total serum bilirubin, asphyxia, acidosis, hypothermia, sepsis, hypercarbia, hypoglycemia, and drug therapy. Unfortunately, this study did not examine the infants' albumin, bilirubin binding, or serum free bilirubin levels.

Pathology

During the acute stage of bilirubin encephalopathy, the central nervous system usually shows prominent yellow staining of the leptomeninges, and occasionally the brain shows a diffuse icteric tint (155). On sectioning, pigmentation of selected nuclear masses is regularly observed (Table 3); the globus pallidus, subthalamic nucleus, and cornu ammonis of the hippocampus are extremely pigmented (164). Microscopically, these areas exhibit diffuse interstitial pigmentation, yellow staining of neurons and glia, and neuronal changes ranging from chromatolysis to pyknosis Some stained nuclear complexes, such as the dentate and olivary nuclei, may show no neuronal damage.

Examination of the brain later in life reveals atrophic changes in the subthalamic nuclei, hippocampus, and globus pallidus. The yellow pigment disappears after several months, and the early neuronal damage is followed by cell loss, gliosis, and demyelination (155, 164).

Pathophysiology

The mechanism by which unconjugated hyperbilirubinemia in the infant may lead to an acute encephalopathy and a permanent neurological syndrome is still somewhat controversial. Bilirubin is a tetrapyrrole with two proprionic acid side-groups derived from the degradation of heme. At a physiological pH (7.4), unbound bilirubin exists predominantly as an anion (B^{-2}) with only approximately 0.8% in the monobasic form (BH^-) and 0.006% as the acid [BH_2] (165). There are

Table 3. Distribution of Areas of Pigmentation in 35 Cases of Kernicterus

Affected Area	Number of Cases
Basal ganglia	32
Cerebellum	25
Hippocampus	24
Medulla oblongata	24
Subthalamic nuclei (Luysii)	19
Thalamus	18
Corpus striatum	18
Fourth ventricle	18
Dentate nucleus	17
Olivary nuclei	15
Nuclei in floor of fourth ventricle	15
Lentiform nucleus	14
Midbrain	11
Spinal cord	10
Globus pallidus	9
Ependyma	9
Pons	6
Corpora mamillaria	6
Caudate nucleus	6
Cerebral cortex	5

Note —Reprinted with permission from Claireaux AE: Pathology of human kernicterus. In *Kernicterus*. Edited by Sass-Kortsak A. Toronto, University of Toronto Press, 1961.

significant increases in the concentrations of both the monobasic and acid forms when the pH decreases from 7.4 to 7.0, while the anionic concentration remains relatively unchanged.

$$B^{-2} \overset{H^+}{\rightleftarrows} BH \overset{-\ H^+}{\rightleftarrows} BH_2$$

Due to the ability of the bilirubin molecule to rotate around on its central methylene bridge, the acidic form (and to some degree the monobasic form) is capable of forming intramolecular hydrogen bonds which cause the polar groups to be bound within the molecule. This makes the molecule nearly insoluble in water (Fig. 3).

Previous reviews (155, 165-167) documented that the transport of bilirubin in plasma occurs almost exclusively in association with albumin. This albumin-bilirubin interaction occurs primarily on the basis of a single high-affinity binding site, although there is at least one and possibly more weaker

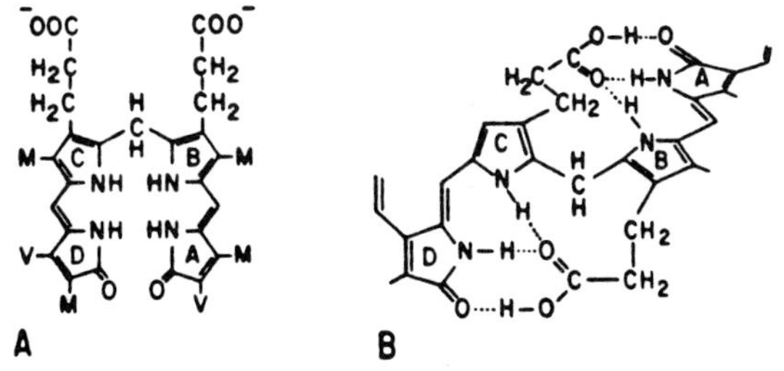

Figure 3. The chemical structure of bilirubin. Bilirubin consists of two dipyrroles connected by a central methylene bridge (*A*). The proprionate groups on the B and C rings are largely dissociated at pH 7.4. Rotation of the molecule about the methylene bridge (*B*) potentiates intramolecular hydrogen bonding of the acid and probably the monobasic forms of bilirubin, producing a water-soluble molecule. (Reprinted with permission from Wennberg RP, Ahlfors CE, Rasmussen LF: The pathochemistry of kernicterus. *Early Hum Dev* 3:353-372, 1979.)

affinity binding sites (165, 166). Since albumin binds both the anionic and acidic forms of bilirubin, the great majority of bound bilirubin in the physiological pH range is as the anion. Recent reports have indicated that within the physiological pH range, hydrogen ion concentration has little if any effect on albumin-bilirubin binding (161, 165, 168). The concentration of unbound bilirubin is a function of the total bilirubin concentration, the total albumin concentration, the albumin-bilirubin binding capacity, and the albumin-bilirubin binding affinity (165). Cashore (166) has recently shown that there is a marked reduction in the albumin-bilirubin binding capacity and affinity with a resultant significantly higher free bilirubin fraction in seriously ill preterm infants (Fig. 4).

In order for bilirubin to cause cellular dysfunction, it must first bind and then alter the function of cellular components. It has been shown experimentally, using both bound and unbound isotopically labeled bilirubin, that accumulation in brain and neurotoxicity result primarily from unbound bilirubin (169). Unlike albumin-bilirubin binding, cellular binding of free bilirubin is greatly enhanced by mild acidosis (165, 168, 170). The concentration of the bilirubin anion changes very little within the physiological pH range while the concentration of the acid changes significantly. Since pH changes have little effect on albumin-bilirubin binding but produce major effects on cellular binding, it has been suggested that the acid form of bilirubin binds to tissues while the anion binds to albumin (165). However not all cell types bind bilirubin with equal affinity (170).

The role of the blood-brain barrier in the pathogenesis of kernicterus has long been a subject of speculation. Initially, bilirubin was thought to gain access to the central nervous system through an "immature" blood-brain barrier. However, there is no convincing evidence to show that the barrier for bilirubin is immature in any species. The blood-brain

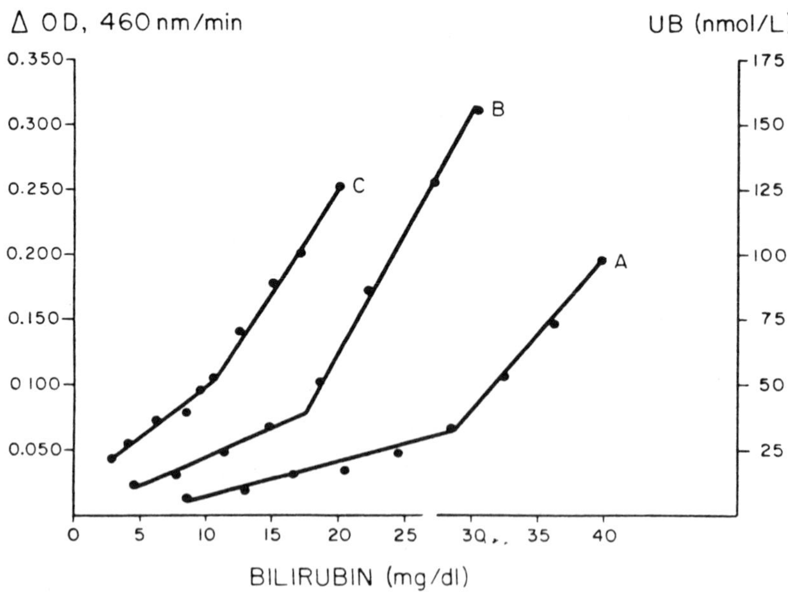

Figure 4. Bilirubin titration curves from three neonatal sera. *Ordinate*: unconjugated bilirubin concentration. *Abscissa (left)*: Δ OD for 1 minute at 460 nm (oxidation rate of free bilirubin); *(right)*: free bilirubin (UB) concentration derived from oxidation rate. *Curve A*: healthy 3055 g term infant. *Curve B*: 32-week infant 1780 g with mild respiratory distress. *Curve C*: 1100 g infant, 29 weeks gestation, with severe respiratory distress and kernicterus. Apparent transition to secondary bilirubin binding occurs at 29, 18, and 11 mg/100 ml for curves A, B, and C, respectively. Upward displacement of curves B and C suggests decreased binding affinity for bilirubin compared to serum A. (Reprinted with permission from Cashore WJ: Free bilirubin concentrations and bilirubin-binding affinity in term and preterm infants. *J Pediatr* 96:521-527, 1980.)

barrier at all ages is effective at excluding ionized polar substances from entry into the central nervous system but is less effective for unionized nonpolar substances. The blood-brain barrier behaves as a lipoid membrane toward lipid-soluble molecules, and the rate of entry into brain is directly proportional to the lipid-to-water partition coefficient at pH 7.4. Thus, for unionized molecules, the rate-limiting factor appears to be the degree of lipid solubility. Proteins and large molecular weight substances are also effectively excluded from entry. These findings suggest that the unbound nonpolar acidic forms of bilirubin are the pigment components which have greatest access to the central nervous system and produce bilirubin encephalopathy.

Several recent reports speculated that bilirubin bound to albumin may be more important in the pathogenesis of kernicterus (159, 160, 171). Reversible osmotic opening of the blood-brain barrier has been shown to allow entry of albumin into the brain (172). Even if this occurred, there is no evidence that bound bilirubin is toxic in brain. In fact, albumin is capable of removing bilirubin from brain with a striking reduction of neurotoxicity and mortality [Fig. 5] (169).

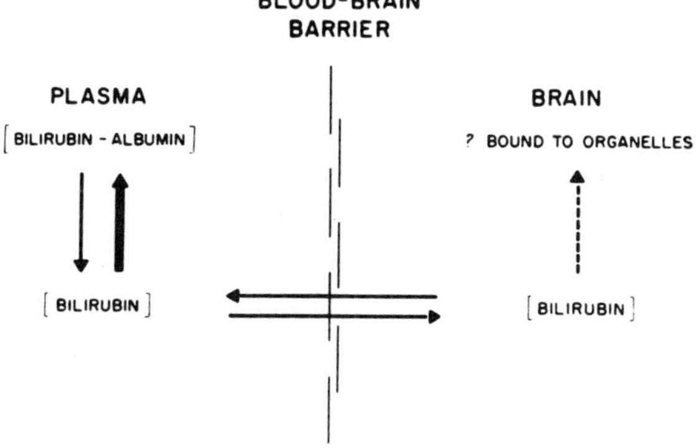

Figure 5. Interaction of bilirubin with albumin in the plasma. The amount of bilirubin transferred into the brain is determined by the magnitude of the unbound pigment fraction. This is in equilibrium with the bound fraction. (Reprinted with permission from Diamond I: Bilirubin encephalopathy (kernicterus). In *Scientific Approaches to Clinical Neurology.* Edited by Goldenshoha ES, Appel SH. Philadelphia, Lea Febiger, 1977, pp 1212-1233)

Although there is little doubt that bilirubin is potentially toxic and is capable of interfering with vital cell functions, the pathogenesis of the cellular toxicity is unclear. Previous reviews have discussed proposed mechanisms which include: uncoupling of oxidative phosphorylation, inhibiting electron transport, promoting potassium and ATP leakage from cells, inhibiting DNA and protein synthesis, and competitively inhibiting phosphofructokinase and other NAD-dependent enzymes (155, 165, 173). In neutrophils unconjugated bilirubin interferes with the hexose-monophosphate shunt (174). This shunt is essential for generating NADPH, which is needed for the detoxification of hydrogen peroxide and amino aldehydes. Although these mechanisms have been clearly demonstrated in vitro, their role in vivo is less clear. Uncoupling of oxidative phosphorylation seen in vitro cannot be demonstrated when brain mitochondria extracted from areas of high pigment concentration are assayed (175).

The pathogenesis of kernicterus appears to depend on the unbound lipophilic bilirubin fraction (Fig. 5). Serum albumin tightly binds bilirubin in equilibrium reactions. Unbound bilirubin must equilibrate with albumin and other components in the body. When the concentration of bilirubin in susceptible cells reaches a critical level, vital metabolic functions are disrupted and cells die. Although the free bilirubin pool has been difficult to measure, recent methodologic advances using peroxidase oxidation, difference spectroscopy, and 2-(4-hydroxybenzene)azobenzoic acid have been helpful in studying bilirubin kinetics (165, 166, 177, 178). Systemic factors which alter bilirubin binding will lead to changes in the free bilirubin level in accord with the laws of mass action. Cashore (166) has shown that both gestational age and the clinical condition of newborn infants influence the albumin-bilirubin binding capacity and binding affinity. Examination of 25 ill preterm infants disclosed 5 with kernicterus at autopsy, and those 5 patients had significantly higher free bilirubin levels (peroxidase method) and significantly lower bilirubin binding capacity and affinity. Similarly, using a fluorometric method for determining the bilirubin-reserve binding capacity of albumin, Brown and coworkers (177) were able to demonstrate that the specific bilirubin binding capacity was greater for infants whose birth weight exceeded 2000 g than for a lower birth weight group. Kozuki and coworkers (175) have shown an increase in bilirubin-albumin binding affinity after correction of neonatal acidosis.

Conjugated bilirubin does not appear to play a role in the pathogenesis of kernicterus. The polarity and water-solubility of conjugated pigments tends to exclude it from gaining access to the central nervous system. Transient unconjugated hyperbilirubinemia develops in the neonatal period because the activity of hepatic glucuronyltransferase is reduced (155). This microsomal enzyme catalyzes the formation of bilirubin glucuronide, which is required for bilirubin excretion. Reduced enzyme activity places the neonate at risk for kernicterus by increasing the pool of free unconjugated bilirubin.

Exchange transfusions over "critical" levels of serum bilirubin have been used to prevent bilirubin encephalopathy. The "critical" level appears to be dependent on the level of free bilirubin which is in turn affected by the binding capacities and affinities of both albumin and tissues for bilirubin. Because of these variables, it is not yet possible to establish an absolute "safe level" from bilirubin in the circulation. Other modes of therapy have been reviewed elsewhere (155, 159, 167).

ACKNOWLEDGMENT

We would like to thank Roberta Carol Webb for editorial assistance.

REFERENCES

1. Reye R, Morgan G, Baral J: Encephalopathy and fatty degeneration of the viscera: a disease entity in childhood. *Lancet* 2:749-752, 1963

2. Corey L, Rubin RJ: Reye's syndrome 1974: an epidemiological assessment. In *Reye's Syndrome.* Edited by Pollack, JD. New York, Grune and Stratten, 1975, pp 179-187

3. Glick TH, Ditchek NT, Saltisky S, et al: Acute encephalopathy and hepatic dysfunction associated with chickenpox in siblings. *Am J Dis Child* 119:68-71, 1970

4. Huttenlocher PR, Trauner DA: Reye's syndrome. In *Handbook of Clinical Neurology*, vol 29, part 3. Edited by Vinken PJ, Bruyn GW. Amsterdam, North Holland, 1977, pp 331-344

5. Hutchison HT, Diamond I: Metabolic disorders. In *Current Neurology*, vol 3. Edited by Appel SH. New York, John Wiley, 1981, pp 204-230

6. Fleirsher G, Schwartz J, Lennette E: Primary Epstein-Barr virus infection in association with Reye syndrome. *J Pediatr* 97:935-937, 1980

7. Chalhub EG, DeVivo DC, Keating JP, et al: Reye syndrome complicated by a generalized herpes simplex type I infection. *J Pediatr* 98:73-76, 1981

8. Sundwall DA, Bergeson ME, Ortiz A: Reye syndrome associated with *Hemophilus influenzae* infection. *Clin Pediatr* 19:357-360, 1980

9. Pitel PA, McCormick KL, Fitzgerald E, et al: Subclinical hepatic changes in varicella infection. *Pediatrics* 65:631-633, 1980

10. Bourgeois CH, Shank RC, Grossman RA, et al: Acute aflatoxin B_1 toxicity in the macaque and its similarities to Reye's syndrome. *Lab Invest* 24:206-215, 1971

11. Tanaka K, Isselbacher KJ: Isovaleric and -methylbutyric acidemias induced by hypoglycin A: mechanisms of Jamaican vomiting sickness. *Science* 175:69-71, 1972

12. Gerber N, Dickinson RC, Harland RC, et al: Reye-like syndrome associated with valproic acid therapy. *J Pediatr* 95:142-144, 1979

13. Young RS, Bergman I, Gang DL, et al: Fatal Reye-like syndrome associated with valproic acid. *Ann Neurol* 7:389, 1980

14. Makela AL, Yrana T, Mattile M: Dosage of salicylates for children with juvenile rheumatoid arthritis. A preliminary report. *Scand J Rheumatol* 4:250-252, 1975

15. Christoffersen P, Faarup P, Geertinger P, et al: Reye's syndrome in a child on long-term salicylate medication. *Forensic Sci* 15:129-133, 1980

16. *Morbid Mortal Week Rep* 29:532, 537-539, 1980

17. Starko KM, Ray CG, Dominquez LB, et al: Reye's

syndrome and salicylate use. *Pediatrics* 66:859-864, 1980

18. Vanholder R, DeReuck J, Sieben-Praet M, et al: Reye's syndrome in an adult. *Eur Neurol* 18:367-372, 1979

19. Atkins JN, Haponik EF: Reye's syndrome in adult patients. *Am J Med* 67:672-678, 1979

20. Huttenlocher P, Trauner D: Reye's syndrome in infancy. *Pediatrics* 62:84-90, 1978

21. Partin JS, McAdams AJ, McLaurin RL, et al: Brain ultrastructure. In *Reye's Syndrome II.* Edited by Crocker JFS. New York, Grune and Stratton, 1979, pp 237-246

22. Hilty MD, McClung HS, Haynes RE, et al: Reye syndrome in siblings. *J Pediatr* 94:576-579, 1979

23. Sullivan-Bolyai JZ, Nelson DB, Morens DM, et al: Reye's syndrome in children less than 1 year old: some epidemiologic observations. *Pediatrics* 65:627-629, 1980

24. Huttenlocher PR: Reye's syndrome: relation of outcome to therapy. *J Pediatr* 80:845-850, 1972

25. Lovejoy FH, Smith AL, Bresnan MJ, et al: Clinical staging in Reye syndrome. *Am J Dis Child* 128:36-41, 1974

26. Tomasi L: Treatment of Reye syndrome—importance of clinical staging. *Ann Neurol* 8:201-202, 1980

27. Boutros AR, Esfandiari S, Orlowski J, et al: Reye syndrome: a predictably curable disease. *Pediatr Clin North Am* 27:539-552, 1980

28. Trauner DA: Treatment of Reye syndrome—importance of clinical staging—(letter). *Ann Neurol* 8:202, 1980

29. Shaywitz BA, Rothstein P, Venes JL: Monitoring and management of increased intracranial pressure in Reye syndrome: results in 29 children. *Pediatrics* 66:198-204, 1980

30. Teasdale G, Jennett B: Assessment of coma and impaired consciousness. A practical scale. *Lancet* 2:81-83, 1974

31. Coin CG, Pennink M, Gray R, et al: Cerebral computed tomography in Reye syndrome. Case report. *J Comput Assist Tomogr* 3:276-277, 1979

32. Russell EJ, Zimmerman RD, Leeds NE, et al: Reye syndrome: computed tomographic documentation of disordered intracerebral structure *J Comput Assist Tomogr* 3:217-220, 1979

33. Gilboa N: Reye's syndrome and pancreatitis. *Am J Dis Child* 134:903, 1980

34. Chaves-Carballo E, Menezes AH, Bell WE, et al: Acute pancreatitis in Reye's syndrome: a fatal complication during intensive supportive care. *South Med J* 73:152-154, 1980

35. Baliga R, Fleischmann LE, Chang CH, et al: Acute renal failure in Reye's syndrome. *Am J Dis Child* 133:1009-1013, 1979

36. Lansky LL, Linn CR, Mathewson HS, et al: Neurogenic pulmonary edema and intracranial pressure monitoring in severe Reye syndrome. *Ann Neurol* 4:191, 1978

37. Smith P, Green WR, Miller NR, et al: Central retinal vein occlusion in Reye's syndrome. *Arch Ophthalmol* 98:1256-1260, 1980

38. Bentz MS, Cohen C: Periportal hepatic necrosis in Reye's syndrome: one case in a review of eight patients. *Am J Gastroenterol* 73:49-53, 1979

39. Partin JS, Bove K, et al: Liver and muscle ultrastructure in Reye's syndrome. In *Reye's Syndrome II.* Edited by Crocker JFS, New York, Grune and Stratton, 1979, pp 217-232

40. Appelbaum MM, Thaler MM: Reye's syndrome without initial hepatic involvement. *Am J Dis Child* 131:295-296, 1977

41. Faraj BA, Newman SL, Caplan DB, et al: Evidence for hypertyraminemia in Reye's syndrome. *Pediatrics* 64:76-80, 1979

42. Mitchell RA, Arcinue EL: Hepatic monoamine oxidase deficiency in Reye's syndrome. *Pediatrics* 65:673-674, 1980

43. Mitchell RA, Ram ML, Arcinue EL, et al: Comparison of cytosolic and mitochondrial hepatic enzyme alterations in Reye's syndrome. *Pediatr Res* 14:1216-1221, 1980

44. Ansevin CF: Reye syndrome: serum-induced alterations in brain mitochondria function are blocked by fatty-acid free albumin. *Neurology* 30:160-166, 1980

45. Robinson B: Preservation of mitochondrial enzymes in brain and muscle in Reye's syndrome. *Pediatr Res* 13:869, 1979

46. Partin JS: Preservation of mitochondrial enzymes in brain and muscle in Reye's syndrome (letter). *Pediatr Res* 13:868, 1979

47. Lloyd KG, Davidson L, Price K, et al: Catecholamine and octopamine concentrations in brains of patients with Reye's syndrome. *Neurology* 27:985-989, 1977

48. Shaywitz BA, Venes J, Cohen DJ, et al: Reye syndrome: monoamine metabolites in ventricular fluid. *Neurology* 29:467-472, 1979

49. Aprille JR, Austin J, Costello CE, et al: Identification of the Reye's syndrome "serum factor." *Biochem Biophys Res Commun* 94:381-389, 1980

50. Trauner DA: Effects of sodium octanoate on intracranial pressure in rabbits. *Ann Neurol* 8:233, 1980

51. Chaves-Carballo E, Ellefson RD: Tissue lipids in hyperammonemic encephalopathies of childhood. *Arch Neurol* 37:165-167, 1980

52. Chapoy PR, Angelini C, Brown WJ, et al: Systemic carnitine deficiency—a treatable inherited lipid-shortage disease presenting as Reye's syndrome. *N Engl J Med* 303:1389-1394, 1980

53. Glasgow AM, Eng G, Engel AG: Systemic carnitine deficiency stimulating recurrent Reye syndrome. *J Pediatr* 96:889-891, 1980

54. Hinshaw Jr WB, Glenn JL, Hatch KM: Serum carnitine in Reye's syndrome. *N Engl J Med* 302:1423, 1980

55. Willner JH, Chutorian AM, DiMauro S: Tissue carnitine in Reye syndrome. *Ann Neurol* 4:468-469, 1978

56. Dusheiko G, Kew MC, Joffe BI, et al: Recurrent hypoglycemia associated with glutaric aciduria type II in an adult. *N Engl J Med* 301:1405-1409, 1979

57. Robinson BH, Oei J, Sherwood WG, et al: Hydroxymethylglutaryl CoA lyase deficiency: features resembling Reye syndrome. *Neurology* 30:714-718, 1980

58. Huttenlocher PR, Schwartz AD, Klatskin G: Reye's syndrome: ammonia intoxication as a possible factor in the encephalopathy. *Pediatrics* 43:443-454, 1969

59. Trauner DA: Treatment of Reye syndrome. *Ann Neurol* 7:2-4, 1980

60. Hahn JF: Cerebral edema and neurointensive care. *Pediatr Clin North Am* 27:587-592, 1980

61. McGraw CP, Alexander R Jr, Howard G: Effects of dose and dose schedule on the response of intracranial pressure to mannitol. *Surg Neurol* 10:127-130, 1978

62 Botterell EH, Lougheed WM, Scott JW, et al: Hypothermia and interruption of carotid or carotid vertebral circulation in the surgical management of intracranial aneurysms. *J Neurosurg* 13:1-42, 1956

63. Marshall LF, Shapiro HM, Rauscher A, et al: Pentobarbital therapy for intracranial hypertension in metabolic coma—Reye's syndrome. *Crit Care Med* 6:1-5, 1978

64. Pettegrew JW, Payne H, Blaw ME: Physostigmine in Reye's syndrome. *Ann Neurol* 5:105, 1979

65. Dobyns WB, Gunderson CB, Deering WM: Unsuccessful physostigmine therapy in Reye syndrome. *Ann Neurol* 6:141, 1979

66. Knott LJ: Safety of intravenous dimethyl sulphoxide. *Lancet* 13:1299, 1980

67. Duvojny M, Barraneuvo PJ, Decastro SC, et al: Protective effects of methylprednisolone and dimethyl sulfoxide in experimental middle artery embolectomy. *J Neurosurg* 49:508-516, 1978

68. de la Torre JC, Surgeon JW: Dexamethasone and DMSO in experimental transorbital cerebral infarction. *Stroke* 7:577-583, 1976

69. Brown FD, Johns LM, Mullan S: Dimethyl sulfoxide in experimental brain injury with comparison to mannitol. *J Neurosurg* 53:58-62, 1980

70. Brunner RL, O'Grady DJ, Partin JC et al: Neuropsychological consequences of Reye syndrome. *J Pediatr* 95:706-711, 1979

71. Zieve L: Hepatic encephalopathy: summary of present knowledge with an elaboration on recent developments. *Prog Liver Dis* 6:327-341, 1979

72. Rogers EL, Rogers MC: Fulminant hepatic failure and hepatic encephalopathy. *Pediatr Clin North Am* 27:701-713, 1980

73. Battistin L, Zauchin G: The role of amino acids in hepatic encephalopathy. *Prog Clin Biol Res* 39:315-326, 1980

74. Bucci L, Chiaverelli R: Hepatic encephalopathy, EEG and octopamine. *J Clin Psychiatry* 41:175-177, 1980

75. Hill DM, Warren SE, Mitas JA, et al: Hepatic coma after open heart surgery. *South Med J* 73:906-908, 1980

76. Marchesini G, Zoli M, Dondi C, et al: Prevalence of subclinical hepatic encephalopathy in cirrhosis and relationship to plasma amino acid imbalance. *Dig Dis Sci* 25:763-768, 1980

77. Gilberstadt SJ, Gilberstadt H, Zieve L, et al: Psychomotor performance defects in cirrhotic patients without over encephalopathy. *Arch Intern Med* 140:519-521, 1980

78. Conomy J, Swash M: Reversible decerebrate and decorticate postures in hepatic coma. *N Engl J Med* 278:876-879, 1968

79. Cartlidge N, Bates D, Jones R: Prognostic value of oculovestibular reflex. *Br Med J* 1:1346, 1978

80. Rai G, Buxton-Thomas M, Scanlon M: Ocular bobbing in hepatic encephalopathy. *Br J Clin Pract* 30:202-205, 1976

81. Caplan LR, Scheiner D: Dysconjugate gaze in hepatic coma. *Ann Neurol* 8:328-329, 1980

82. MacGillivary BB: The EEG in liver disease. In *Handbook of Electroencephalography and Clinical Neurophysiology*, vol 15. Edited by Redmond A. Amsterdam, Elsevier, 1976, pp 26

83. Tanaka S, Yano Y, Sakamoto H, et al: Recovery after prolonged flat EEG in hepatic coma. *Lancet* 2:1379, 1980

84. Blitzer BL: Fulminant hepatic failure: a rare but often lethal coma syndrome. *Postgrad Med* 68:153-162, 1980

85. Silk DBA, Hanid MA, Trewby PN, et al: Treatment of fulminant hepatic failure by polyacrylonitrile-membrane hemodialysis. *Lancet* 2:1-3, 1977

86. Hanid MA, Davies M, Mellon PJ, et al: Clinical monitoring of intracranial pressure in fulminant hepatic failure. *Gut* 21:866-869, 1980

87. Oei LT, Kuys J, Lombarts AJPF, et al: Cerebrospinal fluid glutamine levels and EEG findings in patients with hepatic encephalopathy. *Clin Neurol Neurosurg* 81:59-63, 1979

88. Derr RF, Zieve L: Effect of fatty acids on the disposition of ammonia. *J Pharmacol Exp Ther* 197:675-680, 1976

89. Teychenne PF, Walters I, Claveria LE, et al: The encephalopathic action of five-carbon-atom fatty acids in the rabbit. *Clin Sci Mol Med* 50:463-477, 1976

90. Watanabe A, Takesue A, Higashi T, et al: Serum

amino acids in hepatic encephalopathy—effects of branched-chain amino acid infusion on serum aminogram. *Acta Hepatogastroenterol (Stuttg)* 26:346-357, 1979

91. Editorial: Biochemical monitoring of encephalopathy in liver failure. *Lancet* 2:783-784, 1980

92. Oldendorf WH: Brain uptake of radiolabeled amino acids, amines and hexoses after arterial injection. *Am J Physiol* 221:1629, 1971

93. James JH, Escourrou J, Fischer JE: Blood-brain neutral amino acid transport activity is increased after portacaval anastamosis. *Science* 200:1395-1397, 1978

94. Knell A: Serum methionine in liver failure. *Lancet* 2:1036, 1980

95. Riederer P, Jellinger K, Kleinberger G, et al: Oral and parenteral nutrition with L-valine: mode of action. *Nutr Metab* 24:209-217, 1980

96. Cuilleret G, Pomier-Layrargues G, Pons F, et al: Changes in brain catecholamine levels in human cirrhotic hepatic encephalopathy. *Gut* 21:565-569, 1980

97. Young SN, Lal S: CNS tryptamine metabolism in hepatic coma. *J Neural Transm* 47:153-161, 1980

98. Capocaccia L, Cangiano C, Cascino A, et al: Influence of phenylethanolamine on octopamine plasma determination in hepatic encephalopathy. *Clin Chim Acta* 93:371-376, 1979

99. Wardle EN, Williams R: Depressed uptake of serotonin by platelets in hepatic encephalopathy. *Biochem Med* 24:223-227, 1980

100. Jouvet M: Biogenic amines and the states of sleep. *Science* 163:301-306, 1969

101. Marchesini G, Zoli M, Forlani G: The role of insulin and glucagon in the plasma amino acid imbalance of chronic hepatic encephalopathy. *Z Gastroenterol* 17:469-476, 1979

102. Marchesini G, Forlani G, Angiolini A, et al: Oral glucose in cirrhotics: effects on plasma amino acid patterns and the role of insulin and glucagon. *Diabete Metab* 5:135-139, 1979

103. James JH, Ziparo V, Jeppsson B, et al: Hyperammonemia, plasma amino acid imbalance and blood-brain amino acid transport: a unified theory of portal-systemic encephalopathy. *Lancet* 2:772-775, 1979

104. Challenger F, Walshe JM: Methyl mercaptan in relation to foetor hepaticus. *Biochem J* 59:372-375, 1955

105. McClain CJ, Zieve L, Doizaki WM, et al: Blood methanethiol in alcoholic liver disease with and without hepatic encephalopathy. *Gut* 21:318-323, 1980

106. Chong TMS, Lister C: Analysis of possible toxins in hepatic coma, including the removal of mercaptan by albumin-collodion charcoal. *Int J Artif Organs* 3:108-112, 1980

107. Gundermann KJ, Lie TS: Treatment of acute hepatic failure by hemoperfusion over baboon and human livers: alpha fetoprotein levels in serum. *Artif Organs* 4:27-29, 1980

108. Fiaccadori F, Ghinelli F, Pelosi G, et al: Selective amino acid solutions in hepatic encephalopathy treatment (a preliminary report). *Ric Clin Lab* 10:411-422, 1980

109. Freund H, Yoshimura N, Fischer JE: Chronic hepatic encephalopathy. Long-term therapy with a branched-chain amino-acid-enriched elemental diet. *JAMA* 242:347-349, 1979

110. Herlong HF, Maddrey WC, Walser M: The use of ornithine salts of branched-chain ketoacids in portal-systemic encephalopathy. *Ann Intern Med* 93:545-550, 1980

111. Michel H, Solere M, Granier P, et al: Treatment of cirrhotic hepatic encephalopathy with L-dopa. A controlled trial. *Gastroenterology* 79:207-211, 1980

112. Uribe M, Farca A, Marquez MA, et al: Treatment of chronic portal-systemic encephalopathy with bromocriptine: a double-blind controlled trial. *Gastroenterology* 76:1347-1351, 1979

113. Morgan MY, Jakobouits AW, James IM, et al: Successful use of bromocriptine in the treatment of chronic hepatic encephalopathy. *Gastroenterology* 78:663-670, 1980

114. Marzio L, Lanfrauchi GA: Bromocriptine for chronic portal-systemic encephalopathy. *Gastroenterology* 78:1661-1662, 1980

115. Uribe M: Bromocriptine to treat "intractable" portal-systemic encephalopathy. *Gastroenterology* 79:603, 1980

116. Morgan MY: Bromocriptine to treat "intractable" portal-systemic encephalopathy—a reply. *Gastroenterology* 79:603, 1980

117. Schenker S, Desmond PV, Speeg KV, et al: Cryptic nature of bromocriptine therapy in portal systemic encephalopathy. *Gastroenterology* 78:1094-1096, 1980

118. Satran R, Griggs RC: Metabolic encephalopathies. In *Current Neurology* vol 3. Edited by Appel SH, John Wiley, New York, 1981, pp 240-241

119. Okita K, Matsuda S, Hata K, et al: Clinical use of glucagon and insulin in therapy of fulminant hepatic failure. *Gastroenterol Jpn* 14:453-457, 1979

120. Depew W, Boyer T, Omata M, et al: Double-blind controlled trial of prednisolone therapy in patients with severe acute alcoholic hepatitis and spontaneous encephalopathy. *Gastroenterology* 78:524-529, 1980

121. Wilson SAK: Progressive lenticular degeneration: a familial nervous disease associated with cirrhosis of the liver. *Brain* 34:295-509, 1912

122. Hall HC: *La Degenerescence Hepatico-Lenticulaire, Maladie de Wilson-Pseudosclerose,* Paris, Masson and Cie, 1921

123. Sternlieb I: Copper and the liver. *Gastroenterology* 78:1615-1628, 1980

124. Dobyns WB, Goldstein NP, Gordon H: Clinical spectrum of Wilson's disease (hepatolenticular degeneration). *Mayo Clin Proc* 54:35-42, 1979

125. Fleming CR, Dickson ER, Wahner HW, et al: Pigmented corneal rings in non-Wilsonian liver disease. *Ann Intern Med* 86:285-288, 1977

126. Fleming CR, Dickson ER, Hollenhorst RW, et al: Pigmented corneal rings in a patient with primary biliary cirrhosis. *Gastroenterology* 69:220-225, 1975

127. Kaplinsky C, Sternlieb I, Javitt N, et al: Familial cholestatic cirrhosis associated with Kayser-Fleischer rings. *Pediatrics* 65:782-788, 1980

128. Schoenberger M, Ellis PP: Disappearance of Kayser-Fleischer rings after liver transplantation. *Arch Ophthalmol* 97:1914-1915, 1979

129. Gadoth N, Liel Y: Transient external ophthalmoplegia in Wilson's disease. *Metab Pediatr Ophthalmol* 4:71-72, 1980

130. Wiebers DO, Wilson DM, McLeod RA, et al: Renal stones in Wilson's disease. *Am J Med* 67:249-254, 1979

131. Haggstrom G, Hirschowitz BI: Disordered esophageal motility in Wilson's disease. *J Clin Gastroenterol* 2:273-275, 1980

132. Werlin SL, Grand RJ, Perman JA, et al: Diagnostic dilemmas of Wilson's disease: diagnosis and treatment. *Pediatrics* 61:47-51, 1978

133. Gibbs K, Walshe JM: A study of the caeruloplasmin concentrations found in 75 patients with Wilson's disease, their kinships and various control groups. *Q J Med* 48:447-463, 1979

134. Perman JA, Welin SL, Grand RJ, et al: Laboratory measures of copper metabolism in the differentiation of chronic active hepatitis and Wilson's disease in children. *J Pediatr* 94:564-568, 1979

135. Spechler SJ, Koff RS: Wilson's disease: diagnostic difficulties in the patient with chronic hepatitis and hypoceruloplasminemia. *Gastroenterology* 78:803-806, 1980

136. Sternleib I, Scheinberg IH: The role of radiocopper in the diagnosis of Wilson's disease. *Gastroenterology* 77:138-142, 1979

137. Edwards CQ, Williams DM, Cartwright GE: Hereditary hypoceruloplasminemia. *Clin Genet* 15:311-316, 1979

138. Nelson RF, Guzman DA, Grahavac Z, et al: Computerized cranial tomography in Wilson's disease. *Neurology* 29:866-868, 1979

139. Harik SI, Post MJ: Computed tomography in Wilson's disease. *Neurology* 31:107-110, 1981

140. Fujita M, Hosoki M, Miyazaki M: Brain stem auditory evoked responses in spinocerebellar degeneration and Wilson's disease. *Ann Neurology* 9:42-47, 1981

141. Chan WY, Cushing W, Coffman MA, et al: Genetic expression of Wilson's disease in cell culture: a diagnostic marker. *Science* 208:299-300, 1980

142. Stromeyer FW, Ishak KG: Histology of the liver in Wilson's disease: a study of 34 cases. *Am J Clin Pathol* 73:12-24, 1980

143. Malamud N, Hiran O: *Atlas of Neuropathology*, 2nd ed. Berkeley, University of California Press, 1974, pp 402

144. Vallat JM, Dumas M, Leboutet MS, et al: Ultrastructure of nerve biopsy in Wilson's disease (letter). *Muscle Nerve* 2:504-505, 1979

145. Gibbs K, Walshe JM: Biliary excretion of copper in Wilson's disease. *Lancet* 2:538-539, 1980

146. Epstein O, Sherlock S: Is Wilson's disease caused by a controller gene mutation resulting in perpetuation of the fetal mode of copper metabolism into childhood? *Lancet* 303-305, 1981

147. Brown CE, Antholine WE: Evidence that carnosine and anserine may participate in Wilson's disease. *Biochem Biophys Res Commun* 92:470-477, 1980

148. Haggstrom GD, Hirschowitz BE, Flint A: Long-term penicillamine therapy for Wilson's disease. *South Med J* 73:530-531, 1980

149. Borthwick TR, Benson GD, Schugar HJ: Copper chelating agents: a comparison of cupriuretic responses to various tetramines and D-penicillamine. *J Lab Clin Med* 95:575-580, 1980

150. Haslam RHA, Sass-Kortsak A, Stout W, et al: Treatment of Wilson's disease with triethylene tetramine dihydrochloride. *Dev Pharmacol Ther* 1:318-324, 1980

151. Hoogenraad TU, Koevoet R, de Ruyter Korver EGWM: Oral zinc sulphate as long-term treatment in Wilson's disease (hepatolenticular degeneration). *Eur Neurol* 18:205-211, 1979

152. Schouwink G: *De Hepato-cerebrale Degeneratie. Met een Onderzoek van de Zinkstofwisseling; Academishch Proefschrift*. Amsterdam, Van der Wiel, Arnhem, 1961

153. Orth J: Veber das Vorkommen von bilirubinkrystallen bein neugeborenen kindern. *Virchows Arch [Path Ana]* 63:447, 1875

154. Schmorl G: Zur kinntnis des ikterus neonctorum, insbesondere der dabei auftretenden gehirnveranderungen. *Verh Dtsch Ges Pathol* 6:109, 1903

155. Diamond I: Bilirubin encephalopathy (kerniturus). In *Scientific Approaches to Clinical Neurology*. Edited by Goldenshohn ES, Appel SH. Philadelphia, Lea and Febiger, 1977, pp 1212-1233

156. Perlstein MA: The clinical syndrome of kernicterus. In *Kernicterus and Its Importance in Cerebral Palsy*. Edited by Swinyard CA. Springfield, Charles C. Thomas, 1961

157. Hsia DY-Y, Allen FH, Gellis SS, et al: Erythroblastosis fetalis. VIII. Studies of serum bilirubin in relation to kernicterus. *N Engl J Med* 247:668-671, 1952

158. Stern L, Denton RL: Kernicterus in small premature infants. *Pediatrics* 35:483-485, 1965

159. Harper RG, Sia CG, Kierney CMP: Kernicterus

1980: problems and practices viewed from the perspective of the practicing clinician. *Clin Perinatol* 7:75-92, 1980

160. Levine RL: Bilirubin: worked out years ago? *Pediatrics* 64:380-385, 1979

161. Lucey JF: The unsolved problem of kernicterus in the susceptible low birth weight infant. *Pediatrics* 49:646-647, 1972

162. Pearlman MA, Gartner LM, Lee K-S, et al: The association of kernicterus with bacterial infection in the newborn. *Pediatrics* 65:26-29, 1980

163. Turkel SB, Guttenberg ME, Moynes DR, et al: Lack of identifiable risk factors for kernicterus. *Pediatrics* 66:502-506, 1980

164. Claireaux AE: Pathology of human kernicterus. In *Kernicterus*. Edited by Sass-Kortsak A. Toronto, University of Toronto Press, 1961

165. Wennberg RP, Ahlfors CE, Rasmussen LF: The pathochemistry of kernicterus. *Early Hum Dev* 3:353-372, 1979

166. Cashore WJ: Free bilirubin concentrations and bilirubin-binding affinity in term and preterm infants. *J Pediatr* 96:521-527, 1980

167. Brodersen R: Bilirubin transport in the newborn infant, reviewed with relation to kernicterus. *J Pediatr* 96:349-356, 1980

168. Nelson T, Jacobsen J, Wennberg RP: Effects of pH on the interaction of bilirubin with albumin and tissue culture cells. *Pediatr Res* 8:963-967, 1974

169. Diamond I, Schmid R: Experimental bilirubin encephalopathy. The mode of entry of bilirubin-^{14}C into the central nervous system. *J Clin Invest* 45:678-689, 1966

170. Wennberg RP, Rasmussen LF: Factors determining the cellular uptake of bilirubin. *Pediatr Res* 12:536, 1978

171. Wible KL: Bilirubin, albumin, and the risk of kernicterus. *J Pediatr* 9:1038, 1980

172. Chiveh CC, Sun CL, Kopin IJ, et al: Entry of [^{3}H] norepinephrine, [^{125}I] albumin and Evans Blue from blood into brain following unilateral osmotic opening of the blood-brain barrier. *Brain Res* 145:291-301, 1978

173. Karp WB: Biochemical alterations in neonatal hyperbilirubinemia and bilirubin encephalopathy: a review. *Pediatrics* 64:361-368, 1979

174. Thong YH: Is kernicterus due to inhibition of brain hexose monophosphate shunt activity by bilirubin? *Med Hypotheses* 5:297-302, 1979

175. Kozuki K, Cashore WJ, Widness J, et al: Increase in bilirubin-albumin binding affinity with correction of neonatal acidosis. *Acta Pediatr Scand* 68:213-217, 1979

176. Diamond I, Schmid R: Oxidative phosphorylation in experimental bilirubin encephalopathy. *Science* 155:1288-1289, 1967

177. Brown AK, Eisinger J, Blumberg WE, et al: A rapid fluorometric method for determining bilirubin levels and binding in the blood of neonates: comparisons with a Diazo method and with 2-(4-hydroxybenzene)azobenzoic acid dye binding. *Pediatrics* 65:767-776, 1980

178. Ash KO, Hentschel WM, Chan GM, et al: Reserve bilirubin binding capacity assessed by difference spectroscopy: assay statistics and results on newborn sera. *Clin Chim Acta* 104:309-318, 1980

6

Dietary Precursors of Neurotransmitters: Treatment Strategies

John H. Growdon and Candace J. Gibson

This review summarizes current knowledge regarding the relationship between synthesis of certain neurotransmitters and dietary-induced changes in the plasma concentrations of their precursors. It describes the ways in which changes in the plasma concentrations of tryptophan, tyrosine, and choline cause parallel changes in the rates at which neurons synthesize and release serotonin, the catecholamines—dopamine and norepinephrine, and acetylcholine, respectively. These experimental observations lead to the suggestion that naturally occurring dietary constituents that are precursors for neurotransmitter synthesis could be used as drugs to treat brain diseases associated with deficient serotonergic, catecholaminergic, or cholinergic neurotransmission (1). Dietary precursor therapy takes advantage of the brain's normal mechanisms for regulating neurotransmitter synthesis; it does not imply that nutritional deficiencies exist in any of the diseases under treatment. The use of tryptophan, tyrosine, and choline to treat specific brain diseases is still experimental and limited to research protocols. Nonetheless, the sound scientific basis for dietary precursor administration and encouraging results in clinical trials indicate that this mode of treatment will become more prevalent and that investigators will continue to test these compounds in additional diseases in which neurotransmitter deficiencies are believed to exist. The principles of dietary precursor therapy and some preliminary results in clinical trials have been sum-marized elsewhere (2); this review considers recent data regarding the biochemical, physiological, and behavioral effects of tryptophan, tyrosine, and choline and describes their current experimental applications and potential utilities in neurological and psychiatric diseases.

TRYPTOPHAN AND SEROTONIN BIOSYNTHESIS

The initial step in the synthesis of brain serotonin involves the 5-hydroxylation of the amino acid tryptophan in a reaction catalyzed by the enzyme tryptophan hydroxylase (Fig. 1). Tryptophan hydroxylase is confined to those brain neurons that synthesize and contain serotonin (3), and its net activity determines the overall rate of serotonin synthesis. Tryptophan hydroxylase is normally unsaturated with respect to its substrates tryptophan and oxygen; the K_m for this reaction is 50–60 μM, and the usual brain tryptophan concentration is 20 μM (4, 5). Oxygen and tetrahydropterine are necessary cofactors for this reaction, and their interaction with tryptophan may affect the affinity of tryptophan hydroxylase for its substrates (6, 7). The hydroxylation product, 5-hydroxy-tryptophan, is rapidly decarboxylated to form serotonin in the presence of the enzyme aromatic acid decarboxylase (8). The major catabolic product of serotonin metabolism in the brain is 5-hydroxyindoleacetic acid (5-HIAA). It is formed by the sequential actions

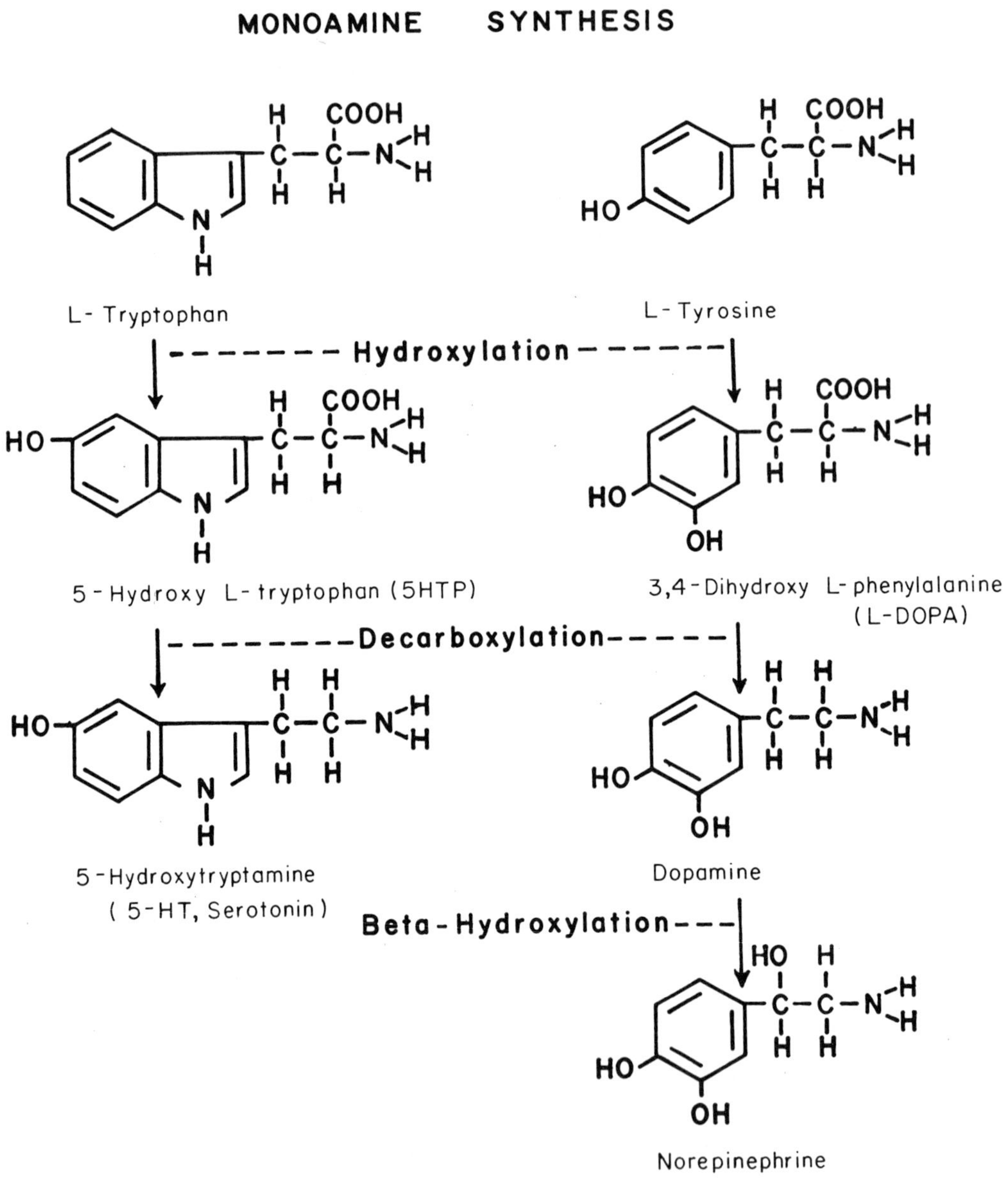

Figure 1. Monoamine biosynthetic pathways in mammalian central nervous system. The dietary amino acid precursors tryptophan and tyrosine are converted to L-5-hydroxytryptophan (5-HTP) and L-3,4-dihydroxyphenylalanine (L-dopa) in the presence of tryptophan hydroxylase and tyrosine hydroxylase, respectively. The rate at which this initial step proceeds determines the rate of the entire reaction. L-5-HTP and L-dopa, once formed, are immediately decarboxylated by aromatic amino acid decarboxylase to form the neurotransmitters 5-hydroxytryptamine (serotonin) and dopamine. Neurons that contain dopamine β-hydroxylase can convert dopamine further to form norepinephrine.

of aldehyde dehydrogenase and monoamine oxidase.

Serotonin was the first neurotransmitter that was shown to be influenced by the availability of a dietary precursor. Tryptophan is an essential amino acid and cannot be made in the body; hence tryptophan consumed as part of dietary protein is the only source of tryptophan for serotonin synthesis. Tryptophan is absorbed from the gut into the bloodstream where it is distributed between two compartments: ten to twenty percent circulates as the free amino acid, and the remainder is bound to serum albumin (9). Both fractions are available for uptake into the brain. Under most physiological conditions, total plasma tryptophan levels correlate best with brain tryptophan concentrations (10, 11), since tryptophan has a greater affinity for the blood-brain barrier transport system than for albumin (12, 13). There are some other instances in which the reverse occurs, and brain tryptophan concentrations have been reported to correlate best with the amount of free tryptophan in plasma. Some of these conditions include stress immobilization, prolonged fasting, or administration of drugs, such as salicylates and probenecid, that alter the affinity of tryptophan for albumin (14–16).

Plasma tryptophan levels, as well as the levels of most other amino acids, characteristically fluctuate during each 24-hour period in a pattern dependent upon food intake. Plasma tryptophan levels are lowest between 2:00 and 5:00 AM and increase 50%–80% to reach a plateau in the late morning or early afternoon (17, 18). Ingestion of the pure amino acid causes a rapid rise in plasma levels of free and total tryptophan that occurs within 2 hours of ingestion and lasts 6–8 hours (19). Tryptophan administration also significantly increases tryptophan and 5-HIAA levels in the cerebrospinal fluid (CSF), indicating that tryptophan hydroxylase is not fully saturated with its substrate in humans (19, 20). Tryptophan is transported into the brain by a specific uptake system at the blood-brain barrier that it shares with other neutral amino acids, including phenylalanine, tyrosine, leucine, isoleucine, and valine (21, 22).

The amount of tryptophan that actually enters the brain depends upon the tryptophan ratio, defined as the ratio of the plasma-free (20, 23) or total tryptophan concentration (10, 11) to the sum of the plasma concentrations of the competing neutral amino acids. This transport system is not fully saturated with its substrates under physiological conditions, and increases in the plasma tryptophan ratio are likely to cause parallel increases in tryptophan's entry into the brain and nerve cells. Since tryptophan hydroxylase is not fully saturated with tryptophan, increased amounts of this precursor substrate would be expected to increase the amounts of product serotonin that are synthesized.

Fernstrom and Wurtman (24) originally conducted a series of experiments to define the conditions under which tryptophan availability influenced serotonin synthesis. They first showed that physiological amounts of tryptophan increased plasma tryptophan, brain tryptophan, and brain serotonin levels in rats. There was a parallel increase in 5-HIAA levels indicating that tryptophan administration increased serotonin metabolism as well (25). In separate experiments (26, 27), they injected rats with insulin or fed them a meal with a high carbohydrate content to elicit insulin secretion. Insulin lowered the plasma concentrations of most neutral amino acids but did not affect tryptophan because of its unique binding to albumin; thus, the tryptophan ratio increased, and brain serotonin levels increased. Colmenares and coworkers (28) measured the rate at which 5-hydroxytryptophan accumulated during carbohydrate consumption and showed that the elevation in serotonin levels was due to increased synthesis. Surprisingly, a high protein meal did not increase brain serotonin levels (10). Dietary protein contains less than 1% of tryptophan and much larger amounts of the competing neutral amino acids. Plasma tryptophan levels increased, but the plasma tryptophan ratio actually decreased. This observation further confirmed the importance of the tryptophan ratio for predicting brain levels of tryptophan and serotonin.

Increased serotonin levels induced by tryptophan probably cause increased serotonin release since brain levels of 5-HIAA in rats rise in parallel with serotonin (10). Gillman and coworkers (20) have obtained the most direct evidence for tryptophan-induced serotonin release in humans. They infused 15 mg/kg/hr of tryptophan into patients who were undergoing neurosurgical operations and collected samples of frontal cortex, ventricular CSF, and lumbar CSF. They reported that tryptophan administration significantly increased tryptophan concentrations in all three compartments and also significantly increased 5-HIAA concentrations in both ventricular and lumbar CSF.

CLINICAL USES OF TRYPTOPHAN

Pharmacological amounts of the purified amino acid L-tryptophan have been tested as treatments for such disparate conditions as depression, myoclonus, migraine headache, sleep disorders, and Parkinson's disease. The results of clinical trials with tryptophan in these conditions have been reviewed recently (2): the use of tryptophan as an antidepressant remains controversial; tryptophan has suppressed myoclonus in a few patients with post-hypoxic intention myoclonus but is not as effective as 5-hydroxytryptophan (5-HTP) or clonazepam; tryptophan apparently is an effective hypnotic in some patients; and the utility of tryptophan in Parkinson's disease and migraine remain to be proved. The following sections review new data regarding the use of tryptophan in depression and describe the uses of tryptophan in pain syndromes and as an adjunct to appetite control.

Endogenous Depression

The monoamine theory of depression originally proposed by Coppen (29) postulated that there was a defect in central serotonergic neurotransmission. This was based on biochemical analyses of brain tissue obtained at postmortem examinations from patients with depression (30, 31), from CSF studies (32, 33), and from the proposed actions of antidepressant drugs (34). These observations stimulated clinical investigators to test tryptophan, alone or in combination with standard antidepressant therapies, in patients with endogenous depression. Despite extensive clinical trials (2, 35), the results are inconclusive: at least 8 studies report an antidepressant effect, but an equal number found no benefit from tryptophan administration alone, although it is beneficial in combination with monoamine oxidase inhibitors (36). Several factors have been described that may account for these conflicting reports and possibly indicate ways to resolve the controversy. Accumulating evidence indicates that depression is not a single homogeneous biochemical entity, and that there are at least 2 subsets of patients with monoamine lesions: 1 serotonergic and 1 noradrenergic (37). Neurons that synthesize acetylcholine may be involved as well, since cholinergic agonists can produce depression and have been used to treat the symptoms of mania (38). Accepting the fact that even this division is probably overly simplistic, tryptophan administration might improve depression in those patients with an underlying serotonergic deficit but probably would not affect patients with noradrenergic or cholinergic abnormalities. Secondly, it is necessary to treat patients for at least 1 month, to segregate patients into unipolar and bipolar affective groups, and to use an appropriate dose of tryptophan. Recent evidence suggests that there is an optimal dose range for tryptophan. Young and Sourkes (35) reviewed published reports in which tryptophan was an effective antidepressant and noted that the mean dose was 6 g/day, whereas it was 8.7 g/day in studies in which tryptophan was ineffective. Co-administration of a pyrolase inhibitor such as nicotinamide would permit a further reduction in the optimal dose of tryptophan (39), and the optimal dose of tryptophan may be less in patients with unipolar and more in patients with bipolar depressions. Finally, the transport of tryptophan into the brain and its subsequent hydroxylation may be decreased in a subset of depressed patients (40, 41). Some investigators reported decreased levels of tryptophan in plasma and in spinal fluid (42), whereas others reported normal (43) or even higher than normal levels (44). The ratio of plasma tryptophan to its neutral amino acid competitors may provide a more accurate basis for guiding treatment with tryptophan. Moller and coworkers (45) measured the plasma tryptophan ratio in 32 patients with depression; 12 improved during tryptophan ingestion. Eighty percent of those had low plasma tryptophan ratios, whereas those with high tryptophan ratios did not improve during treatment. In another study, the plasma tryptophan ratio was inversely correlated with the severity of depression; the lower the ratio, the greater the depression (46). These data indicate that plasma amino acid determinations may be used to predict a patient's response to treatment.

Pain Syndromes

Serotonergic neurons that originate in the raphé nucleus and descend in the dorsal lateral funiculus of the spinal cord to terminate in the dorsal horn (47) have been implicated in modulating the perception of noxious stimuli (48–50). Although tryptophan itself is not an analgesic agent, treatments that decrease brain serotonin levels enhance the perception of pain, whereas treatments that increase serotonin levels can decrease painful sensations. Lytle and coworkers (51) fed rats a corn-based diet that was deficient in tryptophan to deplete brain levels of serotonin. They reported that these animals showed lower thresholds to noxious stimuli than untreated rats and that refeeding with a complete amino acid diet or administering tryptophan alone restored thresholds to control values.

Analgesia induced by narcotics or electrical stimulation of the periaqueductal and periventricular gray matter is thought to be mediated by a common mechanism that involves serotonin (48). Electrical stimulation of the periventricular region in humans has been used to treat cases of intractable pain (52), but the therapeutic utility of this procedure is often limited since tolerance develops to both electrical stimulation and to opiate administration. Hosobuchi found that 3 g/day of trytophan could reverse tolerance to electrical stimulation (53) and chronic opiate administration (54) and restore relief from pain. Rhizotomies and cordotomies are additional surgical approaches to treating intractable pain. These procedures relieve pain and also produce anesthesia in the area supplied by the severed sensory afferents. In some patients, however, the areas of anesthesia contract with time, and pain recurs after a few months or years. King (55) reported that 2 g/day of tryptophan restored anesthesia and full pain relief in 5 patients whose pain recurred after rhizotomy or cordotomy. Similar results were obtained in 6 patients with recurrent face pain after denervation operations. Tryptophan administration did not relieve pain in patients with peripheral nerve injuries. These data are all consistent with the notion that tryptophan's ability to relieve pain is best related to conditions such as direct electrical stimulation, chronic opiate administration, or postsurgical lesions, in which serotonergic neurons are activated.

Appetite Control

The experimental use of tryptophan in appetite control is based on the suggestion that serotonergic neurons act as sensors for plasma amino acid concentrations (10, 24). Consumption of a meal that contains a large amount of carbohydrate but little protein increases the plasma tryptophan ratio, increases brain tryptophan levels, and stimulates serotonin synthesis (26). Consumption of a high protein meal would reverse this effect, and brain serotonin levels would not increase. Since serotonergic neurons detect changes in plasma amino acid concentrations, they are ideally suited to influence mechanisms that control appetite. Wurtman and Wurtman (56) gave drugs that enhance serotonergic transmission to rats and found that they decreased carbohydrate and caloric consumption without affecting protein intake. Reduction in carbohydrate consumption would be desirable in clinical conditions such as diabetes mellitus or in obese subjects with irresistable carbohydrate cravings. Wurtman and coworkers (57) tested the effects of 2.4 g/day of tryptophan and 45–60 mg/day of D,L-fenfluramine in 24 obese patients with carbohydrate craving according to a double-blind protocol. Fenfluramine administration decreased the number of carbohydrate snacks in 6 of 9 subjects, and tryptophan significantly decreased carbohydrate snacking in 3 of 8 subjects. Placebo administration did not affect carbohydrate intake in the remaining 7 patients. These observations indicate that increasing serotonergic neurotransmission affects caloric intake and should be tested further in clinical disorders of eating.

TYROSINE AND CATECHOLAMINE BIOSYNTHESIS

Tyrosine is the physiological precursor for the catecholamines: dopamine, norepinephrine, and epinephrine (Fig. 1). The initial biosynthetic step involves the addition of an hydroxyl group to the aromatic ring of tyrosine in a reaction catalyzed by the enzyme tyrosine hydroxylase (58). The product of this reaction, L-dihydroxyphenylalanine or L-dopa, is rapidly decarboxylated by aromatic l-amino acid decarboxylase to form the catecholamine dopamine (8). A third enzyme, dopamine β-hydroxylase, is located within vesicles of noradrenergic brain neurons and catalyzes the formation of norepinephrine (59). A small number of neurons in the brain apparently synthesize epinephrine; they contain the enzyme, phenylethanolamine-*N*-methyl transferase (60). Homovanillic acid (HVA) is the major metabolite of dopamine (61); 3-methoxy-4-hydroxyphenylglycol (MHPG) and its sulfated conjugate are the major metabolites of norepinephrine in the brain (62).

There are many similarities between the ways in which tyrosine influences catecholamine biosynthesis and the effects of tryptophan on serotonin synthesis. In both instances, the brain cannot synthesize sufficient amounts of the precursor amino acid and must therefore extract them from the systemic circulation. Plasma tyrosine levels normally vary two- to fourfold during the day, and tyrosine from protein ingestion is an important source of plasma tyrosine (17, 18). The essential amino acid phenylalanine can also be converted to tyrosine in the liver (63). Tyrosine is transported into the brain by an unsaturated uptake system located at the blood-brain barrier that it shares with the other neutral amino acids including tryptophan (21, 22). The tyrosine ratio, which is the ratio of the plasma concentration of tyrosine to the sum of the plasma concentrations of the competing neutral amino acids, is the best predictor of brain tyrosine concentrations (11). Since the uptake system is greatly unsaturated, fluctuations in the plasma concentrations of tyrosine and in the tyrosine ratio will cause parallel changes in brain tyrosine concentrations. Tyrosine and tryptophan do not act as neurotransmitters but must be enzymatically converted to their transmitter products. In both instances, their hydroxylation is the rate-limiting biosynthetic step; both hydroxylases are normally unsaturated with their precursor amino acids. Tyrosine hydroxylase, like tryptophan hydroxylase, requires molecular oxygen and a pteridine cofactor for full activity. Under normal conditions, tyrosine hydroxylase is saturated with its oxygen substrate (7) but may not be fully saturated with respect to the pterin cofactor (64). Finally, increased tyrosine or tryptophan availability increases the rates at which neurons synthesize catecholamines and serotonin, respectively (65).

There are some important differences between these two monoaminergic systems. Tryptophan administration increases brain levels of serotonin, whereas tyrosine administration does not increase brain levels of the catecholamines; this fact obscured the relationship between tyrosine availability and catecholamine biosynthesis. Wurtman and coworkers (66) first showed that tyrosine administration increased the rate at which catecholaminergic neurons synthesized the catechol, L-dopa. Carlsson and Lindquist (65) subsequently reported that tyrosine hydroxylase in the rat brain was only 75%–80% saturated with its amino acid precursor and that intraperitoneal injections of tyrosine increased dopa accumulation particularly in the limbic forebrain. Gibson and Wurtman (67) also found a similar amount of tyrosine hydroxylase saturation in fed animals and reported an even greater increase in dopa accumulation when tyrosine was given to fasted rats with dietary-induced decreases in brain tyrosine levels.

Although tyrosine administration does not produce increases in brain catecholamine levels, it will increase the rate of catecholamine synthesis and turnover in some conditions. Scally and coworkers (68) measured HVA levels (a measure of dopamine release) in striata of rats injected with haloperidol alone or with tyrosine in combination with haloperidol. A single injection of haloperidol activated dopaminergic neurons by blocking the postsynaptic receptor sites. They reported a greater increase in striatal HVA levels in animals treated with tyrosine plus haloperidol than in animals treated with haloperidol alone. Hefti and coworkers (69) confirmed the importance of firing rate in the ability of tyrosine to enhance dopaminergic neurotransmission. They reported that lesions in the nigrostriatal tract increased the rate of dopamine turnover in the residual neurons; tyrosine administration caused further increases in HVA levels within the striatum (70). Pharmacological experiments provide additional evidence that tyrosine administration can increase dopamine synthesis and release. Sved and coworkers (71) injected rats with reserpine to induce hyperprolactinemia and contrasted the effects of levodopa and tyrosine on prolactin levels. They found that tyrosine administration significantly decreased plasma prolactin levels although levodopa was more potent.

Tyrosine administration also increases norepinephrine release in nonadrenergic neurons that are discharging rapidly. Gibson and Wurtman (72) measured $MHPG\text{-}SO_4$ accumulation in the brains of rats subjected to cold stress and found that it increased significantly after tyrosine administration. These data indicate that increased availability of tyrosine will increase dopamine and norepinephrine turnover in conditions in which the rate-limiting enzyme tyrosine hydroxylase has been activated. The exact mechanism for this is unknown but may involve a conformational change in the enzyme that causes changes in the affinity for substrates or cofactors. These data also suggest that tyrosine availability will have its major effect on those neurons in which catecholaminergic turnover is already increased (usually by a pathological condition). Quiescent catecholaminergic neurons that are firing at a normal rate will be less influenced by increased amounts of tyrosine. This observation suggests that tyrosine administration will selectively increase transmission at damaged synaptic sites and, in contrast to other drugs that enhance dopamine transmission such as levodopa and bromocriptine, avoid effects at normal synapses. Selectivity is most clearly seen in experiments on the effects of tyrosine on blood pressure regulation by noradrenergic neurons in the central and peripheral autonomic nervous systems (Fig. 2). Norepinephrine released from peripheral sympathetic nerves and the adrenal medulla tend to elevate blood pressure while that released from brain stem loci tend to lower blood pressure (73). Sved and coworkers (74) reported that a single intraperitoneal injection of tyrosine significantly lowered blood pressure in rats with spontaneous hypertension. There was also a concomitant rise in $MHPG\text{-}SO_4$ levels in the brain stem. The authors postulated that tyrosine-induced increases in norepinephrine turnover decreased blood pressure by a central mechanism, possibly by inhibiting sympathetic neuronal outflow from the spinal cord. The addition of tyrosine to normal diets increased plasma tyrosine and brain tyrosine levels and significantly decreased blood pressure in spontaneously hypertensive rats (75). The concurrent administration of valine to block tyrosine entry into the brain blunted the hypotensive effects (74). Tyrosine placed directly into the ventricular system of the brain lowered blood pressure (76). Bresnahan and coworkers (77) confirmed the ability of tyrosine to lower blood pressure in animals with hypertension induced by administering deoxycorticosterone acetate and salt and also in rats with the Goldblatt kidney preparation. In all three models of hypertension, α-adrenergic neurons in the brain stem are presumably firing rapidly and therefore sensitive to increased amounts of tyrosine. Hemorrhagic shock is the reverse situation in which peripheral sympathetic and adrenal medullary neurons are firing rapidly. Conley and coworkers (78) produced hemorrhagic shock in rats and found that intra-arterial tyrosine administration significantly increased blood

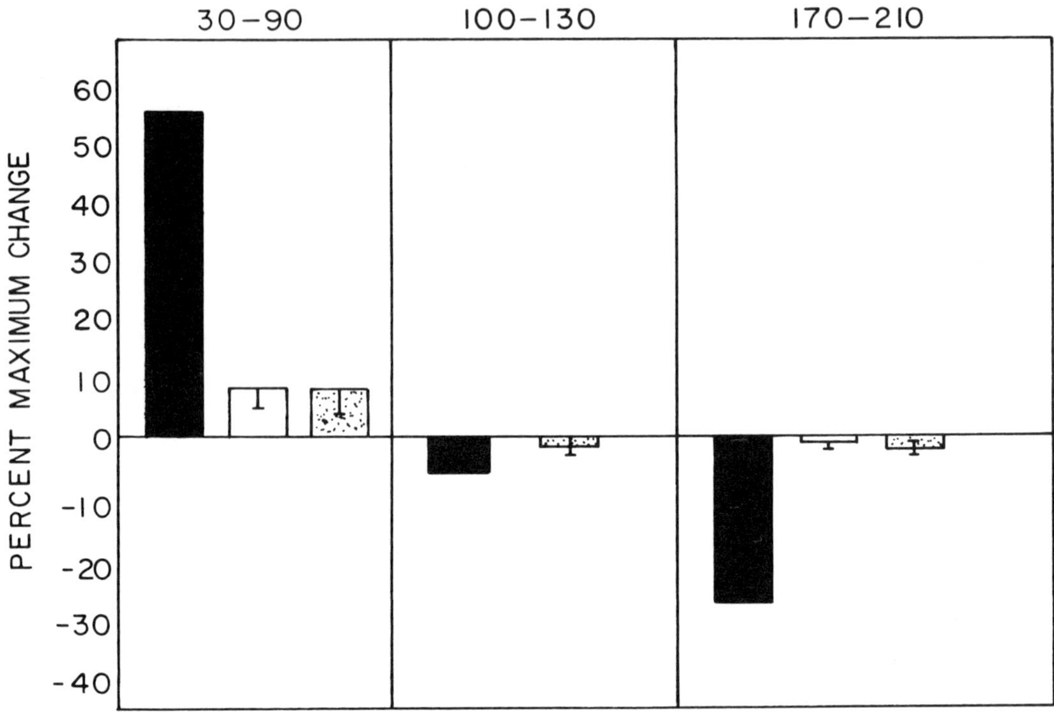

Figure 2. The effect of tyrosine on blood pressure is shown in hypotensive, normotensive, and hypertensive rats. The range of the initial blood pressures is indicated at the *top* of each panel. Rats were injected with 100 mg/kg of tyrosine *(black bars)*, 100 mg/kg of valine *(white bars)*, and saline *(stippled bars)*. Blood pressure was measured 15 minutes *(first panel)* and 2 hours *(second and third panels)* later. Results are expressed as percent change in blood pressure. Tyrosine significantly increased blood pressure in hypotensive rats *(first panel)*; had no effect on normotensive rats *(second panel)*; and decreased blood pressure in spontaneously hypertensive rats [*third panel*] (74, 78).

pressure. No clinical studies have been published in which tyrosine has been tested either in hypertension or shock.

Tyrosine has other centrally-mediated cardiovascular effects that are distinct from those on blood pressure. Scott and coworkers (79) studied ventricular arrhythmias in intact dogs and reported that tyrosine administration significantly increased the electrical stimulus necessary to induce ventricular fibrillation. Coadministration of valine to impede tyrosine's entry into the brain antagonized this effect. These data suggest that tyrosine administration may be useful in treating a variety of cardiac arrhythmias, including those which occur after myocardial infarction. This new potential use of tyrosine awaits clinical application.

CLINICAL USES OF TYROSINE

Clinical studies with tyrosine have just begun. There are published reports regarding the effects of tyrosine on plasma tyrosine levels in normal subjects and preliminary reports regarding the use of tyrosine in patients with Parkinson's disease and in patients with depression.

Glaeser and coworkers (80) studied plasma tyrosine responses to a single dose of 100 mg/kg or 150 mg/kg of tyrosine in 12 healthy young subjects. Plasma tyrosine levels increased within 1 hour and remained significantly elevated for 6 hours; there was a two- to threefold increase in the plasma tyrosine ratio and a similar increase in catecholamines and their metabolites excreted in the urine (81). In a separate study, Melamed and co-workers (82) gave a 113 g/day high protein diet to 11 normal subjects and measured plasma tyrosine and neutral amino acid levels on separate days before and during ingestion of 100 mg/kg/day of tyrosine (Fig. 3). They found that tyrosine administration significantly increased the tyrosine ratio, although the rise was slightly less than that obtained in the fasting state due to the diet-induced increase in the plasma levels of the competing neutral amino acids. Tyrosine administration increased urinary catecholamine excretion of dopamine, norepinephrine, and epinephrine in these same subjects (83). These studies

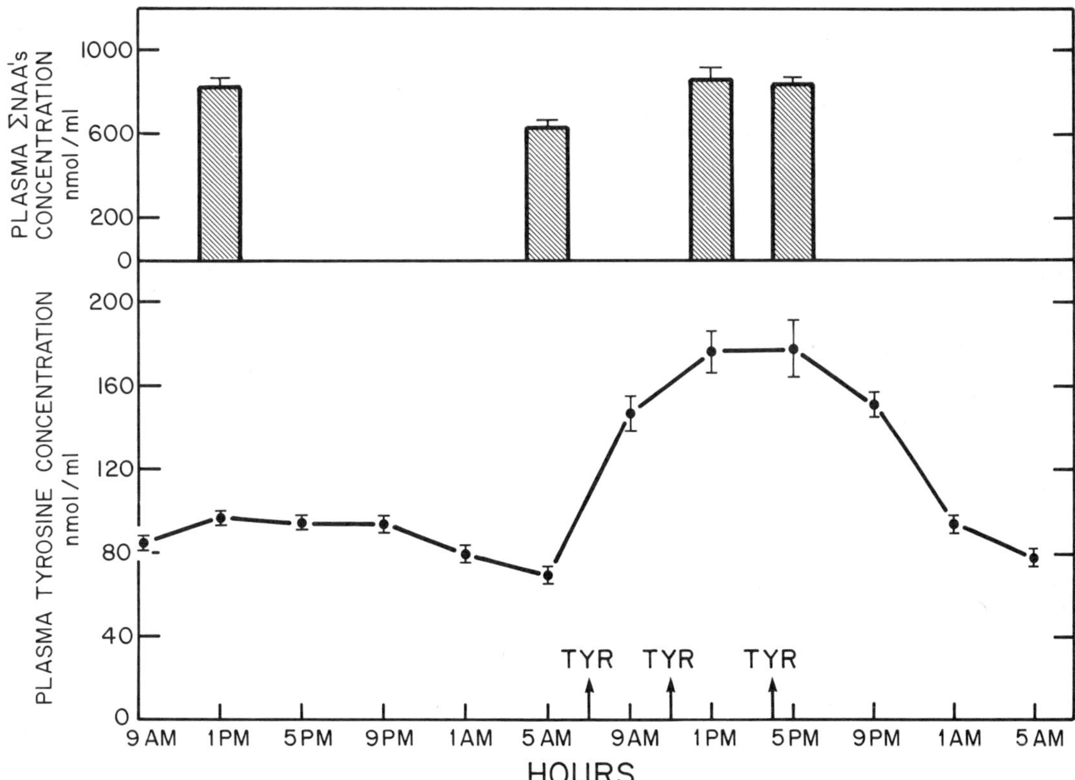

Figure 3. Plasma tyrosine and neutral amino acid levels are shown in fed subjects during tyrosine administration. Diurnal variations in plasma tyrosine levels *(lower part)* and in the sums of the plasma concentrations of the large neutral amino acids valine, leucine, isoleucine, methionine, phenylalanine, and tryptophan *(upper part)* in 11 normal human subjects ingesting protein-containing meals alone (day 1 of the study) or with tyrosine supplementation (day 2 of the study). Identical meals, each containing 38 g of protein, were consumed at 8 AM, 12 noon, and 5 PM on the 2 consecutive days of the study. On day 2, tyrosine was administered orally 1 hour before each meal at a dose of 33 mg/kg body weight. All amino acid levels are expressed in nmols/ml, and the vertical bars represent standard errors of the mean (82).

indicated that pharmacological doses of tyrosine were well tolerated in human subjects, significantly increased the plasma tyrosine ratio, and could be tested as a treatment for disease in which physicians wish to increase catecholaminergic neurotransmission.

Parkinson's Disease

Parkinson's disease is a degenerative neurological disorder characterized by rigidity, tremor, bradykinesia, and postural instability. Most of the signs and symptoms of parkinsonism are believed to result from decreased dopaminergic transmission in the nigrostriatal pathway (84). Levodopa, alone or in combination with a peripheral decarboxylase inhibitor (Sinemet), increases dopamine levels in the striatum and produces clinical improvement in about 75% of patients with Parkinson's disease. It remains the most effective treatment for Parkinson's disease. Levodopa is converted to dopamine within the striatum, but it is also converted to dopamine in sites that ordinarily do not synthesize catecholamines, including glia, blood vessels, and serotonergic neurons (85). The widespread increase in dopamine levels throughout the brain may account for some of the side effects that occur during levodopa administration. In theory, tyrosine should be a more specific anti-parkinsonian therapy, since it is converted to dopamine only in those neurons that normally synthesize the neurotransmitter. To test this hypothesis, Growdon and Melamed (86) measured tyrosine and HVA levels in the CSF of 8 patients with Parkinson's disease before and during 100 mg/kg/day of tyrosine. Tyrosine administration doubled CSF tyrosine levels and significantly increased HVA levels in 7 of 8 patients. These observations indicate that tyrosine administration increased dopamine turnover in patients with Parkinson's disease just as it did in experimental animals with lesions in the nigrostriatal pathway (70). In a separate clinical study, Growdon (87) gave 100 mg/kg/day of tyrosine in three equally divided doses to a group of 33 patients that included all stages of Parkinson's disease. He found that tyrosine administration improved 10 of the mildly affected patients; rigidity, bradykinesia, and handwriting improved most, but tremor was generally unaffected. Tyrosine administration did not improve patients with more advanced stages of parkinsonism. This preliminary study is consistent with previous reports (88, 89) and suggests that tyrosine should be tested further as an alternate treatment to levodopa or Sinemet in patients with early or mild stages of Parkinson's disease.

Depression

The catecholamine theory of depression (90) postulated that there was decreased noradrenergic transmission in brains of patients with endogenous depression. Levels of norepinephrine are normal (30) but MHPG levels are decreased (91) in brains of depressed patients. Urinary levels of MHPG are thought to reflect a portion of norepinephrine released in the brain. They are decreased in patients with bipolar depression (92–94) and changes in urinary MHPG levels appear to precede mood swings (95). Patients with bipolar depression also have decreased levels of MHPG in their spinal fluid (96). The data are not as conclusive in patients with unipolar depression in whom there are reports of decreased, normal, or increased MHPG excretion. It is known that urinary MHPG excretion can be influenced by mental stress, anxiety, diet, and drugs (97–99) and that activity can affect CSF levels (100). Some of these factors may explain discrepancies regarding the value of MHPG measurements. In general, patients with low levels of MHPG respond better to antidepressant drugs such as desimipramine (101) or amphetamines (102) than those patients with normal MHPG levels.

Altered tyrosine metabolism in the periphery or decreased tyrosine transport into the brain may occur in some patients with depression (40, 103); the normal fluctuation in plasma tyrosine levels may be reduced in these patients as well (41, 104). Even if these metabolic changes were not primary factors in the genesis of depression, decreases in plasma tyrosine levels or in the plasma tyrosine ratio could aggravate existing defects in norepinephrine neurotransmission. Gelenberg and coworkers (105) gave 100 mg/kg/day of tyrosine in three equally divided doses to a young woman with recurrent depressions according to a double-blind crossover protocol. They found that she improved during tyrosine ingestion and deteriorated during placebo administration on three separate trials. The ability of tyrosine to improve depression was subsequently confirmed by Goldberg (106) who reported significant improvement in 2 patients who had previously responded to amphetamine administration. In a subsequent report, Gibson and Gelenberg (107) found that 3 of 5 patients with unipolar depression improved significantly after 4 weeks of tyrosine administration, whereas only 1 of 4 patients improved during placebo conditions. Clinical improvement was measured by a decrease in the Hamilton depression score and was significantly correlated with the percentage increase in fasting plasma tyrosine levels. Urinary MHPG levels increased in 4 of 5 patients during tyrosine ingestion.

CHOLINE, LECITHIN, AND THE BIOSYNTHESIS OF ACETYLCHOLINE

The following discussion summarizes the evidence currently available indicating that plasma choline levels normally influence the synthesis of acetylcholine in brain neurons. Acetylcholine is synthesized in a reaction catalyzed by the enzyme choline acetyltransferase (CAT) in which a molecule of choline combines with a molecule of acetyl coenzyme

A (Fig. 4). The K_m of choline acetyltransferase for choline (0.4 mM) and the K_m acetyl coenzyme A (18 mM) are both well above the normal brain concentrations of these substances, and changes in the brain level of either of the precursors for acetylcholine might be expected to modify the rate at which the neurotransmitter is synthesized. Acetyl coenzyme A is a product of aerobic glucose metabolism. Acetylcholine synthesis has been shown to decrease with brain hypoxia or hypoglycemia (108, 109), but choline availability is the major determinant for acetylcholine synthesis under normal physiological conditions.

Brain choline used for acetylcholine synthesis derives from at least three sources: a small amount of choline is synthesized de novo in the brain (110, 111), some comes from the breakdown of phosphatidylcholine in membranes (112, 113), and some comes from the bloodstream. Plasma choline levels vary widely and reflect the quantities of choline (chiefly as lecithin) consumed in the diet (114, 115). The transport of choline into the intact brain is mediated by a low affinity transport system similar to but distinct from that described for the amino acids (22). Deanol and lithium act competitively at this locus (116). A high affinity choline uptake system has also been observed in synaptosomes prepared from cholinergic nerve terminals (117, 118); this carrier is sodium-dependent and is blocked by hemicholinium. The high affinity system may affect the distribution of choline within the brain by preferentially shunting it

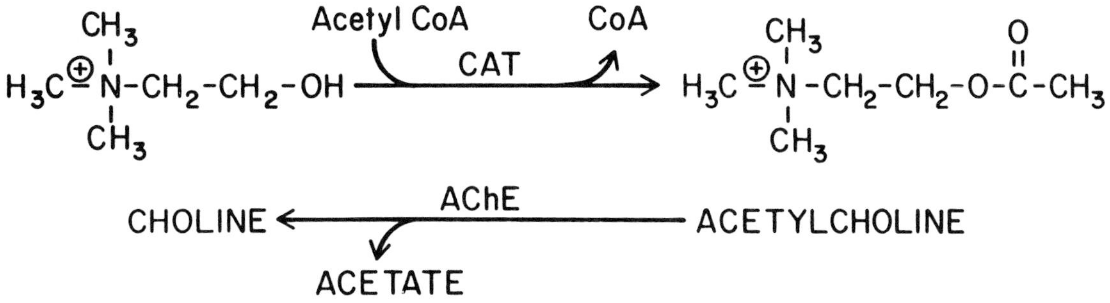

Figure 4. Pictured is acetylcholine biosynthesis. The enzyme choline acetyltransferase (CAT) catalyzes the acetylation of choline, using acetyl coenzyme A as the acetate donor. Acetylcholine is inactivated by the hydrolytic enzyme acetylcholinesterase (AChE); choline may be reutilized for acetylcholine synthesis.

to the locus of acetylcholine synthesis. It also serves to reutilize choline formed from hydrolysis of acetylcholine released into synapses. The K_m of the low affinity system that transports choline into the intact brain is 0.22 mM (22). Since plasma choline levels normally fall below this concentration (119), the uptake system is highly unsaturated, and any significant variation in plasma choline levels should generate corresponding changes in brain choline uptake and ultimately in brain choline levels. When plasma choline levels are low (for example, during a fast), there is a net efflux of choline from brain to blood. When plasma choline levels are high (for example, after a meal containing foods with a high choline content or a therapeutic dose of choline or lecithin), there is a net influx of choline molecules from the bloodstream into the brain.

Cohen and Wurtman (120, 121) and Haubrich and coworkers (122) independently and concurrently reported that choline administration to rats produced sequential increases in plasma choline, brain choline, and brain acetylcholine levels. These findings have been amply confirmed and extended. Choline administration can block atropine-induced decreases in striatal acetylcholine levels (123) and partly restore acetylcholine levels in the caudate nucleus after striatal injections of kainic acid (124). The increase in acetylcholine levels induced by choline administration results from increased de novo synthesis. Cohen and Wurtman (121) gave the acetylcholinesterase inhibitor physostigmine to rats in conjunction with choline. The resulting increase in brain acetylcholine concentration was equal to the sum of either agent alone. This finding suggests that choline acts by stimulating acetylcholine synthesis and not by slowing its degradation. Lecithin, or phosphatidylcholine, is the naturally occurring source of choline; its administration to rats produces similar increments in plasma choline, brain choline, and brain acetylcholine levels (125).

Several experiments have been performed to examine the relationship between precursor-induced increases in acetylcholine levels and the amounts of acetylcholine released into synapses. To determine whether choline-induced increases in neuronal acetylcholine levels accumulated within inactive metabolic pools or were available for release, Ulus and coworkers (126) measured biochemical changes in cells that are postsynaptic to the cholinergic neuron. They found that choline administration induced tyrosine hydroxylase activity and stimulated catecholamine synthesis in rat striata (126) and adrenal medulla (127). The striatal effects were blocked by atropine, a muscarinic antagonist, and the adrenal effects were blocked by prior transection of the cholinergic splanchnic nerve to the adrenal medulla. They also found that the effects of choline administration on the adrenal medullary response were heightened when the splanchnic nerve was caused to fire rapidly (128). These data indicate that increased levels of acetylcholine induced by choline can result in an increased flow of information across cholinergic synapses. Bierkamper and Goldberg (129) studied the relationship between choline availability and acetylcholine release in an isolated rat vagus nerve-diaphragm preparation. They measured the amount of acetylcholine released as a function of various choline concentrations and found that increasing choline concentrations had a slight effect on the release of acetylcholine when the nerve was in a resting state but had a major influence on the amount of acetylcholine released when the nerve was electrically stimulated. Jenden and coworkers (130, 131) reported similar results in profused cortical rat brain slices incubated with various concentrations of choline. They found that increasing the rate of neuronal firing by increasing potassium concentrations in the medium dramatically increased choline's influence on acetylcholine release. Physiological experiments also indicate that increased choline availability can produce increased acetylcholine release. Löeffelholz and coworkers (132) found that choline administration increased cholinergic transmission in the vagus nerve to the chicken heart. In clinical observations, Gelenberg and coworkers (133) detected parkinsonian signs of bradykinesia, rigidity, and tremor in some patients with tardive dyskinesia who were being treated with choline or lecithin. These biochemical, physiological, and clinical observations all indicate that choline administration can increase the synthesis and release of acetylcholine molecules. Choline itself may act as a direct acetylcholine agonist in some brain regions and has been reported to be one-tenth as potent as acetylcholine (134).

Clinical investigators have begun to study choline and lecithin metabolism in humans. Plasma choline levels derive from two sources: choline synthesized in the liver by the stepwise methylation of ethanolamines (135, 136) and choline that is obtained from dietary sources. Most foods contain very little free choline but larger amounts of lecithin, which

is the naturally occurring dietary source of choline. Plasma choline levels vary in accordance with the choline content of the most recently ingested meal. Plasma choline levels do not increase in subjects who fast or who consume diets that contain very little choline (114, 115). Diets that contain larger amounts of choline produce small increases in plasma choline levels but ingestion of purified phosphatidylcholine is much more effective (Fig. 5). Lecithin administration increases plasma choline levels in humans more effectively than choline salts. Wurtman and coworkers (137) gave equimolar doses of choline as choline chloride or lecithin to 10

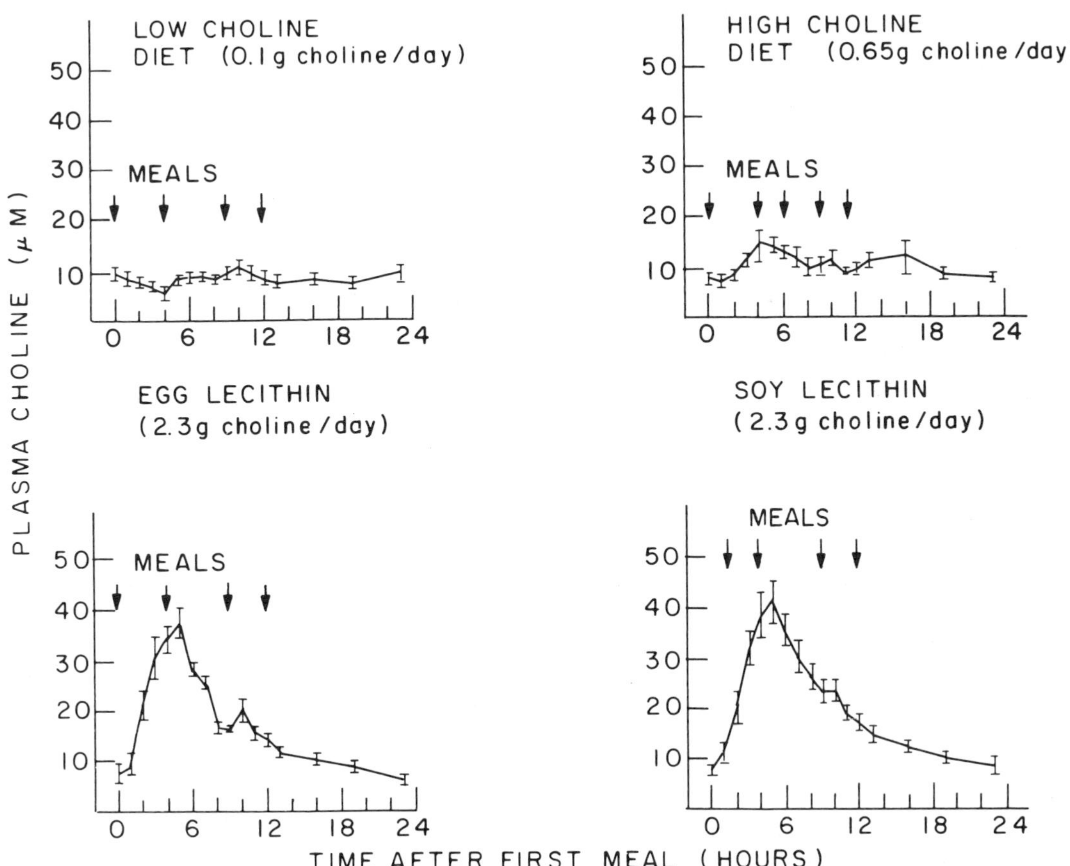

Figure 5. Pictured is plasma choline response to ingested choline and lecithin in which 6 adult human subjects ingested each of four diets (common foods high in choline, common foods low in choline, low-choline diet plus breakfast supplement of 25 g 80% pure egg lecithin, and low-choline diet plus breakfast supplement of 25 g 80% pure soy lecithin). Plasma samples were obtained at regular intervals and assayed for choline. Meal times are indicated by *arrows*. Data are expressed as mean ± SD (115).

healthy subjects and measured plasma choline levels. Lecithin administration produced higher and more prolonged increases in plasma choline levels than choline chloride.

Choline salts are readily available and were initially used in clinical drug trials; they imparted a bitter taste to food and produced a fishy aroma in the breath, sweat, and urine. Lecithin has largely supplanted choline as the favored acetylcholine precursor since it elevates plasma choline levels more efficiently and does not impart a fishy odor. A quirk in the United States Codex defines lecithin as any compound that contains a mixture of phospholipids, but to chemists and physicians, lecithin refers to the specific phospholipid, phosphatidylcholine. Commercial lecithin that is used to emulsify foods and that is sold in health food stores may contain as little as 10% phosphatidylcholine; the other 90% is never identified. Most investigators therefore prefer to use highly purified phosphatidylcholine with a fully analyzed chemical content (138). This reduces the volume and caloric load imposed by lecithin administration and also minimizes potential side effects from other impurities. Unfortunately, highly purified phosphatidylcholine is expensive, and current supplies are limited.

CLINICAL USES OF CHOLINE AND LECITHIN

Tardive Dyskinesia

Tardive dyskinesia is a hyperkinetic choreic movement disorder characterized by buccal-lingual-masticatory facial movements; the extremities and trunk may be involved as well (139). It usually occurs in susceptible patients who have taken large doses of antipsychotic medications for 6 months or longer (140). The results of pharmacological testing indicate that tardive dyskinesia results from an imbalance in the postulated reciprocal relationship between dopamine and acetylcholine in the basal ganglia (141–143). Thus, drugs that block catecholamine synthesis, deplete monoamine stores, or that antagonize dopamine's actions on synaptic receptors often suppress tardive dyskinesia whereas drugs that increase dopaminergic transmission

usually exacerbate these movements (144). Drugs that alter cholinergic transmission also affect tardive dyskinesia. Physostigmine, given to increase the amount of acetylcholine within brain synapses, suppresses tardive dyskinesia, and anticholinergics, such as scopolomine, exacerbate it (145, 146). Despite these leads, a standard effective treatment for tardive dyskinesia is still lacking. Drugs that diminish catecholaminergic tone cause unwanted side effects, and oral cholinomimetic drugs are not available for general use.

The discovery that choline administration increased brain acetylcholine levels in rats made it possible for the first time to test the long-term effects of cholinergic stimulation in patients with tardive dyskinesia. Shortly after the initial report that choline admininstration to rats increased brain acetylcholine levels, Davis and coworkers (147) reported that 16 g/day of choline chloride suppressed the facial movements in a single patient with tardive dyskinesia. These authors subsequently reported that oral doses of 16–20 g/day of choline chloride suppressed tardive dyskinesia in 4 patients treated according to a placebo-controlled protocol (148). Numerous studies have confirmed these initial reports (Table 1). Tamminga and coworkers (149) gave choline chloride to 4 patients; 2 patients improved and 2 could not take adequate doses of choline due to intercurrent depression. Growdon and coworkers (150) reported a large clinical trial in which 20 patients with permanent tardive dyskinesia took 8–20 g/day of choline chloride for 2 weeks according to a double-blind crossover protocol. Choline administration significantly increased plasma choline levels in all patients and suppressed tardive dyskinesia in 9 of 20 patients. Placebo administration did not alter plasma choline levels nor improve any patient. Subsequent single-blind studies confirmed choline's efficacy in treating tardive dyskinesia. Barbeau (151) reported that 10 g/day of choline chloride suppressed tardive dyskinesia in 1 of 2 patients, and Yahr (152) also stated that choline suppressed tardive dyskinesia, whereas it was ineffective in other hyperkinetic disorders such as Huntington's disease.

Table 1. Effect of Choline and Lecithin Administration on Tardive Dyskinesia: A Summary of 10 Studies

Investigators	Treatment	Patients Improved/Patients Treated
Davis and coworkers (147)	Choline	1/1
Davis and coworkers (148)*	Choline	4/4
Tamminga and coworkers (149)	Choline	2/4
Growdon and coworkers (150)*	Choline	9/20
Barbeau (151)	Choline	1/2
Growdon and coworkers (153)	Lecithin	3/3
Gelenberg and coworkers (154)	Choline, Lecithin	5/5
Barbeau (155)	Lecithin	4/4
Jackson and coworkers (156)*	Lecithin	6/6
Branchey and coworkers (157)*	Lecithin	4/7†

*Double-blind or placebo controlled.
†The number of tardive dyskinesia movements counted decreased substantially in 4/7.

Recent studies have explored the use of lecithin in tardive dyskinesia. Growdon and coworkers (153) found that lecithin administration increased plasma choline levels and suppressed tardive dyskinesia in 3 of 3 patients. Gelenberg and coworkers (154) compared sequentially the effects of choline chloride and lecithin in 5 patients with tardive dyskinesia. Both lecithin and choline significantly increased plasma choline levels and improved abnormal movements in all 5 patients. In another single-blind study, Barbeau (155) gave lecithin to 4 patients with tardive dyskinesia and reported a mean of 52% improvement in their movements. Jackson and coworkers (156) conducted a double-blind crossover study of lecithin administration to 6 patients with tardive dyskinesia. They contrasted the effects of 50 g of 60% phosphatidylcholine content to a placebo and reported significant improvement in all 6 patients during lecithin treatment. Branchey and coworkers (157) apparently failed to demonstrate a beneficial effect of lecithin administration on tardive dyskinesia. They rated the patient's clinical response to lecithin by the AIM and Simpson dyskinesia rating scales; they also counted choreic movements. They reported that lecithin administration did not significantly affect the rating scale scores. Their own observations, however, indicated that there was a major reduction in mean frequency counts of abnormal movements in 4 of 7 patients during treatment with lecithin.

Their study differed from previously published studies in several important ways. Branchey and coworkers used lecithin derived from egg, whereas other investigators used lecithin derived from soya. Egg lecithin contains predominantly saturated fatty acids whereas soya lecithin contains a high percent of unsaturated fatty acids. Although egg and soya lecithins produce comparable increases in plasma choline levels (115), their effects on brain choline levels, prostaglandin synthesis, and neuronal membrane composition are probably different. Branchey and coworkers gave a single dose of lecithin and did not measure plasma choline levels to determine the adequacy of this dose or its presumed duration of action. Most other investigators gave multiple daily doses of lecithin and also measured plasma choline levels. Thus, the bulk of published evidence to date indicates that choline or lecithin administration suppresses choreic movements in many patients with tardive dyskinesia. Additional careful double-blind studies are necessary to establish conclusively the optimal dose and composition of lecithin for treating tardive dyskinesia.

Huntington's Disease

Huntington's disease is another choreic movement disorder in which acetylcholine transmission is reduced (84). Clinically, Huntington's disease is characterized by memory loss, personality changes, involuntary muscular contractions (chorea), and postural instability. Many of these features result from pathological changes in the basal ganglia. The small Golgi type II interneurons in the caudate nucleus are especially affected, and CAT activity (a marker for cholinergic neurons) is greatly reduced. These observations suggested that central cholinergic tone may be deficient in Huntington's disease and stimulated clinical investigators to devise rational replacement therapies. Davis and coworkers (148) reported that 12–20 g/day of choline chloride suppressed choreic movements in 2 of 4 patients with Huntington's disease. Growdon and coworkers (158) treated 10 Huntington's patients with 8–20 g/day of choline chloride. Choline administration significantly increased plasma choline and CSF choline levels but did not produce lasting benefit in any patient. The number of choreic movements actually increased in 2 patients during choline administration but reverted to pretreatment ranges once the choline was discontinued. Aquilonius and Eckernas (159) gave choline chloride to 5 patients. They reported minor changes in chorea during choline ingestion but concluded that choline did not significantly suppress these movements.

The failure of choline administration to suppress chorea in the majority of patients with Huntington's disease stands in contrast to its success in tardive dyskinesia, but it is unlikely that this difference is due to inadequate acetylcholine synthesis. In a proposed animal model of Huntington's disease, systemic administration of choline significantly increased acetylcholine levels in striata previously injected with kainic acid (124). The ineffectiveness of choline in Huntington's disease probably results from more widespread neuronal damage than occurs in tardive dyskinesia, since local circuit neurons within the basal ganglia that contain glutamic acid decarboxylase, substance P, enkephalin, and angiotensin converting enzyme are also damaged (160–163). Furthermore, the number of postsynaptic cholinergic muscarinic receptor sites in the basal ganglia is reduced (164) so that acetylcholine, even if it

were formed and released in increased amounts, would not restore neurotransmission.

Gilles de la Tourette Syndrome

Tourette syndrome is another hyperkinetic movement disorder in which choline and lecithin have been tested; clinical results are still inconclusive, and haloperidol remains the treatment of choice (84). Evidence for a cholinergic deficit stems from observations, such as that made by Stahl and Berger (165), that physostigmine administration can suppress tics. Barbeau (155) initially reported that 33 g/day of 20% phosphatidylcholine did not suppress tics in 2 of 2 patients but later found that 40–50 g/day of 20% phosphatidylcholine produced lasting benefit in 3 other patients (166). Polinsky and coworkers (167), however could not confirm these results. They gave 45 g/day of 55% phosphatidylcholine for 4 weeks to 6 patients with Tourette syndrome according to a double-blind crossover protocol and found no improvement. Hanin and coworkers (168) reported that red blood cell choline levels were significantly elevated in patients with Tourette syndrome, but the clinical significance of this observation remains unclear. Perhaps red cell choline determinations might provide a biochemical basis for deciding which patient might respond to choline or lecithin treatment.

Alzheimer's Disease

Alzheimer's disease is a degenerative neurological disorder characterized by progressive memory loss. Aphasias, apraxias, and difficulties with visual-spatial orientation also occur. The experimental use of choline and lecithin in Alzheimer's disease rests on three independent observations. (1) Neurochemical analyses of brain tissue obtained from brain biopsy or at postmortem examination indicate that there is a selective decrease in CAT activity (169–173) with preserved muscarinic binding (171, 174). The distribution of CAT activity probably indicates a presynaptic cholinergic lesion that limits acetylcholine synthesis and release. In contrast to Huntington's disease, postsynaptic muscarinic receptors are preserved in Alzheimer's disease (171, 174), and it is likely that attempts to increase acetylcholine neuro-transmission might modify some clinical aspects of Alzheimer's disease to the extent that cholinergic neurons are involved in its pathophysiology. (2) Pharmacological tests with drugs that affect acetylcholine transmission alter memory in nondemented subjects. Drugs that block acetylcholine receptors, such as scopolamine, induce memory deficits in healthy young subjects similar to those seen in elderly subjects who are not demented (175), whereas these deficits can be reversed by administering physostigmine, a cholinergic agonist that potentiates synaptic effects of acetylcholine (176). Other studies indicate that cholinergic agonists such as physostigmine (177), arecoline (178), and choline (179) can improve some aspects of learning and memory in normal subjects. Comparable experiments in animals have replicated these basic clinical observations (180, 181) and strengthen the cholinergic hypothesis of memory loss. (3) Biochemical studies indicate that choline or lecithin administration increases plasma choline, brain choline, and brain acetylcholine levels in rats (120, 121, 125) and increases plasma choline and CSF choline levels in humans with Alzheimer's disease (182).

There are 11 published studies that report the effects of choline or lecithin administration on selected cognitive tasks used to assess behavior in demented patients (Table 2). Most investigators studied memory, since loss of recent memory is often the initial and chief clinical symptom of Alzheimer's disease. The results of choline administration are mixed, although a few patients apparently did improve. Boyd and coworkers (183) initially reported that 5 g/day of choline chloride for 2 weeks and then 10 g/day for the next 2 weeks did not improve memory in 7 severely demented patients, although they were described as being less irritable. The authors speculated that patients with less severe dementia would be better candidates for choline treatment, and most subsequent studies have been conducted in patients with mild to moderate degrees of dementia.

Etienne and coworkers (184) reported that 8 g/day of choline bitartrate improved performance on the Wexler block design subtest in the 3 least demented of 5 patients with Alzheimer's disease. Signoret and coworkers (185) treated 8 patients with mild to moderate Alzheimer's disease with 9 g/day of choline citrate and found that recall was improved in 3 of 8 patients; there was also an improvement in everyday memory. Smith and coworkers (186) administered 9 g/day of choline bitartrate to 10 patients with Alzheimer's disease but did not detect any improvement on test results; however 3 of 10 patients seemed less confused during treatment. Christie and coworkers (182) treated 12 mild to moderately impaired Alzheimer patients sequentially with choline and lecithin. Neither treatment improved memory, although 2 of 10 had less apraxia; speech and understanding improved in 3 of 10. Fovall and coworkers (187) gave 8–16 g/day of choline bitartrate to 5 patients with mild to moderate Alzheimer's disease and reported improved word recognition. These same authors were unable to replicate this finding in a second larger study (188). Several other studies failed to detect any benefit from choline chloride. Ferris and coworkers (189) gave 12–20 g/day of choline chloride to 14 patients with mild to moderate Alzheimer's disease and were unable to detect any improvement in behavior or in test scores. Renvoize and Jerram (190) gave 15 g/day of choline chloride to 18 moderately severe Alzheimer's patients according to a double-blind crossover protocol and did not detect any improvement.

Although there have been a few reports that lecithin improved some test variables (191, 192), most investigators have failed to detect a convincing or reproducible benefit from treatment. Etienne and coworkers (192) initially reported that 75 g/day of 20% phosphatidylcholine improved paired associate learning in 3 of 7 patients with Alzheimer's disease but could not confirm this finding in a more recent larger study (188). Sullivan and coworkers (193) treated 18 patients with mild to moderate Alzheimer's disease with 20–40 g/day of 80% phosphatidylcholine according

Table 2. Choline or Lecithin Treatment in Alzheimer's Disease: A Summary of 11 Studies

Author	Number of Patients	Severity	Treatment	Test Results	Clinical Observations
Boyd and coworkers (183)	7	Severe	Choline chloride, 10 g/day	No improvement	Less irritable
Etienne and coworkers (184)*	3	Moderate	Choline bitartrate, 8 g/day	1/3 improved block design	No improvement
Smith and coworkers (186)*	10	. . .	Choline bitartrate, 9 g/day	No improvement	3/10 less confused
Signoret and coworkers (185)	8	Mild-moderate	Choline citrate, 9 g/day	3/8 improved recall	Everyday memory improved
Etienne and coworkers (192)	7	Mild-moderate	Lecithin 20% PC, 75 g/day	3/7 improved paired associate learning	More cooperative; improved understanding of instructions
Christie and coworkers (182)	10	Mild-moderate	Choline chloride, 5 g/day Lecithin 20% PC, 28–100 g/day	2/10 less apraxia	3/10 improved speech and understanding
Renvoize and Jerram (190)*	18	Moderate	Choline chloride, 15 g/day	No improvement	No improvement
Ferris and coworkers (189)	14	Mild-moderate	Choline chloride, 12–20 g/day	No improvement	No improvement
Fovall and coworkers (187)*	5	Mild-moderate	Choline bitartrate, 8–16 g/day	Improved word recognition	. . .
Hu and coworkers (191)*	11	Mild-severe	Lecithin 53% PC, 35 g/day	7/11 improved verbal recall	. . .
Sullivan and coworkers (193)*	18	Mild-moderate	Lecithin 80% PC, 20–40 g/day	No improvement	4/18 improved alertness and cooperation

*Double-blind or placebo controlled.

to a double-blind crossover protocol. They found that lecithin administration reliably increased plasma choline levels but did not significantly improve memory in any patient.

Several serious problems confront investigators who conduct drug trials with lecithin in patients with Alzheimer's disease. There is no method available (aside from brain biopsy) to distinguish patients with a predominant cholinergic deficit from those who may have lesions in neurons that synthesize other transmitters (194). Neurochemical heterogeneity is likely in Alzheimer's disease, and cholinergic precursors would not be expected to improve memory in patients, for example, whose dementia resulted from deficient central serotonergic tone. Secondly, there is no consensus regarding the extent to which objective measures of memory predict functionally significant changes in the patient's activities of daily living. Finally, the high cost, difficulty in preparation, and general unavailability of highly purified phosphatidylcholine have precluded its widespread use in clinical investigations. Currently available data indicate that short-term lecithin administration alone does not restore deficits in memory (188, 195). There are as yet no published studies that tested the ability of lecithin administered for 6–12 months to retard the progression of Alzheimer's disease. Lecithin administration in conjunction with other cholinergic drugs, such as physostigmine (196) or piracetam (197) may be more effective than either treatment alone and will certainly be tested further.

Ataxia

The report that physostigmine administration produced benefit in some patients with Friedreich's ataxia (198) stimulated investigators to test acetylcholine precursors in this disease. The suggestion (199) that there was a defect in pyruvate dehydrogenase complex and therefore diminished acetylcholine synthesis in patients with Friedreich's ataxia provided additional rationale for precursor therapy. The studies published to date report conflicting results, and the use of choline or lecithin in ataxic states remains inconclusive. Barbeau gave choline (151) or lecithin (155) to patients with Friedreich's ataxia and patients with spastic spinocerebellar degeneration of the Pierre-Marie type. He reported that 30 g/day of 20% phosphatidylcholine improved performance scores by a mean of 35% in 10 patients with Friedreich's ataxia and seemed to slow the progression of symptoms. Choline administration was also effective. Neither choline nor lecithin improved the 6 patients with spastic ataxia. Several other case reports indicated improvement with choline chloride (200, 201). In contrast to these reports, Lawrence and coworkers (202) conducted a placebo-controlled study of choline administration to 13 patients with a variety of ataxic diseases and found that choline administration significantly improved mobility and hand movement in only 1. Philcox and Kies (203) reported that 4 g/day of choline chloride did not improve familial ataxia in 5 South African patients. Reding and coworkers (204) treated 1 patient with spinal ataxia and 1 patient with cerebellar ataxia with 20 g/day of lecithin according to a double-blind crossover protocol and reported that neither patient improved. Chamberlain and coworkers (205) treated 4 Friedreich's patients with 50–100 g/day of 22% phosphatidylcholine. Plasma choline levels rose in all 4, but none experienced clinical improvement. Pentland and coworkers (206) treated 12 patients with Friedreich's ataxia with 25 g/day of 96% phosphatidylcholine according to a double-blind crossover protocol. Individual responses varied, but no patient showed any consistent improvement during treatment.

Myasthenia Gravis

Pharmacological doses of choline and lecithin have not been tested in myasthenia gravis. It is known that plasma choline levels are normal in patients with this disorder (207). There is a single report of choline administration to a patient with the myasthenic syndrome, in whom 120 mg/kg/day of choline chloride produced significant improvement in neuromuscular transmission (208). Electrophysiological studies conducted during oral choline administration indicated a significant increase in muscle contraction after nerve stimulation, and the authors estimated that this was consistent with a 40% increase in acetylcholine release. Further studies are necessary to establish choline's place in the treatment of myasthenia gravis or myasthenic syndrome.

Epilepsy

There is a single report on choline administration to patients with epilepsy. McNamara and coworkers (209) gave 12–16 g/day of choline chloride to 4 patients with complex partial seizures and reported that plasma choline levels increased in 3 of 4 during choline ingestion. These same 3 patients improved during treatment. There was a slight increase in seizure frequency, but the attacks were briefer and caused less post-seizure fatigue. These preliminary results require further confirmation before choline can be accepted as an anticonvulsant drug.

Parkinson's Disease

Many symptoms of Parkinson's disease are believed to result from inadequate dopaminergic transmission and a relative preponderance of cholinergic tone. Choline administration is therefore counterintuitive since it might be expected to exacerbate the motor symptoms of Parkinson's disease. At the present time, choline is being tested in two specific clinical situations: attempts to suppress levodopa-induced dyskinesias and attempts to reduce emergent symptoms of dementia.

Papavasiliou and Rosal (210) gave 200–300 mg/kg/day of choline chloride to 8 patients with levodopa-induced dyskinesias according to a double-blind protocol. They found that choline administration significantly decreased dyskinesia in 2 of 8 patients but that both patients experienced increased bradykinesia and rigidity. Choline administration worsened parkinsonian symptoms in 1 additional patient and had no effect in the other 5. Barbeau (155) gave 20 g/day of 20% phosphatidylcholine to 10 parkinsonian patients with levodopa-induced dyskinesias and obtained similar results. Although lecithin administration decreased the number of involuntary movements, it also produced deterioration in motor performance.

The use of lecithin to treat dementia in patients with Parkinson's disease is based on similarities with Alzheimer's dementia. In a preliminary study, Garcia and coworkers (211) gave 30 g/day of 25% phosphatidylcholine to 8 patients with Parkinson's disease and reported that they improved on six of eight cognitive tests. There was also significant improvement on a memory test. Eight additional parkinsonian patients received a lecithin placebo. They improved on only one of the eight cognitive tests. Further studies are necessary to confirm the utility of this mode of therapy for dementia in Parkinson's disease.

PSYCHIATRIC DISORDERS

Choline administration has been reported to induce depression in psychiatric patients (149). This observation prompted speculation that choline or lecithin may be used to treat mania. The well-described ability of intravenously administered physostigmine to reduce acute manic symptoms further supported this hypothesis (38). In addition, lithium apparently potentiates the effects of choline administration (212). Lithium competes with choline for transport in red blood cells (213) and also across the blood-brain barrier. The effects of lithium are apparently greater on efflux of choline than in influx (214). These data suggested that a combination of lecithin plus lithium might be a more effective way to treat mania than either drug alone. The preliminary results of Cohen and coworkers (215) tend to support this hypothesis. They gave 15 and 30 g of 90% phosphatidylcholine to 4 patients with acute manic symptoms. In addition to lecithin, 2 patients received lithium, and the other 2 received both lithium and a neuroleptic drug. All 4 patients improved; manic symptoms reappeared in 3 of 4 after lecithin was discontinued.

There is some evidence to suggest that deficient cholinergic transmission may contribute to schizophrenia (216, 217). Davis (218) treated 9 schizophrenic patients with up to 20 g/day of choline chloride but found no improvement.

SUMMARY

The use of naturally-occurring dietary constituents that are precursors for neurotransmitter synthesis constitutes a new mode of drug therapy for brain diseases in which there are specific neurotransmitter abnormalities. All neurotransmitters do not exhibit precursor control, but the best studied and clinically most important ones do, including serotonin, the catecholamines, and acetylcholine. Neurotransmitters that are influenced by precursor availability share certain common features: plasma levels of tryptophan, tyrosine, and choline vary in relation to the amounts ingested; the brain cannot make adequate quantities of the precursor and relies on its uptake from the blood stream by an unsaturated transport system; and the precursor is converted to the transmitter product by an enzyme that is unsaturated with its substrate. In each instance, administering pharmacological amounts of a precursor will increase its plasma level, facilitate its entry into the brain, and increase its availability for conversion to the parent neurotransmitter. The demonstration in animals that precursor administration increased the rates at which certain neurons synthesized their neurotransmitter led to their use in the experimental clinical studies reviewed in this chapter. It is likely that tryptophan, tyrosine, and choline will continue to be tested in clinical conditions in which physicians wish to increase serotonergic, catecholaminergic, or cholinergic transmission.

The therapeutic use of dietary constituents that are precursors for neurotransmitters has several advantages over currently available synthetic drugs. Tryptophan, tyrosine, and choline are naturally occurring substances that normally circulate in the blood; the body already has a capacity to metabolize them. Furthermore, they are water-soluble compounds, and toxic levels are therefore unlikely to accumulate in body tissues. Precursor administration increases synthesis only in those neurons that normally convert the precursor to its neurotransmitter product. Other forms of precursor therapy lack this specificity. For example, L-dopa is converted to dopamine throughout the brain in sites that do not ordinarily synthesize or release dopamine, whereas tyrosine is converted to dopamine only in those neurons that contain tyrosine hydroxylase and that normally synthesize catecholamines. Finally, precursor administration permits a selectivity and lack of side effects that few synthetic drugs can match. Neurons that synthesize serotonin, the catecholamines, and acetylcholine are most sensitive to precursor availability when they are firing rapidly. This may occur for example as a result of neuronal destruction (e.g., a degenerative process such as Parkinson's disease or Alzheimer's disease), during attempts to compensate for a primary remote neuronal dysfunction (e.g., spontaneous hypertension), or as a result of previous drug administration (e.g., neuroleptic-induced tardive dyskinesia). Precursor administration would be expected to increase neurotransmission primarily at the affected synapses and would have relatively little effect on uninvolved normally discharging neurons. Synthetic drugs designed as neurotransmitter agonists lack this presynaptic selectivity and increase transmission at all synapses regardless of need.

REFERENCES

1. Growdon JH, Cohen EL, Wurtman RJ: Treatment of brain disease with dietary precursors of neurotransmitters. *Ann Intern Med* 86:337–339, 1977

2. Growdon JH: Neurotransmitters in the diet: their use in the treatment of brain disorders. In *Nutrition and the Brain,* vol 3. Edited by Wurtman RJ, Wurtman JJ. New York, Raven Press, 1979, pp 117–181

3. Joh TH, Shikimi T, Pickel VM, et al: Brain tryptophan hydroxylase: purification of, production of antibodies to, and cellular and ultrastructural localization in serotonergic neurons of rat midbrain. *Proc Natl Acad Sci USA* 72:3575–3579, 1975

4. Tong JH, Kaufman S: Tryptophan hydroxylase purification and some properties of the enzyme from rabbit hindbrain. *J Biol Chem* 250:4152–4158, 1975

5. Friedman PA, Kappelman AJ, Kaufman S: Partial purification and characterization of tryptophan hydroxylase from rabbit hindbrain. *J Biol Chem* 247:4165–4173, 1972

6. Katz, IR: Interaction between the oxygen and tryptophan dependence of synaptosomal tryptophan hydroxylase. *J Neurochem* 37:447–451, 1981

7. Davis JN, Carlsson A, MacMillan V, et al: Brain tryptophan hydroxylation: dependence on arterial oxygen tension. *Science* 182:72–74, 1973

8. Lovenberg W, Weissbach H, Udenfriend S: Aromatic l-amino acid decarboxylase. *J Biol Chem* 237:89–93, 1962

9. McMenamy RH, Oncley JL: The specific binding of L-tryptophan to serum albumin. *J Biol Chem* 233:1436–1447, 1958

10. Fernstrom JD, Wurtman RJ: Brain serotonin content: physiological regulation by plasma neutral amino acids. *Science* 178:414–416, 1972

11. Fernstrom JD, Faller DV: Neutral amino acids in the brain: changes in response to food ingestion. *J Neurochem* 30:1531–1538, 1978

12. Wurtman RJ, Pardridge WM: Summary: circulating tryptophan, brain tryptophan and psychiatric disease. *J Neural Transm [Suppl]* 15:227–236, 1979

13. Yuwiler A, Oldendorf WH, Geller E, et al: Effect of albumin binding and amino acid competition on tryptophan uptake by brain. *J Neurochem* 28:1015–1023, 1977

14. Curzon G, Joseph MH, Knott PJ: Effects of immobilization and food deprivation on rat brain tryptophan metabolism. *J Neurochem* 19:1967–1974, 1972

15. Tagliamonte A, Biggio G, Bargin L, et al: Free tryptophan in serum controls brain tryptophan level and serotonin synthesis. *Life Sci* 12:277–287, 1973

16. Korf J, VanPragg HM, Sebens JB: Serum tryptophan decreased, brain tryptophan increased and brain serotonin synthesis unchanged after probenecid loading. *Brain Res* 42:239–242, 1972

17. Wurtman RJ, Rose CM, Chou C, et al: Daily rhythms in the concentrations of various amino acids in human plasma. *N Eng J Med* 279:171–175, 1968

18. Fernstrom JD, Wurtman RJ, Hammarshom-Wiklund B, et al: Diurnal variations in plasma concentrations of tryptophan, tyrosine, and other neutral amino acids: effect of dietary protein intake. *Am J Clin Nutr* 32:1912–1922, 1979

19. Eccleston D, Ashcroft GW, Crawford TBB, et al: Effect of tryptophan administration on 5-HIAA in cerebrospinal fluid in man. *J Neurol Neurosurg Psychiatry* 33:269–272, 1970

20. Gillman PK, Bartlett JR, Bridges PK, et al: Indolic substances in plasma, cerebrospinal fluid, and frontal cortex of human subjects infused with saline or tryptophan. *J Neurochem* 37:410–417, 1981

21. Blasberg R, Lajtha A: Heterogeneity of the mediated transport systems of amino acid uptake in brain. *Brain Res* 1:86–104, 1966

22. Pardridge WM, Oldendorf WH: Transport of metabolic substrates through the blood-brain barrier. *J Neurochem* 28:5–12, 1977

23. Perez-Curet J, Chase TN, Murphy DL: Dietary regulation of brain tryptophan metabolism by plasma ratio of free tryptophan and neutral amino acids in humans. *Nature* 248:693–695, 1974

24. Fernstrom JD, Wurtman RJ: Nutrition and the brain. *Sci Am* 230:84–91, 1974

25. Fernstrom JD, Wurtman RJ: Brain serotonin content: physiological dependence on plasma tryptophan levels. *Science* 173:149–152, 1971

26. Fernstrom JD, Wurtman RJ: Brain serotonin content: increase following ingestion of carbohydrate diet. *Science* 174:1023–1025, 1971

27. Fernstrom JD, Wurtman RJ: Elevation of plasma tryptophan by insulin in rat. *Metabolism* 21:337–342, 1972

28. Colmenares JL, Wurtman RJ, Fernstrom JD: Effects of ingestion of a carbohydrate-fat meal on the levels and synthesis of 5-hydroxyindoles in various regions of the rat central nervous system. *J Neurochem* 25:825–829, 1975

29. Coppen A: The biochemistry of affective disorders. *Br J Psychiatry* 113:1237–1265, 1967

30. Bourne JR, Bunney WE, Colburn RW, et al: Noradrenaline, 5-hydroxytryptamine and 5-hydroxyindole acetic acid in hindbrains of suicidal patients. *Lancet* 2:805–808, 1968

31. Lloyd KJ, Farley IJ, Deck JHN: Serotonin and 5-hydroxyindole acetic acid in discrete areas of the brainstem of suicide victims and control patients. *Adv Biochem Psychopharmacol* 11:387–397, 1974

32. Asberg M, Thoren P, Traskman L, et al: Serotonin depression: a biochemical subgroup with the affective disorders? *Science* 191:478–480, 1976

33. VanPraag HM: Central monoamine metabolism in depressions. I. Serotonin and related compounds. *Comp Psychiatry* 21:30–43, 1980

34. Bopp B, Biel JH: Antidepressant drugs. *Life Sci* 14:415–423, 1974

35. Young SN, Sourkes TL: Tryptophan in the central nervous system: regulation and significance. *Adv Neurochem* 2:133–191, 1977

36. Glassman AH, Platman SR: Potentiation of a monoamine oxidase inhibitor by tryptophan. *J Psychiatr Res* 1:83–88, 1969

37. Maas JW: Biogenic amines and depression: bio-

chemical and pharmacological separation of two types of depression. *Arch Gen Psychiatry* 32: 1357–1361, 1977

38. Janowsky DS, El-Yousef MK, Davis JM, et al: Cholinergic reversal of manic symptoms. *Arch Gen Psychiatry* 28:542–547, 1973

39. Chouinard G, Young SN, Annable L, et al: Tryptophan-nicotinamide combination in the treatment of newly admitted depressed patients. *Commun Psychopharmacol* 2:311–318, 1978

40. Gaillard JM, Tissot R: Blood-brain movements of tryptophan and tyrosine in manic-depressive illness and schizophrenia. *J Neural Transm [Suppl]* 15: 189–196, 1979

41. Kishimoto H, Hama Y: The level and diurnal rhythm of plasma tryptophan and tyrosine in manic-depressive patients. *Yokohama Med Bull* 27:89–97, 1976

42. Coppen A, Brooksbank BWL, Peet M: Tryptophan concentration in the cerebrospinal fluid of depressive patients. *Lancet* 1:1393, 1972

43. Moller SE, Kirk L, Honore P: Free and total plasma tryptophan in endogenous depression. *J Affect Disorders* 1:69–76, 1979

44. Niskanen P, Huttunen M, Tamminen T, et al: The daily rhythm of plasma tryptophan and tyrosine in depression. *Br J Psychiatry* 128:67–73, 1976

45. Moller SE, Kirk L, Honore P: Relationship between plasma ratio of tryptophan to competing amino acids and their response to L-tryptophan treatment in endogenously depressed patients. *J Affect Disorders* 2:47–59, 1980

46. DeMyer MK, Shea PA, Hendrie HC, et al: Plasma tryptophan and five other amino acids in depressed and normal subjects. *Arch Gen Psychiatry* 38:642–646, 1981

47. Fuxe K: Evidence for the existence of monoamine neurons in the central nervous system. IV. Distribution of monoamine nerve terminals in the central nervous system. *Acta Physiol Scand [Suppl]* 64:247, 1965

48. Bogduk N, Lance JW: Pain and pain syndromes, including headache. In *Current Neurology*, vol 3. Edited by Appel SH. New York, John Wiley, 1981, pp 377–419

49. Messing RM, Lytle LD: Serotonin-containing neurons: their possible role in pain and analgesia. *Pain* 4:1–21, 1977

50. Mayer DJ, Price DD: Central nervous system mechanisms of analgesia. *Pain* 2:379–404, 1976

51. Lytle LD, Messing RB, Fisher L, et al: Effects of long-term corn consumption on brain serotonin and the response to electric shock. *Science* 190:692–694, 1975

52. Hosobuchi Y, Adams JE, Linchitz R: Pain relief by electrical stimulation of the central gray matter in humans and its reversal by naloxone. *Science* 197: 183–186, 1977

53. Hosobuchi Y: Tryptophan reversal of tolerance to analgesia induced by central grey stimulation. *Lancet* 1:47, 1978

54. Hosobuchi Y, Lamb S, Bascom D: Tryptophan loading may reverse tolerance to opiate analgesics in humans: a preliminary report. *Pain* 9:161–169, 1980

55. King RB: Pain and tryptophan. *J Neurosurg* 53: 44–52, 1980

56. Wurtman JJ, Wurtman RJ: Fenfluramine and fluoxetine spare protein consumption while suppressing caloric intake by rats. *Science* 198:1178–1180, 1977

57. Wurtman JJ, Wurtman RJ, Growdon JH, et al: Carbohydrate craving in obese people: suppression by treatments affecting serotoninergic transmission. *Int J Eat Dis*, pp 2–15, 1981

58. Nagatsu T, Levitt M, Udenfriend S: Tyrosine hydroxylase: the initial step in norepinephrine biosynthesis. *J Biol Chem* 239:2910–2917, 1964

59. Axelrod J: Dopamine β-hydroxylase: regulation of its synthesis and release from nerve terminals. *Pharmacol Rev* 24:233–243, 1972

60. Saavedra JM, Palkovits M, Brownstein MJ, et al: Localization of phenylthanolamine-*N*-mthyl transferase in the rat brain nuclei. *Nature* 248:695–696, 1974

61. Korf J, Grasdijk L, Westernik BHC: Effect of electrical stimulation of the nigro-striatal pathway of the rat on dopamine metabolism. *J Neurochem* 26: 579–584, 1976

62. Meek JL, Neff NH: The rate of formation of 3-methyoxy-4-hydroxyphenylethyleneglycol sulfate in brain as an estimate of the rate of formation of norepinephrine. *J Pharmacol Exp Ther* 184:570–575, 1973

63. Kaufman S, Levenberg B: Further studies on the phenylalanine hydroxylation cofactor. *J Biol Chem* 234:2683–2688, 1959

64. Kettler R, Bartholini G, Pletscher A: *In vivo* enhancement of tyrosine hydroxylation in rat striatum by tetrahydrobiopterin. *Nature* 249:476–478, 1974

65. Carlsson A, Lindquist M: Dependence of 5-HT and catecholamine synthesis on concentrations of precursor amino acids in rat brain. *Naunyn-Schmiedebergs Arch Pharmacol* 303:157–164, 1978

66. Wurtman RJ, Larin F, Mostafapour S, et al: Brain catechol synthesis: control by brain tyrosine concentration. *Science* 185:183–184, 1974

67. Gibson CJ, Wurtman RJ: Physiological control of brain catechol synthesis by brain tyrosine concentration. *Biochem Pharmacol* 26:1137–1142, 1977

68. Scally MC, Ulus IH, Wurtman RJ: Brain tyrosine level controls striatal dopamine synthesis in haloperidol-treated rats. *J Neural Transm* 41:1–6, 1977

69. Hefti F, Melamed E, Wurtman RJ: Partial lesions of the dopaminergic nigrostriatal system in rat brain: biochemical characterization. *Brain Res* 195:123–137, 1980

70. Melamed E, Hefti F, Wurtman RJ: Tyrosine ad-

ministration increases striatal dopamine release in rats with partial nigrostriatal lesions. *Proc Natl Acad Sci USA* 77:4305–4309, 1980

71. Sved AF, Fernstrom JD, Wurtman RJ: Tyrosine administration decreases serum prolactin levels in chronically reserpinized rats. *Life Sci* 25:1293–1300, 1979

72. Gibson CJ, Wurtman RJ: Physiological control of brain norepinephrine synthesis by brain tyrosine concentration. *Life Sci* 22:1399–1406, 1978

73. Van Zwieten PA: Antihypertensive drugs with a central action. *Prog Pharmacol* 1:1–63, 1975

74. Sved AF, Fernstrom JD, Wurtman RJ: Tyrosine administration reduces blood pressure and enhances brain norepinephrine release in spontaneously hypertensive rats. *Proc Natl Acad Sci USA* 76:3511–3514, 1979

75. Osumi Y, Tauaka C, Takaori S: Levels of tyrosine and tryptophan in the plasma and brain of spontaneously hypertensive rats. *Jpn J Pharmacol* 24:715–720, 1974

76. Yamori Y, Fujiwara M, Horie R, et al: The hypotensive effect of centrally administered tyrosine. *Eur J Pharmacol* 68:201–204, 1980

77. Bresnahan MR, Hatzinikolaou P, Brunner HR, et al: Effects of tyrosine infusion in normotensive and hypertensive rats. *Am J Physiol* 239:4206–4211, 1980

78. Conlay LA, Maher TJ, Wurtman RJ: Tyrosine increases blood pressure in hypotensive rats. *Science* 212:559–560, 1981

79. Scott NA, DeSilva RA, Lown B, et al: Tyrosine administration decreases vulnerability to ventricular fibrillation in the normal canine heart. *Science* 211:727–729, 1981

80. Glaeser B, Melamed E, Growdon JH, et al: Elevation of plasma tyrosine after a single oral dose of L-tyrosine. *Life Sci* 25:265–272, 1979

81. Alonso R, Gibson CJ, Wurtman RJ, et al: Elevation of urinary catecholamines and their metabolites following tyrosine administration in humans. *Am J Psychiatry*. In press, 1982

82. Melamed E, Glaeser B, Growdon JH, et al: Plasma tyrosine in normal humans: effects of oral tyrosine and protein-containing meals. *J Neural Transm* 47:299–306, 1980

83. Agharanya JC, Alonso R, Wurtman RJ: Changes in catecholamine excretion after short-term tyrosine ingestion in normally fed human subjects. *Am J Clin Nutr* 34:82–87, 1981

84. Burke RE, Fahn S: Movement disorders. In *Current Neurology*, vol 3. Edited by Appel S. New York, John Wiley, 1980, pp 92–137

85. Riederer P: L-Dopa competes with tyrosine and tryptophan for human brain uptake. *Nutr Metab* 24:417–423, 1980

86. Growdon JH, Melamed E: Effects of oral L-tyrosine administration on CSF tyrosine and homovanillic acid levels in patients with Parkinson's disease. *Neurology* 30:396, 1980

87. Growdon JH: Tyrosine treatment in Parkinson's disease: clinical effects (abstract). *Am Acad Neurol* 1981, p 134

88. Barbeau A: The pathogenesis of Parkinson's disease: a new hypothesis. *Can Med Assoc J* 87:802–807, 1962

89. Birkmayer W, Mentasi M: Weitere experimentelle untersuchungen uber den catecholaminstoffwechsel bei extrapyramidalen erkrankungen (Parkinsonund chorea-syndrom). *Archiv Psychiatr Nervenkr* 210:29–35, 1967

90. Schildkraut JJ: The catecholamine hypothesis of affective disorders: a review of supporting evidence. *Am J Psychiatry* 122:509–522, 1965

91. Reiderer P, Birkmayer W, Seeman D, et al: 4-Hydroxy-3-methoxyphenylglycol as an index of brain noradrenaline turnover in endogenous depression. *Acta Psych Scand [Suppl]* 280:251–257, 1980

92. Schildkraut JJ, Orsulak PJ, Schatzberg, AF, et al: Toward a biochemical classification of depressive disorders, Part I. *Arch Gen Psychiatry* 35:1427–1433, 1978

93. Jones FD, Mass JW, Dekirmenjian H, et al: Diagnostic subgroups of affective disorders and their urinary excretion of catecholamine metabolites. *Am J Psychiatry* 132:1141–1148, 1975

94. Wehr TA, Muscettola G, Goodwin FK: Urinary 3-methoxy-4-hydroxyphenylglycol circulation rhythm. *Arch Gen Psychiatry* 37:257–263, 1980

95. Jones FD, Maas JW, Dekirmenjian H, et al: Urinary catecholamine metabolites during behavioral changes in a patient with manic-depressive cycles. *Science* 179:300–302, 1973

96. Gordon EK, Oliver J: 3-Methoxy-4-hydroxyphenylethylene glycol in human cerebrospinal fluid. *Clin Chim Acta* 35:145–150, 1971

97. Muscettola G, Wehr T, Goodwin FK: Effect of diet on urinary MHPG excretion in depressed patients and normal control subjects. *Am J Psychiatry* 134:914–916, 1977

98. Sweeney DR, Maas JW, Heninger GR: State anxiety, physical activity, and urinary 3-methoxy-4-hydroxyphenylethylene glycol excretion. *Arch Gen Psychiatry* 35:1418–1423, 1978

99. Izzo JL Jr, Horwitz D, Keiser HR: Reduction in human urinary MHPG excretion by guanethidine: urinary MHPG as index of sympathetic nervous activity. *Life Sci* 24:1403–1406, 1979

100. Post RM, Kotin J, Goodwin FK, et al: Psychomotor activity and cerebrospinal fluid amine metabolites in affective illness. *Am J Psychiatry* 130:67–72, 1973

101. Maas JW, Fawcett JA, Dekirmenjian H: Catecholamine metabolism, depressive illness and drug response. *Arch Gen Psychiatry* 26:252–262, 1972

102. Fawcett J, Maas JW, Dekirmenjian H: Depression and MHPG excretion: response to dextro-amphet-

amine and tricyclic antidepressants. *Arch Gen Psychiatry* 26:246–251, 1972

103. Shaw DM, Tidmarch SF, Johnson AL, et al: Multicompartmental analysis of amino acids. III. Tyrosine in affective disorder. *Psychol Med* 9:117–123, 1979

104. Benkert O, Renz A, Marano C, et al: Altered tyrosine daytime plasma levels in endogenous depressive patients. *Arch Gen Psychiatry* 25:359–363, 1971

105. Gelenberg AJ, Wojcik JD, Growdon JH, et al: Tyrosine in the treatment of depression. *Am J Psychiatry* 137:622–623, 1980

106. Goldbert IK: 1-Tyrosine in depression. *Lancet* 2:364, 1980

107. Gibson CJ, Gelenberg A: Tyrosine in the treatment of depression. In *Management of Depression with Precursor Therapy.* Edited by Van Pragg HM, Mendlewicz J. New York, Marcel Decker. In press, 1982

108. Gibson GE, Blass JP: Impaired synthesis of acetylcholine in brain accompanying mild hypoxia and hypoglycemia. *J Neurochem* 27:37–42, 1976

109. Ksiezak HJ, Gibson GE: Oxygen dependence of glucose and acetylcholine metabolism in slices and synaptosomes from rat brain. *J Neurochem* 37:305–314, 1981

110. Hirata F, Viveros O, Bilberto E, et al: Identification and properties of two methyl-transferases in conversion of phosphatidylethanolamine to phosphatidylcholine. *Proc Natl Acad Sci USA* 75:1718–1720, 1978

111. Blusztajn JK, Zeisel SJ, Wurtman RJ: Synthesis of lecithin (phosphatidylcholine) from phosphatidylethanolanine in bovine brain. *Brain Res* 179:319–327, 1979

112. Browning ET, Schulman MP: (^{14}C) acetylcholine synthesis by cortex slices of rat brain. *J Neurochem* 15:1391–1395, 1968

113. Freeman JJ, Jenden DJ: The source of choline for acetylcholine synthesis in brain. *Life Sci* 19:949–962, 1976

114. Hirsch MJ, Growdon JH, Wurtman RJ: Relations between dietary choline or lecithin intake, serum choline levels and various metabolic indices. *Metabolism* 27:953–960, 1978

115. Zeisel S, Growdon JH, Wurtman RJ, et al: Lecithin therapy in neurologic diseases: plasma choline responses to ingested lecithin. *Neurology* 30:1226–1229, 1980

116. Millington WR, McCall AL, Wurtman, RJ: Deanol acetoamidobenzoate inhibits the blood-brain barrier transport of choline. *Ann Neurol* 4:302–306, 1978

117. Haga T, Noda H: Choline uptake systems of rat brain synaptosomes. *Biochim Biophys Acta* 291:564–575, 1973

118. Yamamura HI, Snyder SH: High affinity transport of choline into synaptosomes of rat brain. *J Neurochem* 21:1355–1374, 1973

119. Schuberth J, Jenden DJ: Transport of choline from plasma to cerebrospinal fluid in the rabbit, with reference to the origin of choline and acetylcholine metabolism. *Brain Res* 84:245–251, 1975

120. Cohen EL, Wurtman RJ: Brain acetylcholine: increase after systemic choline administration. *Life Sci* 16:1095–1102, 1975

121. Cohen EL, Wurtman RJ: Brain acetylcholine, control by dietary choline. *Science* 191:561–562, 1976

122. Haubrich DR, Wang PFL, Herman RL, et al: Increase in rat brain acetylcholine induced by choline or deanol. *Life Sci* 17:975–980, 1975

123. Wecker L, Dettbarn WD, Schmidt DE: Choline administration: modification of the central actions of atropine. *Science* 199:86–87, 1978

124. London ED, Coyle JT: Pharmacological augmentation of acetylcholine levels in kainatelesioned rat striatum. *Biochem Pharmacol* 27:2962–2965, 1978

125. Hirsch MJ, Wurtman RJ: Lecithin consumption elevates acetylcholine concentrations in rat brain and adrenal gland. *Science* 207:223–225, 1978

126. Ulus IH, Wurtman RJ: Choline administration: activation of tyrosine hydroxylase in dopaminergic neurons of rat brain. *Science* 194:1060–1061, 1976

127. Ulus IH, Hirsch MJ, Wurtman RJ: Trans-synaptic induction of adrenal tyrosine hydroxylase activity by choline: evidence that choline administration increases cholinergic transmission. *Proc Natl Acad Sci USA* 74:798–800, 1977

128. Ulus IH, Scally MC, Wurtman RJ: Enhancement by choline of the induction of adrenal tyrosine hydroxylase by phenoxybenazamine, 6-hydroxydopamine, insulin, or exposure to cold. *J Pharmacol Exp Ther* 204:676–682, 1978

129. Bierkamper GG, Goldbert AM: Release of acetylcholine from the vascular perfused rat phrenic nerve-hemidiaphragm. *Brain Res* 202:234–237, 1980

130. Jenden DJ, Weiler MH, Gundersen CB: Choline availability and acetylcholine synthesis. In *Alzheimer's Disease: A Report of Progress in Research.* Edited by Corkin S, Davis KL, Growdon JH, et al. New York, Raven Press. In press, 1982

131. Swartz BE, Jenden DJ: Acetylcholine dynamics in rat hippocampal slices (abstract). *Soc Neurosci* 6:151, 1980

132. Löeffelholz K, Lindmar R, Weide W: Relationship between choline and acetylcholine release in the autonomic nervous system. In *Nutrition and the Brain,* vol 5. Edited by Barbeau A, Growdon JH, Wurtman RJ. New York, Raven Press, 1979, pp 233–241

133. Gelenberg AJ, Doller-Wojcik JC, Growdon JH: Choline and lecithin in the treatment of tardive dyskinesia: preliminary results from a pilot study. *Am J Psychiatry* 136:772–776, 1979

134. Krnjevic K, Reinhardt W: Choline excites cortical neurons. *Science* 206:1321–1323, 1979

135. Asell GB, Spanner S: The source of choline for

acetylcholine synthesis. In *Cholinergic Mechanisms and Psychopharmacology*. Edited by Jenden DJ. New York, Plenum, 1978, pp 431–445

136. Bremer J, Greenberg DM: Methyl transferring enzyme system in the biosynthesis of lecithin (phosphatidylcholine). *Biochim Biophys Acta* 46:205–211, 1961

137. Wurtman RJ, Hirsch MJ, Growdon JH: Lecithin consumption raises serum-free choline levels. *Lancet* 2:68–69, 1977

138. Hanin I: Commercially available "lecithin": proposed guidelines for nomenclature and methodology. In *Choline and Lecithin in Brain Disorders*, vol 5, *Nutrition and the Brain*. Edited by Barbeau A, Growdon JH, Wurtman RJ. New York, Raven Press, 1979, pp 443–446

139. Crane G: Tardive dyskinesia in patients treated with major neuroleptics: a review of the literature. *Am J Psychiatry* 124:40–48, 1968

140. Food and Drug Administration Task Force, American College of Neuropsychopharmacology: Neurological syndromes associated with antipsychotic drug use: a special report. *Arch Gen Psychiatry* 28:463–467, 1973

141. Davis KL, Hollister LE, Berger PA, et al: Cholinergic imbalance hypotheses of psychoses and movement disorders: strategies for evaluation. *Commun Psychopharmacol* 1:533–543, 1975

142. Klawans HL: The pharmacology of tardive dyskinesia. *Am J Psychiatry* 130:82–86, 1973

143. Baldessarini RJ, Tarsy D: Dopamine and the pathophysiology of dyskinesias induced by antipsychotic drugs. *Annu Rev Neurosci* 3:23–41, 1980

144. Kobayashi RM: Drug therapy of tardive dyskinesia. *N Engl J Med* 296:257–260, 1977

145. Gerlach J, Reisby N, Randrup A: Dopaminergic hypersensitivity and cholinergic hypofunction in the pathophysiology of tardive dyskinesia. *Psychopharmacologia* 34:21–35, 1974

146. Klawans HL, Rubovits R: Effects of cholinergic and anticholinergic agents on tardive dyskinesia. *J Neurosurg Psychiatry* 27:941–947, 1974

147. Davis KL, Berger PA, Hollister LE: Choline for tardive dyskinesia. *N Engl J Med* 293:152, 1975

148. David KL, Hollister LE, Barchas JD, et al: Choline in tardive dyskinesia and Huntington's disease. *Life Sci* 19:1507–1519, 1976

149. Tamminga CA, Smith RC, Erickson SE, et al: Cholinergic influences in tardive dyskinesia. *Am J Psychiatry* 134:769–774, 1977

150. Growdon JH, Hirsch MJ, Wurtman RJ, et al: Oral choline administration to patients with tardive dyskinesia. *N Engl J Med* 297:524–527, 1977

151. Barbeau A: Emerging treatments: replacement therapy with choline or lecithin in neurological disease. *Can J Neurol Sci* 5:157–160, 1978

152. Yahr M: Choline and lecithin administration to patients with tardive dyskinesia. *Trans Am Neurol Assoc* 103:98–99, 1978

153. Growdon JH, Gelenberg AJ, Doller J, et al: Lecithin can suppress tardive dyskinesia. *N Engl J Med* 298:1029–1030, 1978

154. Gelenberg AJ, Doller JC, Growdon, JH: Choline and lecithin in the treatment of tardive dyskinesia: preliminary results from a pilot study. *Am J Psychiatry* 136:6, 1979

155. Barbeau A: Lecithin in movement disorders. In *Choline and Lecithin in Brain Disorders*, vol 5. *Nutrition and the Brain*. Edited by Barbeau A, Growdon JH, Wurtman RJ. New York, Raven Press, 1979, pp 263–271

156. Jackson IV, Nuttall EA, Ibe LO, et al: Treatment of tardive dyskinesia with lecithin. *Am J Psychiatry* 136:1458–1462, 1979

157. Branchey MH, Branchey LB, Bark NM, et al: Lecithin in the treatment of tardive dyskinesia. *Commun Psychopharmacol* 3:303–307, 1979

158. Growdon JH, Cohen EL, Wurtman RJ: Huntington's disease: clinical and chemical effects of choline administration. *Ann Neurol* 1:418–422, 1977

159. Aquilonius SM, Eckernas SA: Choline therapy in Huntington's chorea. *Neurology* 27:887–889, 1977

160. McGeer PL, McGeer EG, Fibiger HC: Choline acetylase and glutamic acid decarboxylase in Huntington's chorea. *Neurology* 23:912–917, 1973

161. Bird ED, Iversen LL: Huntington's chorea: postmortem measurement of glutamic acid decarboxylase, choline acetyltransferase and dopamine in basal ganglia. *Brain* 97:457–472, 1974

162. Kanazawa I, Bird ED, Gale JS, et al: Substance P: decrease in substantia nigra and globus pallidus in Huntington's disease. In *Advances in Neurology*, vol 23. *Huntington's Disease*. Edited by Chase TN, Wexler NS, Barbeau A. New York, Raven Press, 1979, pp 495–504

163. Arregui A, Bennett JP, Bird ED, et al: Huntington's chorea: selective depletion of activity of angiotensin converting enzyme in the corpus striatum. *Ann Neruol* 2:294–298, 1977

164. Enna SJ, Bird ED, Bennett JF, et al: Huntington's chorea: changes in neurotransmitter receptors in brain. *N Engl J Med* 294:1305–1309, 1976

165. Stahl SM, Berger PA: Cholinergic treatment in the Tourette syndrome. *N Engl J Med* 302:1311, 1980

166. Barbeau A: Cholinergic treatment in the Tourette syndrome. *N Engl J Med* 302:1310–1311, 1980

167. Polinsky RJ, Ebert MH, Caine ED, et al: Cholinergic treatment in the Tourette syndrome. *N Engl J Med* 302:1310, 1980

168. Hanin I, Merikangas JR, Merikangas KR, et al: Red-cell choline and Gilles de la Tourette syndrome. *N Engl J Med* 301:661–662, 1979

169. Bowen DM, Smith CB, White P, et al: Neurotransmitter related enzymes and indices of hypoxia in senile dementia and other abiotrophies. *Brain* 99:459–496, 1976

170. Davies P, Maloney AJF: Selective loss of central cholinergic neurons in Alzheimer's disease. *Lancet* 2:1903, 1976

171. Perry EK, Perry RH, Blessed G, et al: Necropsy evidence of central cholinergic deficits in senile dementia. *Lancet* 1:189, 1977

172. Spillane JA, White P, Goodhardt MJ, et al: Selective vulnerability of neurons in organic dementia. *Nature* 7:558–559, 1977

173. Terry RD, Davies P: Dementia of the Alzheimer type. *Annu Rev Neurosci* 3:77–95, 1980

174. Bowen DM, Spillane JA, Curzon G, et al: Accelerated aging or selective neuronal loss as an important cause of dementia? *Lancet* 1:11–14, 1979

175. Drachman DA, Leavitt J: Human memory and the cholinergic system. *Arch Neurol* 30:113–121, 1974

176. Drachman DA: Memory and cognitive function in man: does the cholinergic system have a specific role? *Neurology* 27:783–790, 1977

177. Davis KL, Mohs RC, Tinkleberg JR, et al: Physostigmine: improvement of long-term memory processes in normal humans. *Science* 201:272–274, 1978

178. Sitaram N, Weingartner H, Gillin JC: Human serial learning: enhancement with arecholine and choline and impairment with scopolamine. *Science* 201:274–276, 1978

179. Sitaram N, Weingartner H, Caine ED, et al: Choline: selective enhancement of serial learning and encoding of low imagery words in man. *Life Sci* 22:1555–1560, 1978

180. Bartus RT, Dean RL, Goas AJ, et al: Age related changes in passive avoidance retention. Modulation with dietary choline. *Science* 209:301–303, 1980

181. Bartus RT, Dean RL, Beer B: Memory deficits in aged Cebus monkeys and facilitation with central cholinomimetics. *Neurobiol Aging* 1:145–152, 1980

182. Christie JE, Blackburn IM, Glen IA, et al: Effects of choline and lecithin on CSF choline levels and cognitive functions in patients with presenile dementia of the Alzheimer type. In *Choline and Lecithin in Brain Disorders,* vol 5, *Nutrition and the Brain.* Edited by Barbeau A, Growdon JH, Wurtman RJ. New York, Raven Press, 1979, pp 377–387

183. Boyd, WD, Graham-White J, Blackwood G, et al: Clinical effects of choline in Alzheimer's senile dementia. *Lancet* 2:711, 1977

184. Etienne P, Gauthier S, Johnson G, et al: Lecithin in Alzheimer's disease. *Lancet* 2:837, 1978

185. Signoret JL, Whiteley A, Lhermitte F: Influence of choline on amnesia in early Alzheimer's disease. *Lancet* 2:837, 1978

186. Smith CM, Swash M, Easton-Smith A, et al: Choline therapy in Alzheimer's disease. *Lancet* 2:318, 1978

187. Fovall P, Dysken MW, Lazarus LW, et al: Choline bitartrate treatment of Alzheimer-like dementias. *Commun Psychopharmacol* 4:141–143, 1980

188. Zeisel S, Reinstein D, Corkin S, et al: Meeting report: international study group on the pharmacology of memory disorders associated with aging. *Neurobiol Aging.* In press, 1982

189. Ferris SH, Sathananthan G, Reisberg B, et al: Long-term choline treatment of memory-impaired elderly patients. *Science* 205:1039–1040, 1979

190. Renvoize EB, Jerram T: Choline in Alzheimer's disease. *N Engl J Med* 301:330, 1979

191. Hu R, Vroulis G, Smith RC: Effects of lecithin on memory and behavior in Alzheimer's type dementia (abstract). Paper presented at the meeting of the Gerontology Society of America, San Diego, November 21–25, 1980

192. Etienne P, Gauthier S, Dastoor D, et al: Lecithin in Alzheimer's disease. *Lancet* 2:1206, 1978

193. Sullivan EV, Shedlack KJ, Corkin S, et al: Physostigmine and lecithin in Alzheimer's disease. In *Alzheimer's Disease: A Report of Progress in Research.* Edited by Corkin S, Davis K, Growdon JH, et al. New York, Raven Press. In press, 1982

194. Adolfsson R, Gottfries CG, Oreland L, et al: Reduced level of catecholamines in the brain and increased activity of monoamine oxidase in platelets in Alzheimer's disease. In *Alzheimer's Disease: Senile Dementia and Related Disorders.* Edited by Katzman R, Terry RD, Bick KL. New York, Raven Press, 1978, pp 441–451

195. Garcia CA, Tweedy JR, Blass JP, et al: Lecithin and parkinsonian dementia. In *Alzheimer's Disease: A Report of Progress in Research.* Edited by Corkin S, Davis K, Growdon JH, et al. New York, Raven Press. In press, 1982

196. Peters BH, Levin HS: Effects of physostigmine and lecithin on memory in Alzheimer's disease. *Ann Neurol* 6:219–221, 1979

197. Friedman E, Sherman KA, Ferris SH, et al: Clinical response to choline plus piracetam in senile dementia: relation to red-cell choline levels. *N Engl J Med* 304:1490–1491, 1981

198. Kark PA, Blass J, Spence MA: Physostigmine in familial ataxias. *Neurology* 27:70–72, 1977

199. Barbeau A, Butterworth RF, Ngo T, et al: Pyruvate metabolism in Friedreich's ataxia. *Can J Neurol Sci* 3:379–388, 1976

200. Legg NJ: Oral choline in cerebellar ataxia. *Br Med J* 2:1403–1404, 1978

201. Livingstone IR, Mastaglia FL: Choline chloride in the treatment of ataxia. *Br Med J* 2:939, 1979

202. Lawrence GM, Millac P, Stout GS, et al: The use of choline chloride in ataxic disorders. *J Neurol Neurosurg Psychiatry* 43:452–545, 1980

203. Philcox DV, Kies B: Choline in hereditary ataxia. *Br Med J* 2:613, 1979

204. Reding MJ, Blass JP, Stern PH, et al: Lecithin in hereditary ataxia. *Neurology* 31:363–364, 1981

205. Chamberlain S, Robinson N, Walker J, et al: Effect of lecithin on disability and plasma free choline levels in Friedreich's ataxia. *J Neurol Neurosurg Psychiatry* 43:843–845, 1980

206. Pentland B, Martyn C, Steer CR, et al: Lecithin treatment in Friedreich's ataxia. *Br Med J* 282:1197–1198, 1981

207. Stein C, Moore W, Weinreich D, et al: Choline levels in plasma of myasthenia gravis patients and normal individuals. *Ann Neurol* 4:290–291, 1978

208. Kranz H, Caddy DJ, Williams AM, et al: Myasthenic syndrome: effect of choline, plasmapheresis, and tests for circulating factor. *J Neurol Neurosurg Psychiatry* 43:483–488, 1980

209. McNamara JO, Carwile S, Hope V, et al: Effects of oral choline on human complex partial seizures. *Neurology* 30:1334–1336, 1980

210. Papavasiliou PS, Rosal V: Effects of choline in patients with levodopa-induced dyskinesia. In *Choline and Lecithin in Brain Disorders*. Edited by Barbeau A, Growdon JH, Wurtman RJ. New York, Raven Press, 1979, pp 335–341

211. Garcia CA, Tweedy JR, Blass JP, et al: Lecithin and parkinsonian dementia. In *Alzheimer's Disease: A Report of Progress in Research*. Edited by Corken S, Davis K, Growdon JH, et al. New York, Raven Press. In press, 1982

212. Millington WR, McCall AL, Wurtman RJ: Lithium and brain choline levels. *N Engl J Med* 300:196–197, 1978

213. Jope RS, Jenden DJ, Ehrlich BE: Choline accumulates in erythrocytes during lithium therapy. *N Engl J Med* 299:833–834, 1978

214. Cornford EM, Braun LD, Oldendorf WH: Carrier mediated blood-brain barrier transport of choline and certain choline analogs. *J Neurochem* 30:299, 1978

215. Cohen BM, Miller AL, Lipinski JF, et al: Lecithin in mania: a preliminary report. *Am J Psychiatry* 137:242–243, 1980

216. Rosenthal R, Bigelow L: The effects of physostigmine in phenothiazine resistant schizophrenic patients. *Compr Psychiatry* 14:489–494, 1973

217. Davis KL, Berger PA, Hollister LE, et al: Cholinergic involvement in mental disorders. *Life Sci* 22:1865–1872, 1978

218. Davis KL, Hollister LE, Berger PA: Choline chloride in schizophrenia. *Am J Psychiatry* 136:1581–1584, 1979

7

Recent Issues in Neuroendocrinology and Neuropeptides

Gajanan Nilaver and Earl A. Zimmerman

In our last review of neuroendocrinology, we dealt with some aspects of the progress made in the basic science of the neuroendocrine system. We discussed the anatomical organization of the corticotropin-β-endorphin system, the concept of a common precursor for the different peptides of this group, and the controversy regarding the source of some of these peptides in the brain. We had also briefly described how the hypothalamic paraventricular nucleus could, by virtue of its peptidergic projections to the various regions of the brain stem and spinal cord, orchestrate the various responses of the autonomic nervous system. In the last section of the chapter, we had briefly outlined some new therapeutic approaches to the pituitary tumors and the pharmacodynamics of some of the new analogues of vasopressin and luteinizing hormone-releasing hormone (LH-RH) that are currently in use in therapy.

Our present chapter is also divided into three sections. The first deals with the controversy surrounding the role of vasopressin as a corticotropin-releasing factor (CRF). The second section discusses the results of various studies supporting the existence of a renin-angiotensin system intrinsic to the brain, analogous to that present in the periphery. Although controversial, these are two active areas of ongoing research (1, 2) and are considered fertile grounds for additional discoveries in the near future. The third section deals with some of the pathophysiological aspects of altered spinal cord func-

tion, specifically with reference to pain and spasticity. While these two problems are frequently encountered in neurology and rehabilitation medicine, until recently recourse to their therapy was limited. A search for rational and successful methods of treatment had resulted in a better understanding of the underlying inhibitory mechanisms in the cord and their pharmacology. It has also provided us with new concepts on neuronal regeneration and reorganization, and the increasing realization that peptides are probably implicated in the pathophysiology of these conditions even more than initially suspected. Further knowledge of the anatomical organization of the peptidergic systems in the spinal cord has also led to a better understanding of the basic mechanisms of some of the therapeutic procedures used in alleviating pain and spasticity.

VASOPRESSIN AND CRF

Historical Background

Nearly 30 years ago, based on studies in animals with experimental diabetes insipidus (3, 4), it was proposed that vasopressin may act as a CRF. Although it was shown that administration of vasopressin released adrenocorticotropic hormone (ACTH) in animals, and despite its use in clinical medicine as a test for anterior pituitary hypofunction (5), enthusiasm for vasopressin as a CRF waned over the next decade. The hypothalamus did not appear to contain enough vasopressin, and the hormone appeared much less potent than some other extractable hypothalamic substances in releasing ACTH (6). Although first sought after because of its importance in sustaining life, the chemical characterization of CRFs other than vasopressin remained elusive (7, 8). Part of the problem involved the apparent lability of CRF activity as well as problems with bioassay methods (1). In the meantime, two peptide hormone releasing factors [thyrotropin releasing hormone, TRH; luteinizing hormone-releasing hormone, LH-RH] (8, 9) and growth hormone inhibiting hormone [somatostatin, ST] (10) were discovered.

Vasopressin Pathways to the Hypophyseal Portal System

New interest in a role for vasopressin in ACTH regulation was stimulated in the mid 1970s by the immunocytochemical demonstration of the hormone and its associated neurophysin in axonal fibers projecting to the hypophyseal portal bed in the zona externa of the median eminence (11). This vasopressin projection, in addition to the one in the posterior pituitary, had been suggested by earlier studies using the Gomori stains (12). It had generally been discarded because zona externa fibers were not demonstrable using these stains, and intervening anatomical studies including electron microscopy showed that the granules in nerve terminals to the hypophyseal portal plexus were smaller than the typical vasopressin granules in the posterior pituitary gland (13). For a considerable time, it was therefore considered that the zona externa was the sole domain of axon terminals containing releasing or inhibiting factors secreted into hypophyseal portal blood. Subsequent application of immunocytochemical methods showed that both these factors (14) as well as vasopressin (11, 15) were present in the smaller granules in different axons in this region. It is now known that there is a specific pathway from the paraventricular nucleus (PVN) of the hypothalamus to the zona externa of the median eminence (11, 16-18) by which vasopressin is secreted into hypophyseal

portal blood in concentrations 100 to 1000 times greater than those found in peripheral blood. At least under the experimental conditions (surgery, anesthesia) in which the portal blood is collected there is more than enough vasopressin to release ACTH. Further evidence that the PVN-median eminence pathway is related to adrenal function was obtained by the effects of adrenalectomy and glucocorticoid replacement, which increased and decreased immunodetectable vasopressin in zona externa, respectively. This suggested that the adrenal cortex inhibits vasopressin secretion at this site as well as at the posterior pituitary (19). The well-known observation that partial diabetes insipidus is made worse by glucocorticoid administration is no doubt due to inhibitory feedback effects on vasopressin neurons.

Retrograde Portal Blood Flow and Short Portal Vessels

Recent anatomical studies have also shown that the posterior pituitary is not the exclusive domain of vasopressin and oxytocin fibers. Axons containing LH-RH (20), ST (14), and dopamine (14, 21) have been described in this region in various animals. This brings us to another important but unresolved issue in current neuroendocrinology, which concerns the recently described vascular connections between posterior and anterior pituitary [short portal vessels] and between the pituitary gland and the hypothalamus [retrograde portal flow] (22). Acute experiments in rats suggest that large concentrations of anterior pituitary hormones and vasopressin travel upward in the hypophyseal portal system (23). Whether this reflects a "short loop" feedback system (24) and an important source of brain ACTH and other anterior pituitary hormones is still unclear. It is complicated by studies demonstrating the production of ACTH and other anterior pituitary hormones (25) in the brain. The posterior pituitary was also considered the major source of the large concentrations of vasopressin in long portal veins in the study mentioned above (22). Removal of the posterior pituitary was reported to produce about a 10-fold reduction in the vasopressin concentrations of the downward flowing blood in the long portal veins (22). However, we repeated these studies and could find no change (26). At the moment, these opposite results are without explanation. The specific pathway from the PVN to the median eminence, because of its anatomical existence, seems more likely to be the important pathway for vasopressin secretion into portal blood. This is further supported by experiments in cats demonstrating release of ACTH upon stimulation of the PVN but not the supraoptic nucleus [SON] (27). This experiment, however, was complicated by some inhibition of ACTH secretion upon stimulation of the SON, suggesting that some other inhibitory factor from SON may also have been released and clouded the results. That the posterior pituitary may yet have important influences on anterior pituitary function via short portal vessels was recently shown in the context of the role of dopamine in prolactin regulation (21). Removal of the posterior pituitary gland in rats resulted in prolonged hyperprolactinemia (21). A similar mechanism may apply for vasopressin and other substances.

Multifactoral CRF

The anatomical studies mentioned above have stimulated further biochemical and physiological studies regarding a possible role for vasopressin in CRF action. Using a more sensitive bioassay system consisting of isolated anterior pituitary cells perfused on a column, Gillies and Lowry (1, 28, 29) have demonstrated that antiserum to vasopressin-inhibited CRF activity in hypothalamic extracts of normal rats, and that CRF activity was markedly reduced in extracts of homozygous Brattleboro rats (DI rats) which cannot produce vasopressin. These studies further showed that the amount of vasopressin with CRF actions in normal hypothalamus was greater than previously appreciated. Chromatographic separation of hypothalamic extracts from normal rats on a BioGel P_2 column revealed three peaks with CRF activity—a major peak co-eluting with vasopressin and two smaller peaks. The three peaks when combined restored full CRF

activity, while the individual peaks only had partial activity (1, 29). Similar chromatography of DI rat hypothalamic extracts revealed only the two minor peaks, and restoration of full CRF activity required the addition of vasopressin (1, 29). These studies support the earlier concept that CRF is multifactorial, with vasopressin as a participant (30).

However, the controversy concerning vasopressin as a CRF continues. Using a different bioassay system, Pearlmutter and colleagues (31) found normal CRF activity in DI rats. The assay system, however, may have been affected by residual vasopressin (1) sequestered in receptors on ACTH cells (32, 33). Although there is considerable evidence of some adrenal insufficiency in DI rats (1, 30, 34, 35), vasopressin is clearly not critical for their survival and therefore constitutes only a part of the CRF. The nature of these factors, other than vasopressin, awaits chemical characterization and may well be reported in the near future. Improved methods of bioassay and the realization that the regulation of ACTH, like that of other anterior pituitary hormones, is probably multifactorial (18), may assist these investigations. Vale and colleagues at the Salk Institute recently reported the structure of a CRF.* CRF is produced by the hypothalamus and releases ACTH and β-endorphin from the pituitary.

BRAIN RENIN-ANGIOTENSIN SYSTEM

Regulation of blood pressure by the central nervous system is of considerable importance to both medicine and neurology. The cause of hypertension, which often results in stroke, remains unknown in many cases. After several years of work on the renal mechanisms of blood-pressure regulation, which have resulted in the elucidation of "renal renin-angiotensin cascade," attention has recently been turned to the central nervous system for new insights. This does not minimize the significance of the progress made in understanding the peripheral mechanisms of

---

* Vale W, Speiess J, Rivier C, et al: Characterization of a 41-residue ovine hypothalamic peptide that stimulates secretion of corticotropin and β-endorphin. *Science* 213:1394-1397, 1981.

blood-pressure regulation; many important therapeutic gains have been realized. Indeed, the recent development of orally active angiotensin-converting enzyme inhibitors which lower blood pressure (36), are results of such research. One of these has recently been released under the name captopril (Squibb).

Clinically, it has long been known that a wide variety of different insults to the brain cause an acute increase in systemic blood pressure. Like respiration and other autonomic functions, blood-pressure control is likely to be complex, involving several levels of the neuraxis from the hypothalamus down to the thoracic spinal cord. Reis (37) has demonstrated that a brain disturbance can produce sustained as well as other forms of hypertension in experimental animals with lesions in the medulla involving the nucleus of the solitary tract. Phillips's experiments (38) with the spontaneously hypertensive strain of rat (SHR) provided evidence for the involvement of a central mechanism in this stroke-prone animal model of essential hypertension. Intracerebroventricular administration of a synthetic peptide-receptor-inhibitor of angiotensin II (saralasin; Sar[1]-Ala[8] angiotensin II) lowered the blood pressure. This work also provided some of the most convincing evidence for an angiotensin II system endogenous to brain, separate from one in the general circulation, since systemic administration of saralasin did not lower the blood pressure in nephrectomized SHR rats. How the angiotensin II is produced, however, and where it may act in the brain is not yet certain and is the subject of considerable current research and controversy (2, 38-40). Also, it is still not certain how many of the so-called intrinsic central angiotensin effects (38) are normally induced by circulating angiotensin II (2). Apparently, all the actions produced by intracerebroventricular administration of the hormone (increase in blood pressure, thirst, and salt appetite and release of vasopressin and ACTH) can be caused by angiotensin II in the circulation (2), acting at circumventricular organs where the blood-brain barrier is deficient. Angiotensin II does not normally appear to cross the blood-brain barrier, except in the hypertensive state. Since peripheral angiotensin II administration raises blood pressure, the experimental effects attributed to circulating angiotensin II on brain may in fact be due to opening of blood-brain barrier in some of the studies (38). Good arguments have been made for both sides of this issue (2, 38). In the long run, both angiotensin systems may well be found to be operative (2).

Considerable evidence has accumulated for the existence of the components of the "renin-angiotensin cascade" in brain since an intrinsic system was proposed 10 years ago (41, 42). Renin, renin substrate, angiotensin I, angiotensin converting enzyme, and to a lesser extent angiotensin II, have been found in the brain (2, 38-43). The issue that brain renin activity was due to cathepsin D has since been resolved by the biochemical and immunochemical identification of renin in brain (44). Both renin and converting enzyme were found in high concentrations in the choroid plexus and anterior pituitary gland (45, 46); negligible amounts of renin could be detected in posterior pituitary gland, compared to large concentrations of converting enzyme in this region. A similar dissociation between these two enzymes was also reported in the rat striatum. After neuronal destruction was induced by injection of ibotenic acid, the converting enzyme was significantly reduced, while renin activity increased (47). Although both enzymes have been found in synaptosomal preparations (40, 48), this initial study suggests that they may not necessarily be found in the same neuronal elements. By assay, renin activity is widely distributed in brain with moderately high levels found in hypothalamus, cerebellum, and amygdala (45). By immunocytochemistry, renin has been found in many neurons all over the brain (49, 50) and in glial elements as well. Converting enzyme activity was reported to be fairly high in corpus striatum, caduate nucleus, substantia nigra, retina, and pituitary (51). It was also reported in medulla and hypothalamus (46). By immunoperoxidase technique, it has been localized in rat choroid plexus and brain blood vessels using antiserum to rabbit lung converting enzyme (46). Recently, we have localized it to nerve terminals on dendrites in human globus pallidus and substantia nigra as well as the choroid plexus with an antiserum to human lung converting enzyme (R. Defendinin, E.A. Zimmerman, and E. Erdos, unpublished observation, 1981). These findings provide further evidence that the converting enzyme is contained in neurons. Depletion of converting enzyme has been reported in the striatum of patients with Huntington's chorea (52) and is the most likely source of the fibers in the globus pallidus and substantia nigra. The function of converting enzyme in these terminals awaits further investigation. It could be involved in the metabolism of enkephalin or substance P (SP) that is present in this region (40), as well as angiotensin I or even other substances. Enzymes with peptidase activity are probably not very specific for a particular substrate, as compared to enzymes of biogenic-amine systems, so that those involved in the "renin-angiotensin cascade" are not necessarily unique markers for the proposed angiotensin II system in the brain. Nevertheless, demonstration of these enzymes and angiotensins in the same neurons would be strong evidence for the existence of such a system in brain. This has not been accomplished so far and will be discussed in the next section. Angiotensinases that could degrade angiotensin II include a diverse group of amino peptidases which are highly concentrated in the brain (4).

The regional distribution of angiotensinogen, the prohormone of renin, was reported for the rat brain (52). It was found to be widely distributed in areas generally reported to contain angiotensin II binding sites (53, 54): higher in thalamus, hypothalamus, midbrain, and medulla and lower in hippocampus, cerebellum, corpus striatum, and cerebral cortex. As discussed by Lewicki and coworkers (52), the wide distribution of angiotensinogen would suggest a more diffuse angiotensin system in brain than the apparently discrete sites sensitive to local angiotensin II administration: subfornical organ or organum vasculosum, supraoptic nucleus, area postrema, and subnucleus medialis (38, 43). The same discrepancy can be discussed with reference to the immuno-histochemical localization of angiotensin II:

high fiber concentrations in the median eminence, amygdala, spinal cord; lesser numbers in the dorsal medial hypothalamus, locus ceruleus, and caudate; and scattered terminals in the preoptic nucleus, periventricular grey, septum, and nucleus tractus solitarius (see 43 for review).

A key missing ingredient in establishing an angiotensin II system intrinsic to brain has been the inability of most investigators to extract significant amounts of angiotensin II from brain (2, 38). This may well be due to rapid turnover or instantaneous inactivation by the ubiquitously high levels of angiotensinases in brain as mentioned above. With the use of the appropriate enzyme inhibitors, it is hoped that this may be accomplished. Meanwhile, the only evidence for angiotensin II in brain is immunocytochemical, a technique, which by its nature, is indirect (55). Immunocytochemistry is an immunological probe, which can at best identify a particular peptide configuration, usually determined by three or more amino acid sequences, but cannot by itself fully identify the chemical nature of the substance in question. We now know that many different brain peptides share similar amino acid sequences. For example β-endorphin contains the five amino acid sequence of methionine-enkephalin. Many antisera to the latter visualize the former, although it is now known that these peptides are contained within different neuronal systems (55). Immunocytochemical methods are the only in situ methods available at present, however, and they are important guides to brain localization.

The only neuronal cell bodies consistently found to react with antiserum to angiotensin II have been those in the supraoptic and paraventricular nuclei (43, 55-57), and the suprachiasmatic nuclei (56) of the hypothalamus. In our own studies, we found that the angiotensin II reactivity was only found in neuronal perikarya which were also reactive to vasopressin (55, 56). Furthermore, the angiotensin reactivity behaved like vasopressin. It was absent or nearly so in homozygous Brattleboro rats lacking vasopressin and increased in zona externa of the median eminence of normal rats, along with vasopressin, after adrenalectomy (56). At the moment we do not know how to interpret these immunocytochemical findings, as well as those of others. One would have expected to visualize angiotensin II in fibers terminating on vasopressin cells, rather than in them, since these vasopressin neurons have receptors for angiotensin II, and the peptide acts directly on them to release vasopressin (58). Many of the extrahypothalamic angiotensin II-like fibers, like those containing vasopressin or oxytocin (16), could originate from the paraventricular nucleus, but this remains to be proven. These cells might yet be shown to generate angiotensin II. Renin has been localized in supraoptic, paraventricular, and suprachiasmatic neurons in the mouse (49), although angiotensin II or vasopressin have not yet been co-localized with renin. With a homogeneous neuroblastoma-glioma cell line in tissue culture, it has been shown that a single cell can contain the entire renin-angiotensin system (59). It is just as likely, however, that another molecule antigenically related to but distinct from angiotensin II has so far been visualized and that the true angiotensin II generating neuron has yet to be found. Intensive ongoing research in this area is likely to provide important additional insights in the near future. Improved techniques of extracting and inhibiting angiotensinase activity and the production of highly specific monoclonal antibodies to the parts of the renin-angiotensin system hold promise as better tools for further investigation of this important problem.

PEPTIDES IN THE SPINAL CORD

Anatomical Organization and Function

Among the major developments in neuroendocrinology and the neurosciences, resulting from the demonstration of peptides in the brain by immunocytochemistry and radioimmunoassay, is the increasing realization that these compounds probably represent a novel class of intercellular messengers or modulators in the brain. Interestingly, of the 24 or so putative peptide neurotransmitter candidates described so far, at least half have been localized in the spinal cord. Elucidation of the roles for these peptides has provided major insights into the functions of the CNS.

The dorsal horn of the spinal cord is particularly rich in neuropeptides. Immunohistochemical techniques have revealed complex inputs of peptide-containing neurons in this region [for a review of the subject see (60)]. Immunoreactive SP, vasoactive intestinal polypeptide (VIP), gastrin/cholecystokinin (CCK), and ST are present in primary sensory neurons (61-63). SP, enkephalin, and neurotensin (NT) are also present in propriospinal neurons or spinal interneurons (64, 65). The bulbo-spinal serotonergic system, with cell bodies in the nucleus raphae magnus of the medulla and descending projections to the ventral horn of the cord, has been also shown to contain SP (66, 67). This system also projects to the dorsal horn via the dorso-lateral funiculus. A descending enkephalinergic system projects to the dorsal horn. Studies from our laboratory (68), as well as those of others (16, 69, 70) have indicated that the magnocellular paraventricular nucleus of the hypothalamus sends vasopressinergic and oxytocinergic projections to the dorsal horn, as well as various autonomic centers in the spinal cord. All these findings suggest an important role for these peptides in the processing of incoming sensory information at the level of the spinal cord.

In this context the position of SP, by virtue of its anatomical location in this region, is very unique. As already pointed out, this peptide is located within three distinct neuronal systems in the cord: (1) within finely myelinated (Aδ) and unmyelinated (C) fibers of the dorsal-nerve root; (2) within perikarya of the dorsal horn of the cord; (3) within the descending bulbo-spinal serotonergic pathway. While iontophoretic studies of SP in the dorsal horn have demonstrated that the peptide functions as an excitatory transmitter in primary sensory neurons (71-73) and is involved in the transmission of nociceptive information within this system, there is also evidence suggesting that the descending SP projection is inhibitory (74) and antinociceptive (75-77). This, then, represents a novel situation wherein the same peptide transmitter, converging on the same marginal neuron system of the dorsal horn from two different sites of origin, exerts opposing physiological effects on the system. Studies demonstrating both excitatory and inhibitory responses to iontophoretically applied SP on cultured spinal neurons (78) tend to further support this novel concept.

The demonstration of opiate receptors in the dorsal horn of the cord and their reduction following dorsal rhizotomy, without any associated change in the overall enkephalin content of this region, has suggested that spinal opiate receptors are located presynaptically on primary afferent terminals. This, combined with the observation that morphine causes a concentration dependent, stereospecific, and naloxone-reversible reduction of SP from slices of rat trigeminal nucleus, but not substantia nigra (79), led Jessel and Iversen to propose a mechanism for the analgesic action of the opiates in the spinal cord. According to this hypothesis, enkephalin interneurons, which exogenously administered opioid peptides and morphine presumably mimic, project presynaptically to terminals of small-diameter (Aδ and C) primary afferent fibers containing SP. Thus, activation of presynaptic opiate receptors, by reducing the amount of SP released, would induce pain relief. Although Mudge and coworkers (72) have demonstrated a similar inhibition of SP release by enkephalin in dispersed-cell cultures of primary sensory neurons, ultrastructural analysis of the dorsal horn to date has failed to demonstrate enkephalin fibers directly terminating on SP axons.

Other peptidergic systems in the dorsal horn may also be involved in the modulation of incoming nociceptive information. Thus, recent studies have shown that vasopressin, upon intraventricular or systemic administration, can exert potent antinociceptive effects (80). DI rats deficient in vasopressin have been shown to exhibit increased sensitivity to foot shock, a condition reversed by the systemic administration of vasopressin (81). Long-lasting antinociceptive effects, not mediated by opiate receptors, have also been reported following the intracisternal administration of neurotensin (82). Thus it is quite

evident that a variety of both opiate and non-opiate peptides can modulate responsiveness to pain and that a major part of such modulation probably occurs at the level of the spinal cord.

Peptides and Spasticity

While it is generally assumed that connections in the spinal cord are laid down during development and remain stable throughout adult life, several lines of evidence have revealed the potential plasticity of such connections (83-88). Employing the Nauta silver technique of staining degenerating fibers, McCouch and coworkers (87) have demonstrated spouting of dorsal-nerve-root fibers in monkeys and cats, following hemisection of the spinal cord. In such studies, axonal sprouts could actually be traced to terminate on the soma and proximal dendrites of spinal neurons, occupying synaptic sites left vacant by the degeneration of the descending tracts. Furthermore, when the results in monkeys were compared to those in cats, it was apparent that species with greater cerebral cortical development and consequently larger numbers of descending fibers had more pronounced evidence of functional sprouting and were, therefore, more spastic. More recently, Hulsebosch and Coggeshall (89) were able to demonstrate and quantitate sprouting of unmyelinated axons in the dorsal horn of the rat following hemisection of the spinal cord at birth. With the demonstration of peptides such as SP, VIP, CCK, and ST in the dorsal-root ganglia, it is logical to assume their involvement in such functional sprouting. However, while the SP system was recently demonstrated to be involved in such sprouting (90), a similar involvement of ST was not seen. Thus, there may be selective involvement of SP in functional sprouting in spinal cord after injuries that result in spasticity. It remains to be seen, however, whether the newly established SP connections are actually responsible for the spasticity. Possible sprouting in other peptide-containing pathways remains to be studied.

If the SP-related sprouting is indeed responsible for the associated spasticity, the basis of certain therapeutic approaches employed in the amelioration of this condition, such as posterior rhizotomies and dorsal-column stimulation, now become quite explainable. Any attempt at reducing spasticity and the pain associated with the mass reflex of spinal cord injuries would necessarily have to limit the afferent sensory input to the anterior horn cells. This is best done by interruption of selected dorsal roots and their freshly sprouted afferents. Indeed, such an approach for the treatment of spasticity is not new; partial posterior rhizotomies as a method of ameliorating spasticity was introduced as early as 1911 by Foerester (91). Its usefulness was forgotten for several decades until it was re-introduced by Gros and coworkers (92) in 1967, and more recently by Austin and coworkers (93). Dorsal rhizotomy has been shown to reduce the amount of immunoreactive SP within the spinal cord (94). The procedure can therefore be expected to be very effective in reducing the increased aberrant SP excitatory input to the anterior horn cells below the level of transection, thereby alleviating spasticity.

Dorsal-column stimulation provides yet another means of reducing excessive sensory input to the ventral horns. Stimulation of the dorsal column has been shown to exert, via gelatinosa cells, a marked inhibitory influence on the soma and proximal dendrites of those marginal cells that are excited by the nociceptive inputs reaching them via the SP-containing Aδ and C fibers of the dorsal-nerve root (95). Such postsynaptic modulation or gating of incoming sensory inputs in the gelatinosa is said to be the basis of the analgesia observed upon stimulation of the dorsal column with implanted electrodes (96). This neurosurgical procedure, over the past 10 years, has gained popularity as an effective method of providing relief from intractable pain. The use of dorsal-column stimulators for pain relief has led to the resurgence of interest in the use of electrical stimulation of the afferent nervous system for the relief of other symptoms. As nociceptive inputs are more effective in initiating firing of α motor neurons in spasticity, it is not surprising that dorsal-column stimulation would be of great

help in the treatment of such disorders. The use of electrical stimulators for the treatment of spasticity, however, is not something that has evolved of late. It had been recommended highly by Duchenne more than 100 years ago (97). Electrotherapy has since been widely used by physiotherapists (98), and gait stimulators with transcutaneous electrodes have become an important appliance in the treatment of spastic-paraparetic patients (99).

Therapeutic Implications

The concept of a peptidergic involvement in spinal cord injury and spasticity may explain the pharmacodynamics of certain drugs such as Lioresal and naloxone that are reported to be beneficial in the treatment of these conditions.

Lioresal

Lioresal (baclofen, β-(4-chlorophenyl)-γ-aminobutyric acid), chemically both a phenylethylamine and a γ-aminobutyric acid (GABA) derivative, has been reported to suppress the spinal monosynaptic and polysynaptic reflexes without affecting the electrical properties of spinal motor neurons in cats (100, 101). This effect is not antagonized by bicuculline or strychnine (102, 103). Lioresal has proven to be very effective in the treatment of spasticity (104-107). Since SP may be an excitatory transmitter of primary afferent neurons, a possible mechanism for the action of Lioresal would be its antagonism of the SP-induced depolarization of spinal neurons. Studies on isolated spinal cords of 7-day-old rats have shown that Lioresal can block SP-induced excitatory transmission at the primary afferent synapse (108), suggesting that it is a specific antagonist of SP. However, in guinea pig ileum and isolated sympathetic ganglia where SP has extremely potent excitatory effects, Lioresal is without specific antagonistic effects (109). This suggests that if the effect of Lioresal in reducing the spasticity in spinal cord injury involves SP, it is brought about by a pharmacological, rather than a physiological antagonism of the peptide's excitatory effects. It must be emphasized that while axonal sprouting, which involves SP, has been demonstrated following spinal transections, and its implication in the resulting spasticity is circumstantially compelling, there is no study to date that has actually established the involvement of SP in the pathogenesis of spasticity.

Naloxone

The role of the opiate compounds in spinal injury is well documented. Recent studies (110, 111) have clearly demonstrated a role for the opiate peptides in the pathogenesis of spinal shock and spasticity resulting from cord transection. Acute transection of the cervical spinal cord in animals results in spinal shock—a state characterized by loss of muscle tone, reflexes, and sensation below the level of the injury (112, 113). The hypotension that accompanies this condition is often not responsive to either pressor therapy (114, 115) or fluid replacement (115, 116). A 10-fold elevation of plasma β-endorphin, accompanied by a 250-fold increase in the cerebrospinal-fluid endorphin level was recently demonstrated in experimental animals with spinal shock produced by cord

injury (116). The increased levels of the peptide were associated with hypotension and decreased spinal cord blood flow. Administration of naloxone was further shown to be effective in reversing not only the hypotensive state and the hemodynamic status of the cord, but it also significantly reduced the pathological changes seen in the spinal cord and had significant beneficial effects on the ultimate neurological outcome. In this context, the effectiveness of corticosteroids in the treatment of shock or spinal injury may be due to their ability to inhibit the release of endorphin from the pituitary (117, 118). In a subsequent study (119), the same investigators further demonstrated that treatment of this condition with the opiate antagonist naloxone, even if delayed by as much as 4 hours, is still capable of ameliorating the subsequent spasticity and improving the ultimate neurological outcome. Taken together, these studies provide strong evidence for the participation of the endorphins in some of the deleterious effects of spinal injury, and opiate antagonists, like naloxone, hold great promise for better treatment of human spinal trauma.

REFERENCES

1. Gillies G, Lowry PJ: Corticotropin releasing hormone and its vasopressin component. In *Frontiers in Neuroendocrinology,* vol 7. Edited by Ganong WF, Martini L. New York, Raven Press, 1982 (in press)

2. Ramsay DJ: Effects of circulating angiotensin II on the brain. In *Frontiers in Neuroendocrinology,* vol 7. Edited by Ganong WF, Martini L. New York, Raven Press. In press, 1982

3. McCann SM, Brobeck JR: Evidence for a role of the supraopticohypophysial system in the regulation of adrenocorticotropin secretion. *Proc Soc Exp Biol Med* 87:318-324, 1954

4. McCann SM: The ACTH releasing activity of extracts of the posterior lobe of the pituitary *in vivo. Endocrinology* 60:664-676, 1957

5. Kreiger DT, Zimmerman EA: The nature of CRF and its relationship to vasopressin. In *Clinical Neuroendocrinology.* Edited by Martini L, Besser GM. New York, Academic Press, 1977, pp 363-391

6. Sirret NE, Purves HD: Assay of corticotropin releasing factor (CRF) in ACTH-primed "grafted" rats. *Neuroendocrinology* 10:83-93, 1972

7. Schally AV, Anderson RN, Lipscomb HS, et al: Evidence for the existence of two corticotropin releasing factors, alpha and beta. *Nature* 188:1192-1193, 1960

8. Schally AV, Arimura A, Kastin AJ: Hypothalamic regulatory hormones. *Science* 179:341-350, 1973

9. Blackwell RE, Guillemin R: Hypothalamic control of adenohypophysial secretions. *Annu Rev Physiol* 35:357-390, 1973

10. Brazeau R, Vale W, Burgus R, et al: Hypothalamic peptide that inhibits the secretion of immunoreactive pituitary growth hormone. *Science* 179:77-79, 1973

11. Zimmerman EA, Stillman MA, Recht LD, et al: Vasopressin and corticotropin releasing factor (CRF): an axonal pathway to portal capillaries in the zona externa of the median eminence

containing vasopressin and its interaction with adrenal steroids. *Ann NY Acad Sci* 297:405-419, 1977

12. Scharrer E, Scharrer B: Hormones produced by neurosecretory cells. *Recent Prog Horm Res* 10:183-240, 1954

13. Knigge KM, Scott DE: Structure and function of the median eminence. *Am J Anat* 129:223-228, 1970

14. Elde R, Hokfelt T: Distribution of hypothalamic hormones and other peptides in the brain. In *Frontiers in Neuroendocrinology*, vol 5. Edited by Ganong WF, Martini L. New York, Raven Press, 1978, pp 1-33

15. Silverman A-J, Zimmerman EA: Ultrastructural immunocytochemical localization of neurophysin and vasopressin in the median eminence and posterior pituitary of the guinea pig. *Cell Tissue Res* 159:291-301, 1975

16. Swanson LW, Sawchenko PE: The paraventricular nucleus: a site for the integration of neuroendocrine and autonomic mechanisms. *Neuroendocrinology* 31:410-417, 1980

17. Zimmerman EA: The organization of oxytocin and vasopressin pathways. In *Neurosecretion and Brain Peptides*. Edited by Martin JB, Reichlin S, Bick KL. New York, Raven Press, 1981, pp 63-75

18. Zimmerman EA, Nilaver G: Neuroendocrinology. In *Current Neurology*, vol 3. Edited by Appel S. New York, John Wiley, 1981, pp 356-376

19. Seif SM, Robinson AG, Zimmerman EA, et al: Plasma neurophysin and vasopressin in the rat: response to adrenalectomy and steroid replacement. *Endrocrinology* vol 1-3:1009-1015, 1978

20. Silverman A-J, Krey LC, Zimmerman EA: A comparative study of luteinizing hormone releasing hormone (LHRH) neuronal net works in mammals. *Bio Reprod* 20:98-110, 1979

21. Peters LL, Hoefer M, Ben-Jonathan N: The posterior pituitary regulation of anterior pituitary prolactin secretion. *Science* 217:659-661, 1981

22. Bergland RM, Page RB: Can the pituitary secrete directly to the brain: (affirmative evidence). *Endocrinology* 102:1325-1328, 1978

23. Oliver C, Michal RS, Porter JC: Hypothalamic-pituitary vasculature: evidence for retrograde flow in pituitary stalk. *Endocrinology* 101:598-604, 1977

24. Martini L: Neurohypophysis and anterior pituitary activity. In *The Pituitary Gland,* vol 3. Edited by Harris GW, Donovan BT. London, Butterworths, 1966, pp 535-577

25. Kreiger DT, Liotta AS, Brownstein MJ, et al: ACTH, β-lipotropin and related peptides in brain, pituitary and blood. *Recent Prog Horm Res* 36:277-344, 1980

26. Recht LD, Hoffman DL, Haldar J, et al: Vasopressin concentrations in hypophysial portal plasma: insignificant reduction following removal of the posterior pituitary gland. *Neuroendocrinology* 33:88-90, 1981

27. Dornhorst A, Carlson D, Seif SM, et al: Control of adrenocorticotropin and vasopressin by supraoptic and paraventricular nuclei. *Endocrinology* 108:1420-1424, 1981

28. Gillies G, Lowry PJ: Corticotropin releasing factor may be modulated vasopressin. *Nature* 278:463-464, 1979

29. Gillies G, Lowry PJ: Corticotropin releasing activity in extracts of the stalk median eminence of Brattleboro rats. *J Endocrinol* 84:65-73, 1980

30. Yates FE, Russell SM, Dallman MF, et al: Potentiation by vasopressin of corticotropin release induced by CRF. *Endocrinology* 88:3-15, 1971

31. Pearlmutter FE, Dokas LA, Loeser B, et al: Properties of CRF from normal and Brattleboro rat median eminence. *Neuroendocrinology* (in press)

32. Chateau M, Marchetti J, Burlet A, et al: Evidence of vasopressin in adenohypophysis: research into its role in corticotrope activity. *Neuroendocrinology* 28:25-35, 1979

33. Lutz-Bucher B, Koch B, Mialhe C: Comparative *in vitro* studies on corticotropin releasing activity of vasopressin and hypothalamic median eminence extract. *Neuroendocrinology* 23:181-192, 1978

34. Wiley MK, Pearlmutter FE, Miller RE: Decreased adrenal sensitivity to ACTH in the vasopressin-deficient rat (Brattleboro). *Neuroendocrinology* 14:257-270, 1974

35. Kenyon CJ, Hargreaves G, Henderson IW: Adrenocortical function in rats with inherited hypothalamic diabetes insipidus (Brattleboro strain). *J Steroid Biochem* 9:345-348, 1978

36. Ondetti MA, Rubin B, Cushman DW: Design of specific inhibitors of angiotensin converting enzyme: a new class of orally active antihypertensive agents. *Science* 196:441-444, 1977

37. Reis DJ: The nucleus tractus solitarius and experimental neurogenic hypertension: evidence for a central neural imbalance hypothesis of hypertensive disease. In *Neurosecretion and Brain Peptides*. Edited by Martin JB, Reichlin S, Bick KL. New York, Raven Press, 1981, pp 409-420

38. Phillips MI: Biological effects of angiotensin in the brain. In *Enzymatic Release of Vasoactive Peptides*. Edited by Gross F, Vogel G. New York, Raven Press, 1980, pp 335-363

39. Reid IA: The brain renin-angiotensin system: a critical analysis. *Fed Proc* 38:2255-2259, 1979

40. Ganten D, Speck G, Schelling P, et al: The brain renin-angiotensin system. In *Neurosecretion and Brain Peptides*. Edited by Martin JB, Reichlin S, Bick KL. New York, Raven Press, 1981, pp 359-372

41. Fischer-Ferraro C, Nahmod VE, Goldstein DJ, et al: Angiotensin and renin in rat and dog brain. *J Exp Med* 133:353-361, 1971

42. Ganten D, Minnich JE, Granger P, et al: Angiotensin-forming enzyme in brain tissue. *Science* 173:64-65, 1971

43. Phillips MI, Weyhenmeyer J, Felix D, et al: Evidence for an endogenous brain renin angiotensin system. *Fed Proc* 38:2260-2266, 1979

44. Hirose S, Yokosawa H, Inagami T: Immunochemical identification of renin in rat brain and distinction from acid proteases. *Nature* 274:392-393, 1978

45. Hirose S, Yokosawa H, Inagami T, et al: Renin and prorenin in hog brain; ubiquitous distribution and high concentration in the pituitary and pineal. *Brain Res* 191:489-499, 1980

46. Rix E, Ganten D, Schull B, et al: Converting-enzyme in the choroid plexus, brain and kidney: immunocytochemical and biochemical studies in rats. *Neurosci Let* 22:125-180, 1981

47. Fuxe K, Ganten D, Kohler C, et al: Evidence for differential localization of angiotensin-I converting enzyme and renin in the corpus striatum of rat. *Acta Physiol Scand* 110:321-323, 1980

48. Husain A, Smeby RR, Litowitz JK, et al: Brain renin: localization in rat brain synaptosomal fractions. *Brain Res.* In press, 1982

49. Celio MR, Clemens DL, Inagami T: Renin in anterior, pineal, and neuronal cells of mouse brain: immunohistochemical localization. *Biomed Res.* In press, 1982

50. Slater EE, Defendini R, Zimmerman EA: Wide distribution of immunoreactive renin in nerve cells of human brain. *Proc Natl Acad Sci USA* 77:5458-5460, 1980

51. Arregui A, Iversen L: Angiotensin-converting enzyme: presence of high activity in choroid plexus of mammalian brain. *Eur J Pharmacol* 52:147-150, 1978

52. Lewicki JA, Fallon JH, Printz MP: Regional distribution of angiotensinogen in rat brain. *Brain Res* 158:359-371, 1978

53. Bennett JP, Snyder SH: Angiotensin II binding to mammalian brain membranes. *J Biol Chem* 251:7423-7430, 1976

54. Sirett NE, McLean AS, Bray JJ, et al: Distribution of angiotensin II receptors in rat brain. *Brain Res* 122:299-312, 1977

55. Zimmerman EA, Krupp L, Hoffman DL, et al: Exploration of peptidergic pathways in brain by immunocytochemistry: a ten year perspective. *Peptides* 1(Suppl):3-10, 1980

56. Kilcoyne MM, Hoffman DL, Zimmerman EA: Immunocytochemical localization of angiotensin II and vasopressin in rat hypothalamus: evidence for production in the same neuron. *Clin Sci* 59:57s-60s, 1980

57. Quinlan JT, Phillips MI: Immunoreactivity for an angiotensin II-like peptide in the human brain. *Brain Res* 205:212-218, 1981

58. Sladek C, Joynt R: Role of angiotensin in the osmotic control of vasopressin release by the organ-cultured rat hypothalamo-neurohypophyseal system. *Endocrinology* 106:173-178, 1980

59. Fishman MC, Zimmerman EA, Slater EE: Renin and angiotensin: the complete system within the neuroblastoma X glioma cell. *Science.* In press, 1982

60. Hokfelt T, Johansson O, Lungdahl A, et al: Peptidergic neurons. *Nature*, 284:515-521, 1980

61. Larsson LI, Rehfeld IF: Localization and molecular heterogeneity of cholecystokinin in the central and peripheral nervous system. *Brain Res* 165:201-218, 1970

62. Hokfelt T, Lundgerg JM, Schultzberg M, et al: Cellular localization of peptides in neural structures. *Proc R Lond (Biol)* 210:63-77, 1980

63. Lundberg JM, Hokfelt T, Nilsson G, et al: Peptide neurons in the vagus, splanchnic and sciatic nerves. *Acta Physiol Scand* 104:499-501, 1978

64. Lungdahl A, Hokfelt T, Nilsson G: Distribution of substance P-like immunoreactivity in the central nervous system of the rat I: cell bodies and nerve terminals. *Neuroscience* 3:861-944, 1978

65. Barber RR, Vaughn JE, Slemmon JR, et al: The origin, distribution and synaptic relationships of substance P axons in rat spinal cord. *J Compar Neurol* 184:331-351, 1979

66. Hokfelt T, Lungdahl A, Steinbusch H: Immunohistochemical evidence of substance P-like immunoreactivity in some 5-hydroxytryptamine-containing neurons in the rat central nervous system. *Neuroscience* 3:517-538, 1978

67. Chan-Palay V, Jonsson G, Palay SL: Serotonin and substance P co-exist in the neurons of the rat's central nervous system. *Proc Natl Acad Sci USA* 75:1582-1586, 1978

68. Nilaver G, Zimmerman EA, Wilkins J, et al: Magnocellular hypothalamic projections to the lower brain stem and spinal cord of the rat. *Neuroendocrinology* 30:150-158, 1980

69. Swanson LW: Immunohistochemical evidence for a neurophysin containing autonomic pathway arising from the paraventricular nucleus of the hypothalamus. *Brain Res* 128:346-353, 1977

70. Swanson LW: Extrahypophysial oxytocin containing pathways in the brain and spinal cord of the rat and monkey (abstract). *Neuroscience* 4:415, 1978

71. Henry JL, Hu JW, Lucier GE, et al: Responses of units in the trigeminal sensory nuclei to oro-facial stimuli and to substance P. In *Pain in the Trigeminal Region.* Edited by Anderson DJ, Matthews B. Amsterdam, Elsevier/North Holland, 1977, pp 295-306

72. Mudge AW, Leeman SE, Fishback GD: Enkephalin inhibits release of substance P from sensory neurons in culture and decreases action potential duration. *Proc Natl Acad Sci USA* 76:526-530, 1979

73. Randik M, Miletic V: Effect of substance P in cat dorsal horn neurones activated by noxious stimuli. *Brain Res* 128:164-169, 1977

74. Fields HL, Basbaum AI, Clanton CH, et al:

Nucleus raphae magnus inhibition of spinal dorsal horn neurons. *Brain Res* 126:441-454, 1977

75. Mayer DJ, Liberskind JC: Pain reduction by focal electrical stimulation of the brain: an anatomical and behavioral analysis. *Brain Res* 68:73-93, 1974

76. Mayer DJ, Wolfe TL, Akil H, et al: Analgesia from electrical stimulation in the brainstem of the rat. *Science* 174:1351-1354, 1971

77. Oliveras J, Besson JM, Guilbaud G, et al: Behavioral and electrophysiological evidence of pain inhibition from midbrain stimulation in the cat. *Exp Brain Res* 20:32-44, 1974

78. Vincent JD, Barker JL: Substance P: evidence for diverse roles in neuronal function from cultured mouse spinal neurons. *Science* 205:1409-1412, 1979

79. Jessel TM, Iversen LL, Cuello AC: Capsaicin-induced depletion of substance P from primary sensory neurons. *Brain Res* 152:183-188, 1978

80. Brentson GG, Berson BS: Antinociceptive effects of intraventricular or systemic administration of vasopressin in the rat. *Life Sci* 26:455-459, 1980

81. Bodnar RJ, Zimmerman EA, Nilaver G, et al: Dissociation of cold water swim and morphine analgesia in Brattleboro rats with diabetes insipidus. *Life Sci* 26:1581-1590, 1980

82. Clineschmidt BV, McGuffin JC: Neurotensin administered intracisternally inhibits responsiveness of mice to noxious stimuli. *Eur J Pharmacol* 46:395-396, 1977

83. Basbaum AI, Wall PD: Chronic changes in the response of cells in adult cat dorsal horn following partial de-afferentiation: the appearance of responding cells in a previously non-responsive region. *Brain Res* 116:181-204, 1976

84. Edds MV, Jr: Collateral nerve regeneration. *Quart Rev Biol* 28:260-276, 1953

85. Freeman LW: Return of function after complete transection of the spinal cord of the rat, cat and dog. *Ann Surg* 136:193-205, 1952

86. Murray JG, Thompson JW: Regeneration by collateral sprouting in the partially denervated superior cervical ganglion of the cat. *J Physiol (Lond)* 131:32P-33P. 1956

87. McCouch GP, Austin GM, Liu CN, et al: Sprouting as a cause of spasticity. *J Neurophysiol* 21:205-216, 1958

88. Liu CN, Chambers WW: Intraspinal sprouting of dorsal root axons. *AMA Arch Neurol Psych* 79:46-61,1958

89. Hulsebosch CE, Coggeshall RE: Quantitation of sprouting dorsal root axons. *Science* 213:1020-1021, 1981

90. Tessler AM, Goldberger ME, Murray M, et al: Lack of plasticity in somatostatin systems in cat lumbar spinal cord (abstract). *Neuroscience* 6:173, 1980

91. Foerster O: Resections of the posterior spinal nerve roots in the treatment of gastric crises and spastic paralysis. *Proc R Soc Med Lond* 4:226-246, 1911

92. Gros C, Ouaknine G, Vlahovitch B, et al: La radicotomie selective posterieure dans le traitement neurochirurgical de l'hypertonie pyramidale. *Neurochirurgie* 13:505-518, 1967

93. Austin GM, McCouch GP, Grant FC: Decrease of spasticity by physiological dorsal root rhizotomy. *Surg Forum* 8:559-562, 1957

94. Takahashi T, Otsuka M: Distribution of substance P in cat spinal cord and alteration following unilateral dorsal root section. *Jap J Pharmacol* 24(Suppl):105, 1974

95. Kerr F: Pain, a central inhibitory balance theory. *Mayo Clin Proc* 50:685-690, 1975

96. Siegfried J: Treatment of spasticity by dorsal column stimulation. *Int Rehabil Med* 2:31-34, 1980

97. Duchenne GB: De l'electrisation localisee et de son application a la pathologie et a la therapeutique. *J B Baillere* 926, 1855

98. Hufschmidt HJ: Die elektrotherapie der spastik. *Med Welt* 47:2613-2616, 1968

99. Pateisky K, Wessely P, Kifhtreiber G: Zur elektrobehandlung der spastischen gangstorung mit einem "Schrittstimulator." *Fortschr Neurol Psychiatr* 14:21-33, 1976

100. Pedersen E, Arlien-Soborg P, Grynderup V, et al: GABA derivative in spasticity (beta-(4-chloro-phenyl)-gamma-aminobutyric acid, Ciba 34, 647-Ba). *Acta Neurol Scand* 46:257-266, 1970

101. Pierau FK, Zimmerman P: Action of a GABA - derivative on postsynaptic potentials and membrane properties of cats' spinal motor neurons. *Brain Res* 54:376-380, 1973

102. Curtis DR, Game CJA, Johnston GAR, et al: Central effects of beta-(p-chlorophenyl)-gamma-aminobutyric acid. *Brain Res* 70:493-499, 1974

103. Davies J, Watkins JC: The action of beta-phenyl-GABA derivatives on neurons of the cat cerebral cortex. *Brain Res* 70:501-505, 1974

104. Tolonen U, Myllya V, Hokkanen E: Treatment of spasticity with Baclofen and salbutamol. *Curr Ther Res* 25:251-259, 1979

105. Sachais BA, Logue JN, Carey MS: Baclofen, a new antispastic drug. A controlled multicenter trial in patients with multiple sclerosis. *Arch Neurol* 34:422-428, 1977

106. Liversedge LA: Treatment and management of multiple sclerosis *Br Med Bull* 33(1):78-83, 1977

107. Feldman RG, Kelley-Hayes M, Conomy JP, et al: Baclofen for spasticity in multiple sclerosis. *Neurology* 28(11):1094-1098, 1978

108. Saito K, Konishi S, Otsuka M: Antagonism between Lioresal and substance P in rat spinal cord. *Brain Res* 97:177-180, 1975

109. Fotherby KJ, Morrish NJ, Ryall RW: Is Lioresal (Baclofen) an antagonist of substance P? *Brain Res* 113:210-213, 1976

110. Faden AI, Holaday JW: Naloxone treatment of endotoxic shock: stereospecificity of physiologic and pharmacologic effects in the rat. *J Pharmocol Exp Ther* 212:441-447, 1980

111. Holaday JW, Faden AI: Naloxone acts at central opiate receptors to reverse hypotension, hypothermia and hypoventilation in spinal shock. *Brain Res* 189:295-299, 1980

112. Tibbs PA, Young B, McAllister RG, et al: Studies on experimental cervical spinal cord transection. *J Neurosurg* 49:558-562, 1978

113. Yaashon D: *Spinal Injury.* New York, Appleton Century Crofts, 1978, pp 248-252

114. Ducker TB, Salcman M, Daniell HB: Experimental spinal cord trauma. III: Therapeutic effect of immobilization and pharmacologic agents. *Surg Neurol* 10:71-76, 1978

115. Faden AI, Jacobs TP, Woods M: Cardioaccelatory sites in the zona intermedia of the cat spinal cord. *Exp Neurol* 61:301-310, 1978

116. Faden AI, Jacobs TP, Mougey E, et al: Endorphins in experimental spinal injury: therapeutic effects of naloxone. *Ann Neurol* 1981 (in press)

117. Faden AI, Jacobs TP, Holaday JW: Opiate antagonist improves neurological recovery after spinal injury. *Science* 211:493-494, 1981

118. Holaday JW, Faden AI: Naloxone reversal of endotoxin hypotension suggests a role of endorphins in shock. *Nature* 275:450-451, 1978

119. Faden AI, Jacobs TP, Holaday JW: Comparison of early and late naloxone treatment in experimental spinal injury (submitted to Neurology).

Figure 2. A schematic representation of the descending pain inhibitory systems. The ventral periaqueductal gray matter (*PAG*) activates the nucleus raphe magnus (*NRM*), which projects through the dorsolateral funiculus (*DLF*) and inhibits nociceptive neurons in the dorsal horn. Serotonin (*S*) is possibly the transmitter involved. The PAG is tonically inhibited by noradrenergic neurons probably arising in the A1-3 nuclei of the medulla. The nucleus reticularis magnocellularis (*NRMc*) inhibits dorsal-horn nociceptive neurons either by a direct spinal projection using an unknown transmitter (*X*), possibly noradrenalin, or by a secondary connection to noradrenergic neurons (*N*) projecting from such sites as locus ceruleus (*LC*), the parabrachial nuclei (*PBN*), the A1-3 nuclei, or nucleus reticularis lateralis (*NRL*). The mesencephalic lateral reticular formation (*LRF*) also inhibits spinal nociceptive transmission but its connections are not known. The PAG and NRM are activated by ascending nociceptive fibers in either the spinothalamic (*STT*) or spino-reticulothalamic (*SRTT*) tracts through either direct collaterals, or collaterals which relay in the nucleus reticularis gigantocellularis (*NRGc*). Nociceptive fibers also inhibit the dorsal raphe nucleus (*DRN*) thereby removing its inhibitory influence on the PAG.

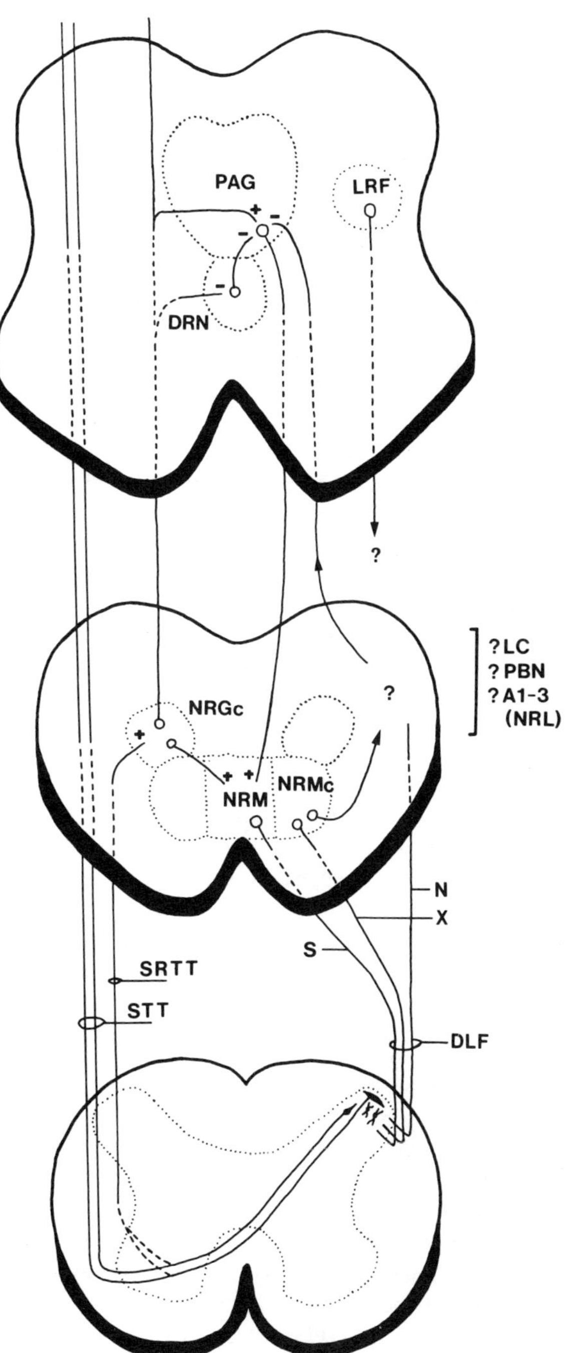

An inhibitory noradrenergic innervation of the NRM has been described such that the injection of α-antagonists into the NRM produces hypalgesia (32, 33). The origin of this noradrenergic innervation is not known. It is apparently not the locus ceruleus but may be among the A1-3 nuclei of the medulla (33).

The inhibitory effects of electrical stimulation of the PAG and NRM on medullary dorsal-horn units in the trigeminal subnucleus caudalis have been studied in detail (17), as has the effect of NRM stimulation on lumbosacral spinothalamic-tract neurons (34). At both trigeminal and lumbosacral levels, wide dynamic-range and nociceptive-specific neurons were inhibited, and, as well, trigeminal low-threshold mechanoreceptive neurons were inhibited.

However, the effect of PAG or NRM stimulation is not nociceptive specific. The responses of both wide dynamic-range and low-threshold mechanoreceptive neurons to innocuous stimuli are also inhibited (17, 34) as too are dorsal-column neurons (31, 34, 35). Thus the PAG-NRM system may not be a specific nociceptive negative-feedback loop but part of a more general sensory-discriminating system.

While the capacity of electrical stimulation of the PAG-NRM system to inhibit pain is well accepted, it is the pharmacology of this system which has been most severely challenged in recent studies. In particular its role in morphine analgesia and the involvement of serotonin as a transmitter has been questioned. Duggan and coworkers (36) found that the effect of intravenous morphine on dorsal-horn nociceptive activity was more potent when spinal-cord conduction was blocked by cooling. These authors found that morphine does not inhibit pain transmission at the dorsal horn by activating descending inhibition.

Other studies have challenged the role of the PAG-NRM system in morphine analgesia more specifically. While PAG stimulation inhibits the activity of ascending nociceptive neurons, this effect is not reversed by naloxone nor is it altered by systemic administration of morphine (37). These results indicate that the PAG system inhibits nociceptive transmission by a means which does not necessarily involve endogenous opiates. While the injection of morphine into the NRM excites some of the neurons therein, the concurrent response of dorsal-horn neurons to noxious stimuli remains unaffected (38).

Destruction of the NRM by electrolysis or anesthetizing it with tetracaine produces hyperalgesia, which is consistent with a tonic pain inhibitory function for the nucleus. Neither procedure interferes with the analgesic effect of systemic morphine (39). Thus, the NRM modulates pain through a system other than that which mediates opiate analgesia. Although intravenous methysergide blocks the pain inhibitory effects of PAG stimulation (40), it does not interfere with morphine analgesia (41).

In contrast to these results, Barton and coworkers (42) have shown that destruction of the dorsolateral fasciculus does interfere with the potency of systemic morphine. Depending on the dose administered, transection of the dorsolateral funiculus reduces the effect of morphine by 30%-60%. Thus the action of morphine comprises both spinal and supraspinal components.

These results (42) appear to contradict the conclusions of Duggan and coworkers (36) who used spinal-cord cooling to block descending inhibition. It may be that spinal-cord cooling affects pathways other than those in the dorsolateral funiculus and thereby conceals the descending inhibitory effect of morphine, thus producing paradoxical results. In order to integrate the results of Barton and coworkers (42) with those studies that challenged specifically the role of the PAG-NRM system in opiate analgesia, it may have to be concluded that other descending systems are involved, for the dorsolateral funiculus transmits brain-stem axons other than those arising in the NRM (1).

The challenge to serotonin being the inhibitory transmitter released by NRM neurons onto dorsal-horn neurons comes mainly from Greirsmith and Duggan in Canberra (43). While many experiments have provided data consistent with the contention that serotonin is the transmitter, direct confirmation of this has not been achieved. Intravenous methysergide reduces both tonic supraspinal inhibition (44) and the inhibitory effects of PAG stimulation (40). Also, serotonin administered into the substantia gelatinosa does inhibit the response of nociceptive lamina V neurons, and this effect can be antagonized by methysergide injected into the same site (45). However, methysergide injected around the cell bodies of nociceptive dorsal-horn neurons, into the substantia gelatinosa, or topically applied to the spinal cord does not interfere with either tonic supraspinal inhibition or with the inhibitory effect of NRM stimulation (43). The antagonistic effects of intravenous methysergide thus appear to occur at supraspinal levels and not in the spinal cord (40, 43). The lack of antagonism at the spinal-cord level is a major limitation to the concept of serotonergically-mediated supraspinal inhibition.

While debate has continued about the pharmacology of the PAG-NRM system, other investigations have concentrated on quite separate descending pain inhibitory pathways. Serotonin depletion abolishes the analgesic effects of PAG and NRM stimulation, but it does not abolish all descending inhibitory controls (46), indicating the persistence of nonserotonergic systems. The search for these pathways has focused on noradrenergic pain inhibitory systems. The capacity of intrathecally injected noradrenalin to inhibit nociception at the spinal-cord level is well established. The inhibitory effect is mediated by α-receptors since α-blockers, but not β-blockers, reverse it (47, 48).

There is still disagreement, however, as to whether enkephalinergic interneurons are involved in noradrenergic inhibition. Some investigators (47) find it not to be reversible by naloxone, while others do (48). This difference may be a function of the experimental model used and the type of noxious stimulus employed. Inhibition of thermal pain by noradrenalin appears to be refractory to naloxone (47), that of pinch appears to be reversible (48).

The origin of descending noradrenergic-pain inhibitory systems is believed to lie in the locus ceruleus or nearby nuclei (49, 50). A locus-ceruleus origin still remains possible, but if so, the system does not mediate morphine analgesia because destruction of the locus ceruleus does not appear to interfere with morphine analgesia (51). Destruction of the nearby parabrachial nucleus, however, does appear to attenuate morphine analgesia, so this nucleus rather than the locus ceruleus itself could be the origin of spinal inhibitory noradrenergic neurons.

A nucleus involved with the descending noradrenergic system is the NRMc. Morphologically, the NRMc is continuous with the NRM (Fig. 2), and the two appear to be one anatomical unit (52); however, physiological studies differentiate the two regions. Electrical stimulation of either nucleus produces analgesia but systemic phenoxybenzamine blocks that is produced from the NRMc while NRM stimulation remains unaffected (53). Conversely, methysergide blocks NRM analgesia but not NRMc analgesia (53,). Naloxone blocks NRMc analgesia but not NRM analgesia (53, 54). The indications are that the NRMc activates an α-adrenergic inhibitory pathway, which possibly involves an enkephalinergic neuron. What is still not known is whether the NRMc inhibitory effect is mediated by the direct spinal connection of the nucleus (Fig. 2). It could also be mediated secondarily through noradrenergic neurons in the lateral reticular nuclei such as the A1 (54, 55) or the parabrachial nuclei (Fig. 2).

An interesting observation has been that, in rats, the capacity of α-adrenergic agonists to produce analgesia persists for at least 3 weeks after spinal transection, but serotonergic analgesia occurs only immediately after spinal transection and cannot be elicited after 7 days (50). These observations indicate that noradrenergic pathways act on intrinsic dorsal-horn neurons, but that serotonergic neurons require a target neuron that is destroyed by spinal transection.

Another pain inhibitory system which has been identified is one located in the mesencephalic lateral-reticular formation (LRF). Electrical stimulation of the LRF induces pain suppression in the dorsal horn, which is different both neurophysiologically and pharmacologically from that produced by PAG stimulation (7, 56). PAG stimulation decreases the slope of the frequency-response curve of dorsal-horn units, whereas LRF stimulation produces a parallel shift to the right. These results have been interpreted as indicating different spatial arrangements in the terminal synapses of the two systems in the dorsal horn. The LRF connections involve spatially separate excitatory and inhibitory synapses, which produce summation of excitatory postsynaptic potentials (EPSPs) and inhibitory postsynaptic potentials (IPSPs). The PAG connections may be adjacent or presynaptic, which produces a multiplicative effect on intensity coding. The anatomy of how the LRF system projects to the spinal cord is not known, but something is known of its pharmacology. Naloxone does not block the effect of LRF stimulation (7, 57), but the effect is partially blocked by α-antagonists. This suggests that enkephalinergic neurons are not involved and that LRF stimulation activates at least some neurons which are noradrenergic. Serotonin depletion does not block the effect of LRF stimulation (40), which excludes serotonin as a transmitter in the system and an association with the NRM.

Further studies are still required to elaborate the anatomical connections of the LRF pain inhibitory system and, indeed, of the noradrenergic system. Also, in view of the controversy surrounding the PAG-NRM system, a question still to be answered is which systems are involved in opiate analgesia.

A broader challenge, however, is the teleological reason for such a multiplicity of pain inhibitory systems. Particularly, in view of the fact that, clinically, pain does not extinguish itself by means of some form of negative feedback loop. In this context we refer to our previous contention (1) and that reiterated by Le Bars and coworkers (46, 58) that the descending inhibitory controls function to provide an inhibitory surround or contrast system which enhances the perception of an incoming painful stimulus.

Inhibition at the Dorsal Horn

The capacity of various drugs and transmitter substances to inhibit nociceptive transmission when injected into the dorsal horn is well known. The actions of serotonin and the debate as to whether it is the transmitter released by the NRM have already been discussed. Noradrenalin facilitates the response of dorsal-horn cells to innocuous stimuli but has an inhibitory effect on responses to noxious stimuli (49).

Electronmicroscopic studies are now disclosing the way in which descending serotonergic and noradrenergic neurons are connected in the dorsal horn. Both islet cells and stalked cells have been found to receive two types of endings which resemble those known to contain noradrenalin and serotonin (22). Thus the inhibitory effect of noradrenalin and serotonin on nociception may well be mediated by these cells. Other studies have focused on enkephalinergic neurons in the dorsal horn. The capacity of systemic morphine to act directly on the dorsal horn, particularly on responses to C fiber activity, has been reaffirmed (59, 60). Similarly, the inhibitory effect on nociceptive transmission of enkephalin injected into the substantia gelatinosa has been confirmed (61). A direct spinal effect of morphine has been demonstrated electrophysiologically in man (62-64).

The data of the inhibitory effect of opiates at the cellular level indicate two possible mechanisms (65). The first is a presynaptic effect causing a decrease in the amount of transmitter released by presynaptic terminals. The second is a postsynaptic effect wherein opiates impede sodium flux. This effect causes a slowing of the rise time of EPSPs, particularly those elicited by C fiber volleys. Either or both of these mechanisms may be active in the dorsal horn. The first would act on primary nociceptive afferents, while the second could act on dendrites of second-order neurons. The direct spinal actions of morphine and the location of enkephalin in the spinal cord indicate the presence of local enkephalinergic neurons. Electronmicroscopic studies have attempted to reveal these and their connections.

Hunt and coworkers (66) identified enkephalin-containing neurons in the substantia gelatinosa that synapsed on local dendrites and cell bodies in laminae I and II. However, they found only one instance of an enkephalin-containing neuron terminating on a primary afferent fiber. This result is surprising for it does not correlate with the high density of opiate receptors found on primary afferent terminals (65-68). Arguments with respect to difference of species and technique may serve to explain this anomaly. Hunt and coworkers (66) relied on the degeneration of primary afferents to identify synapses between them and enkephalin-containing neurons. They studied rats sacrificed 5-72 hours after dorsal rhizotomy. However, in the monkey, degeneration of unmyelinated fibers in lamina II started 2 days after rhizotomy and reached a peak at about 7 days (15). Thus, the failure to observe connections between enkephalin-containing neurons and primary afferents may have been due to the premature sacrifice of the animals.

Another study has revealed that the majority of enkephalin-containing neurons lies in lamina I (69), and the authors inferred that propriospinal (association) marginal neurons, rather than substantia gelatinosa neurons, were the principal enkephalinergic cells of the dorsal horn. Although not studied directly, a variety of possible connections of these cells was postulated (Fig. 1). These included axoaxonic and dendroaxonic synapses with primary nociceptive afferents, axodendritic and dendrodendritic connections between marginal cells, and connections to neurons in deeper laminae of the dorsal horn.

GABA has also been implicated as an inhibitory transmitter in dorsal-horn neurons. The ultrastructure of GABA-containing neurons resembles that of islet cells, which has led to the interpretation that islet cells are inhibitory neurons (22, 23). Significantly both the dendrites and axons of islet cells appear to contain GABA.

A striking aspect of the observed (22) and postulated (69) anatomy of interneurons in the superficial dorsal horn is the large number of dendrodendritic and dendroaxonic synapses they form in addition to their efferent axonic connections (Fig. 1). Each cell receives multiple inputs and has multiple axonic and dendritic efferent connections. Moreover, as postulated by Gobel and coworkers (22), the release of transmitter at different dendrites or the axon probably depends on differing interactions or sum-

mations of EPSPs from the several afferent inputs to the cell. The actions of these interneurons, therefore, are likely to be diverse and complex and they cannot be regarded as simple intercalated neurons responding uniformly and uniquely to one form of stimulus or to one transmitter. The circuitry underlying inhibition in the dorsal horn will probably prove to be very complex. Many more meticulous electron microscope studies, correlating physiological and pharmacological data, are required before the picture is complete.

Substance P and Other Peptides

Several authors have reviewed the evidence favoring the concept that substance P is the transmitter released by nociceptive afferent fibers and that these fibers are subject to presynaptic inhibition by enkephalinergic neurons (67, 68, 70). The concept (Fig. 3) is based on the facts that substance P is contained in small-diameter myelinated and unmyelinated fibers; it is released from these fibers by a Ca^{2+} dependent mechanism, which can be activated by either K+ or stimulation of Aδ and C fibers; opiate receptors are found on primary afferents and morphine or enkephalin inhibit the release of substance P both in vitro and in vivo; and capsaicin, which depletes substance P in primary afferents, produces analgesia (67, 68, 70).

Recent studies have elaborated this concept to the extent that substance P appears to mediate only certain types of pain. In one study (71) depletion of substance P by capsaicin in rats markedly raised their threshold for pressure pain and chemically-induced pain but sometimes lowered or did not change their threshold for heat pain. In another study (72), iontophoretic application of a substance P analogue onto nociceptive dorsal-horn neurons mimicked the effect of intra-arterial bradykinin but not that of noxious pinch. Thus, substance P appears to predominantly mediate both pressure-induced and chemically-induced pain but not that due to pinch or heat.

In contrast to the predominant evidence supporting the role of substance P as a

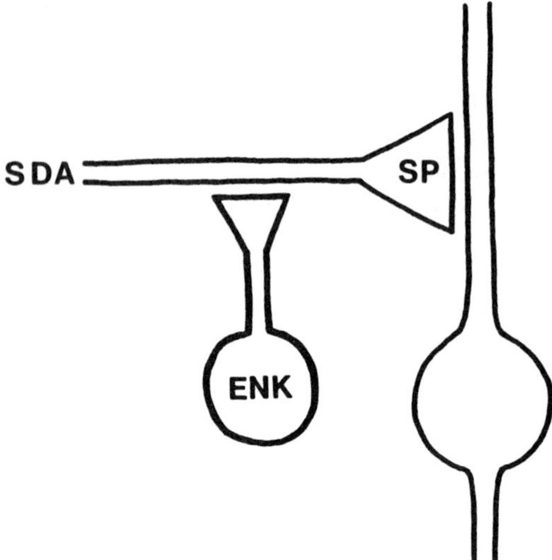

Figure 3. A schematic representation of the proposed interaction between substance P (*SP*) containing neurons and enkephalinergic (*ENK*) neurons. SP neurons excite the dendrites of second-order nociceptive neurons but are subject to presynaptic inhibition by ENK neurons.

nociceptive transmitter substance, challenges to this concept have been raised on three fronts. Anatomically, electronmicroscopic studies have still to demonstrate enkephalin containing terminals synapsing on substance P containing terminals.

Neurophysiologically, it has been argued that since substance P has a slow time course of action, it is unlikely to be a true transmitter substance but more likely a neuromodulator (73). This objection, however, has been countered with the explanation that the slow time course may be a technical artifact due to the low transport number of substance P and a delay in its release from microelectrodes (67). Furthermore, the long duration of action of substance P may be the basis for the prolonged after-discharge exhibited by second-order neurons following C-fiber stimulation (65). Thus substance P still remains a candidate for distinction as a true transmitter.

Pharmacologically, the role of substance P has been challenged because its iontophoretic application in the substantia gelatinosa failed to excite nociceptive lamina V neurons (74). However, contrary evidence has recently become available (61). This evidence however did not completely vindicate a role for substance P because, although it enhanced the response of some nociceptive neurons, it depressed that of others. Thus, the pharmacological evidence about the role of substance P is inconclusive, but it may indicate a role that is more diverse than is currently believed.

Other peptides, such as neurotensin, somatostatin, and vasoactive intestinal peptide, are known to be present in primary afferent fibers (6, 75), but their role in nociception has remained largely unstudied. Neurotensin is distributed in the spinal cord in a manner similar to that of enkephalin. It is a potent analgesic, but this has been established only by using intraventricular injections (76). Cholecystokinin, another peptide found in primary afferents, has been shown to postsynaptically activate neurons in laminae I to VII of the dorsal horn, both in vivo and in vitro. The effect, however, was not nociceptive-specific for it was exerted on all categories of units (77).

THERAPEUTIC APPLICATIONS

Transcutaneous Nerve Stimulation

Each year that passes brings with it further papers attesting to the efficacy of transcutaneous nerve stimulation (TNS) in the treatment of pain. The efficacy of this mode of therapy by now must be recognized but so, too, should its limitations.

TNS is of some benefit in postoperative pain where it decreases the need for analgesics but does not replace them (78-82). It has a comparable efficacy for musculoskeletal pain following acute spinal-cord injury (83). In chronic-pain states results are better when electrodes can be interposed between the site of origin of pain and the neuraxis (79, 84). In other situations, results are less rewarding. Regardless of initial success the efficacy of TNS wanes with continued use. This has been particularly illustrated by Bates and Nathan (85) who reported their 7-year experience using TNS on 235 patients suffering from postherpetic neuralgia, back pain, spinal pain, stump pain, neuropathy, and assorted other "neurological" pains. Irrespective of diagnosis about one-third of their patients failed to receive any benefit from an initial trial of TNS. Of those patients who initially responded to the therapy, 70% were still using their device after 4 weeks, but by 32 weeks only a third and by 2 years only a fifth were still obtaining satisfactory relief. Only a small proportion of patients gave up stimulation because their pain ceased or because of allergic reaction to the electrode adhesives. Results were particularly poor in patients with thalamic syndrome, pain in the face, and painful scars. Long-term results were marginally better than average for patients with postherpetic neuralgia. Bates and Nathan (85) included in their paper a helpful discussion of various practical and technical aspects of the use of TNS. They concluded that about 50% of patients with chronic pain can be expected to obtain relief for about 1-2 weeks, but 25% obtain continuous pain relief to a far greater degree than from any other method of therapy.

The mechanism by which TNS works is still debated. Some favor a peripheral mechanism whereby the excitability and conduction velocity of peripheral nerves are impaired by TNS (86). Others favor a central mechanism, for microneurographic studies of peripheral nerves reveal no significant change in the neurogram during TNS (87). In rats, the analgesic effect of TNS has been shown to be reversible by naloxone and attenuated by either serotonin depletion or spinal cord transection. This indicates both segmental and supraspinal mechanisms of central inhibition (88). In pain-free individuals TNS raises cerebrospinal fluid (CSF) β-endorphin levels, suggesting a possible humoral mechanism or a central nervous system (CNS) effect rostral to the brain stem (89).

Allied to TNS is the use of epidural stimulation with either implanted devices or, as in recent years, percutaneously inserted wires. As with TNS, the efficacy of these devices wanes with time. In one study of amputees with stump pain good results decreased from 54.2% after 2 years to 39% after 5 years (90). In another study results in the treatment of pain in paraplegic patients proved disappointing, but 4 out of 7 patients with pain from a peripheral neuroma

continued to receive satisfying relief after 1 year of stimulation (91). Technical problems are still the major source of failures with epidural stimulation (1). Despite this, it must be viewed as a worthwhile, if only a temporary, therapeutic option for intractable pain.

Brain stimulation at either mesodiencephalic or thalamic sites continues to be evaluated (79), but there have been no major reports since our previous review (1). The trend appears to be that somatic pain such as that due to malignancy responds better to periventricular grey-matter stimulation while central pains such as deafferentation pain (see below) are more responsive to thalamic or internal capsule stimulation (79, 92).

Ablative Neurosurgery

Techniques such as spinothalamic tractotomy are well established as a treatment for pain, particularly in malignancy. Sweet (93) has reviewed a variety of other, and sometimes bewildering, techniques which have been investigated. These include limited frontal leukotomy, thalamotomy (at the centrum medianum or parafascicularis nuclei), pulvinotomy, thalamolaminotomy, amygdalotomy, frontothalamic tractotomy, posteromedial hypothalamotomy, and hypothalamotomy at the periventricular nuclei. Each of these has been reported to achieve noteworthy success rates but without detailed follow-up.

A striking feature of these procedures is that, although chronic pain may be relieved, the lesions do not interfere with somatic sensation nor do they affect perception of new or acute pain. Thus, rather than interrupting a pain transmission pathway, they may well be affecting the neural circuits that mediate the affective, suffering component of chronic pain.

In view of our minimal knowledge about telencephalic involvement in pain, these techniques may appear unsoundly based. Conversely, they may serve to provide insight into the role of higher centers in the pain experience.

Acupuncture

With the explosion of research into pain

physiology, acupuncture has found a potential substrate for its action. The mechanism of acupuncture has been loosely lodged in the maze of descending-pain inhibitory systems and related to opiate analgesia (2, 94). The correlating evidence is that acupuncture raises CSF endorphin levels, and its effect can be blocked by naloxone (79, 94-96) or by lesions in the PAG or limbic system (95). Some investigators view this evidence as circumstantial and unsatisfactory (97). In particular, naloxone reversibility does not necessarily indicate enkephalin or endorphin-mediated mechanisms (98). Moreover, in some instances naloxone does not reverse acupuncture analgesia (99).

Regardless of mechanism, an important aspect of acupuncture is the evaluation of its efficacy and the tempering of exaggerated claims. Wall and Woolf (97) list some of the trials which have revealed only temporary relief. A recent study of acupuncture therapy for low-back pain by a group enthusiastic about its value revealed only a modest reduction in pain compared to controls (100).

Thus acupuncture, which resembles the effect of TNS, is likely to become only another therapeutic modality that may afford some benefit to some patients but that does not have a reliable or predictable success rate.

Epidural Morphine

The discovery, in animal experiments, of a direct spinal action of morphine invited the use of morphine intrathecally or epidurally as a therapeutic technique in man. Epidural application has become the preferred route since it avoids the possible complications and side effects of dural puncture. Reports on the use of epidural morphine have been numerous in the last year, but so too have been warnings about side effects.

Epidural morphine has been successfully used in the treatment of multiple fractured ribs (101), ischemic rest pain (102), and as a perioperative analgesic (103). There are differing reports as to its efficacy in postoperative analgesia. After prostatectomy, epidural morphine produced a longer-lasting analgesia than bupivacaine and

without the complication of hypotension (104). Successful analgesia with epidural morphine has been reported in one case after an orthopedic operation (105) and in 66% of patients undergoing a variety of operations (106). Caudally injected epidural morphine, however, did not relieve postoperative pain in patients undergoing hemorrhoidectomy (106). Epidural or intrathecal morphine seems to be effective in early labor (107, 108) but not in established labor (107, 109, 110), after cesarean section (110), or after hysterectomy (111). In terminal care of patients with malignancy, epidural morphine can be a worthwhile adjunct, but tolerance develops after about 10 days of continued use (112).

One study of a heterogeneous group of patients with pain reported a good result in 56% of patients (113). The most favorable results were obtained in patients with multiple rib fractures and ischemic pain. About one-half of the patients with malignancy or low-back pain responded well enough to allow other analgesics to be withdrawn or considerably reduced. Labor pains during abortion were well relieved. In keeping with the other studies mentioned above, the pains of full-term labor were not. Poor results were obtained in patients with causalgia. Another study (114) described long-lasting relief following 2 mg epidural morphine in 11 patients with assorted painful complaints, mainly postoperative pain. Further observations by the same author (115) established in normal volunteers that the principal action of epidural morphine was at the spinal cord level and that it lacked the side effects of intramuscular morphine.

While some authors have encountered no side effects (106, 114) or an infrequent (5%) incidence of mild side effects (113), there have been reports of serious complications such as respiratory depression (116), a high incidence of nausea and vomiting in obstetric patients (107, 110, 117), and of severe itching (107, 117, 118). Although preservatives were suspected as the cause of this itching, it has also followed the use of preservative-free morphine sulphate (117, 118). A report from Iceland, based on a single case study, maintained that the itching was dose-related (119).

As is the fashion in the field of pain therapy, a promising technique (in this case epidural morphine) after further investigation, finds its application limited to certain conditions and not others. Also, its use is possibly seriously restricted by untoward side effects.

SPECIFIC NEUROLOGICAL CONDITIONS

Deafferentation Pain

Deafferentation pain refers to those pain states produced by destruction of peripheral nerves or pain pathways in the CNS. As we reviewed previously (1), the mechanism of deafferentation pain appears to depend on alteration in the spontaneous activity and responsiveness of neurons which are disconnected from their normal afferent input. Supersensitivity of deafferented neurons to substance P has been postulated as a possible component of this mechanism (70).

Three recent papers have provided further insight into the clinical features and mechanism of deafferentation pain. One of these, a clinical study, examined the features of pain in 275 patients after brachial plexus injury (120). Only 108 of these patients suffered pain, notably those whose avulsion was proximal to the dorsal root ganglion. None of those with avulsions distal to the ganglion complained of pain. The patients reported two types of pain: all were subject to a background pain most commonly described as burning, with some degree of paresthesia or electric-shock sensation; 87 patients had superimposed paroxysms of sharp pain. There was a good correlation between the site of pain and the affected dermatomes. The pains were particularly intractable to drug therapy and various surgical procedures. TNS was of considerable benefit, but only in about one-third of patients. Significantly the pains were worsened by worry and emotional stress, but conversely were lessened by distraction. Absorption in work was the single most effective measure that reduced pain. On the basis of this observation the authors recommended early return to work as a critical component of management.

A form of deafferentation syndrome has been experimentally induced and studied in monkeys. Levitt and Levitt (121) observed that division of a spinothalamic tract produced a syndrome consisting of variable degrees of contralateral hypalgesia coupled with bizarre behavior involving self-mutilation of the affected limb. The behavior was presumed to be evoked by dysesthesias arising in the affected limb. Since the causative injury was located in the spinal cord, the syndrome could not be attributed to peripheral mechanisms such as neuromata, nor could it be ascribed a psychosomatic origin. The onset of the syndrome was about 1 week after injury, a period comparable with that required for orthograde tract degeneration. Accordingly, the authors felt that the syndrome was caused by altered function of relay nuclei such as the ventralis posterolateralis (VPL) nucleus of the thalamus. The syndrome occurred only after contralateral lesions of the spinothalamic tract and not at all after ipsilateral or bilateral lesions, indicating that persistence of ipsilateral pain pathways was necessary for its production.

Tasker and coworkers (92) reviewed various surgical aspects of deafferentation pain in man including the literature indicating denervation supersensitivity at various sites in the CNS. Whereas local anesthetic blockade of nerves proximal to the site of injury nearly always relieved symptoms, subsequent destructive surgical procedures such as neurotomy, cordotomy, and thalamotomy rarely achieved long-lasting relief. On the other hand, neural stimulation appears to offer better prospects of pain control. Stimulation of peripheral nerves, spinal cord, centrocaudal thalamus, or the internal capsule more frequently control deafferentation pain than PAG, mesodiencephalic or NRM stimulation.

From their experience in performing stereotactic procedures on patients with pain, Tasker and coworkers (92) provided new data about the neurophysiological changes that occur in some pain states. In patients with deafferentation pain, various sites were identified in the medial midbrain medial to the neospinothalamic tract, which were four times more sensitive to electrical stimulation than in patients with somatic cancer pain. Electrical stimulation at these sites produced a burning sensation or reproduced the quality of the patients' natural pain. On the basis of these observations, the authors postulated that as a result of deafferentation "mesencephalic-reticulothalamic-cortical circuits become sensitive not only to electrical stimulation but also to natural neural input, causing constant reproduction of the patient's pain."

One consequence of these observations is that neurophysiological correlates can be identified with the often bizarre complaints reported by patients with deafferentation pain. This makes it less acceptable to dismiss the complaints as simply of psychosomatic origin.

Causalgia

The IASP Subcommittee on Taxonomy has defined causalgia as a "syndrome of sustained burning pain after a traumatic nerve lesion combined with vasomotor and sudomotor dysfunction and later trophic changes" (122). Qualitatively, the pain of causalgia is like that of deafferentation pain, but causalgia is distinguished by apparent changes in sympathetic activity. The mechanism of causalgia is believed to be a deafferentation pain in which sympathetic activity sensitizes the endings of intact peripheral nerves, the afferent activity of which facilitates and perpetuates the abnormal activity set up in deafferented neurons (1).

Previous studies have demonstrated the sensitizing effect of noradrenalin and sympathetic activity in causalgia, and Loh and coworkers (123) have further elaborated their observations. Regional intravenous infusion of guanethidine relieved the pain and hyperpathia of 30 patients within about 20 minutes of the infusion, lasting between 3-24 hours. Six of the patients had sustained relief for 6 months or more. Relief of pain did not correlate with changes in peripheral circulation, and the observed vasodilation appeared most likely to be due to a direct effect of the guanethidine rather than to inhibition of vasomotor nerves. Relief of pain was interpreted as being due to the inhibition of

release of noradrenalin onto intact peripheral nerve endings. This was consistent with the sensitizing and facilitating role of the sympathetic nervous system in causalgic states.

Traditionally, causalgia has been a diagnosis reserved for pain following traumatic nerve injury, but many of the clinical features of causalgia occur in other pain states in which nerve injury is absent or not apparent. The latter have been referred to as reflex sympathetic dystrophy or minor causalgia (124) and include conditions such as Sudeck's atrophy and shoulder-hand syndrome. In reflex sympathetic dystrophy, the precipitating trauma appears to be a somatic injury rather than a nerve injury.

Reflex sympathetic dystrophy most commonly affects the limbs, but recently a case of diffuse reflex sympathetic dystrophy has been reported in which symptoms were distributed over the entire body (125). The syndrome was successfully managed using a series of lumbar sympathetic and stellate ganglion blocks.

The association between causalgia and reflex sympathetic dystrophy has been investigated by Tahmoush (124) who studied two groups of patients with burning pain associated with hyperalgesia and allodynia following an episode of trauma proximal to the affected part. One group had suffered the classical injury of causalgia—a penetrating missile injury to a peripheral nerve. The other group had no apparent nerve injury. Subjectively and on testing with the McGill pain questionnaire, both groups gave similar descriptions of their pain, and both had similar behavioral consequences of their pain. So, in this respect, the two groups were indistinguishable. A possible explanation may be that in reflex sympathetic dystrophy deep somatic tissues are deafferented. Another possibility is that a constant nociceptive input physiologically facilitates central neurons in a manner similar to the way in which they are sensitized by cutaneous deafferentation.

Low-Back Pain

Research activities into low-back pain have

been diverse and prolific during the last year. The high prevalence and economic cost of this complaint have been emphasized by several authors (126-129), as have the poor results of surgery in improperly selected patients (129-132). The causes of low-back pain and sciatica have been classified on the basis of their innervation into ventral disorders affecting the intervertebral disks, dorsal disorders affecting tissues innervated by the lumbar dorsal rami, and disorders directly affecting the spinal nerves (133).

The intervertebral disks are innervated by the sinuvertebral nerves, and by branches of the ventral rami and grey rami communicantes (134). Mechanical disorders such as strain of the annulus fibrosus or longitudinal ligaments can cause primary pain mediated by these nerves [see (133)]. Such pains known as discogenic or primary disk pain do not involve compression of the spinal nerve or nerve roots.

Structures innervated by the lumbar dorsal rami can also be a potent source of low-back pain and referred pain in the lower limbs (133, 135). The lumbar zygapophyseal joints are currently the popular nidus for such pains (135, 136).

Although compression of nerve roots has traditionally been held to be the cause of sciatica, Howe (137) and Loeser (129) have both reiterated their earlier collaborative work in which they demonstrated that compression of normal nerve roots did not produce pain. They found that compression of dorsal-root ganglia or damaged nerve roots produced neural activity consistent with their being a source of pain.

On a different but related tack, a pathological study has revealed that spondylolisthesis of a vertebra is always accompanied by a rotatory deformity. The rotation draws a pedicle dorsally, so that it can stretch the subadjacent nerve roots. Such a phenomenon may explain certain myelographic defects, which apparently demonstrate disk protrusion, although laminectomy reveals no such protrusion (138).

A preliminary report was published of a novel procedure for the diagnosis of lumbar radiculopathy (139). Ultrasonic stimulation of lumbosacral nerve roots produced both local pain and pain that radiated to the buttocks of 11 patients who had lumbosacral radiculopathy. In a control group of 13 asymptomatic volunteers only 1 reported radiating pain. Although this technique could not determine the precise segmental level of involvement, the authors felt that it could in the future provide a noninvasive method of screening for lumbar radiculopathy.

An excellent review of diagnostic radiology in low-back pain (136) points out that plain x-rays have little to offer as a screening tool for nonspecific back pain but advocates provocation radiology as an alternative. In these techniques the radiologist, using fluoroscopic control, localizes a stimulus to various structures in the spine and records the characteristics of the pain response. In essence it is as if a needle were substituted for the examining finger to elicit tenderness and pain from impalpable structures.

Structures which can be so investigated include the intervertebral disks and zygapophyseal joints. In patients with primary disk pain, the injection of normal saline or contrast medium into the disk reproduces the patient's pain. Disk lesions diagnosed in this way can then be treated surgically. Significant observations made during the use of this technique have been that symptomatic disks are not necessarily the most abnormal on plain radiographs, and that different disks may be responsible for different components of a patient's complaints (136).

Zygapophyseal joints can be stimulated by injections of hypertonic saline and anesthetized with intra-articular local anesthetic. Exacerbation of pain by hypertonic saline and its relief by local anesthetic strongly implicates the particular joint as the cause of pain. Provocation radiology provides an objective means of assessing the source of a patient's pain. Its disadvantages are that it is time consuming and must be done systematically and meticulously. Its advantages, however, are that the source of a patient's pain can be directly identified and not just inferred. Other investigations, such as myelography, reveal only the morphology and not the source of pain, and have high false-negative and false-positive rates. Although scientifically attractive, what remains to be established is whether provocation radiology can lead to improved therapeutic results.

A controlled trial has shown that dry needling of muscle motor points (a form of acupuncture) improved the status of patients with musculoskeletal back pain and increased their capacity to return to work (140). A limited controlled trial confirmed that hard beds aided low-back pain but that water beds were an alternative (141).

Lumbar medial-branch neurotomy has been advocated as a technique for treating disorders mediated by the medial branches of the lumbar dorsal rami (142). Ignelzi and Cummings (143) obtained an overall success rate of 41.3% in 61 patients treated in this manner. Follow-up at 2 years revealed significant improvement in activity levels and reduced narcotic usage despite a trend towards recurrence of pain. One limitation of this study was that patients were not selected on the basis of local anesthetic blocks of the nerves that indeed mediated the patients' symptoms. Another limitation was the omission of a comparison of the progress of patients who did respond to those who did not. This comparison would exclude the effect of natural progress or resolution of the complaint. Although the authors (143) concluded favorably about their procedure, more thorough clinical trials are required before the value of lumbar medial branch neurotomy can be defended.

The technique of chemonucleolysis has been reviewed by Graham (144) who, on the basis of pooled results, attests to a successful response to 70% of over 14,000 injections. Comparable success rates have also been reported in separate but much smaller series (145, 146). The issue of chemonucleolysis is still contentious, and its use is still not approved in the United States; however, a meticulously designed, multicenter double-blind controlled study is currently being performed, the results of which may finally determine the true efficacy of the technique.

Among negative results have been the failure of sympathetic blocks to influence low-back pain (147) and a sobering study of the use of epidural injections (148). Studying a series of 304 patients who underwent combined injections of local anesthetic and steroids, White and coworkers (148) found an initially high success rate but one which waned rapidly after 2 weeks to the extent that only 7% of patients were still relieved at 6 months. Patients with histories of pain shorter than 2 weeks fared marginally better and those with detectable psychological overlay fared much worse. White and coworkers (148) emphasized the temporary effect of epidural injections, and their study illustrates the importance of thorough continuing evaluation of results in the treatment of low-back pain.

The problem of lumbar adhesive arachnoiditis has again received attention. Since its pathology consists of scarring and ischemia of nerve roots in the absence of skeletal lesions, it may well become a problem more frequently referred to neurologists and neurosurgeons. The clinical features of this condition are persisting low-back pain and radicular pain with variable neurological signs. The most strongly implicated causes are myelography and surgery (1). To date, effective therapy has been lacking.

Benoist and coworkers (149) studied 38 patients in whom massive epidural scarring with no coexistent pathological condition was confirmed at operation. Diagnostically, they found myelography unreliable. Therapeutically, only 19 of their patients responded to excision of the scar tissue. The authors argued that reaccumulation of scar or concomitant subarachnoid adhesions possibly accounted for the failures. Alternatively, injury to the nerve-root axons may have been irreversible. Another possible explanation not considered by the authors is ischemia of the nerve roots. The blood supply to the lumbosacral nerve roots is tenuous and easily damaged during back surgery. No excision of epidural scar tissue will be successful if the blood supply to an ischemic root is not restored.

Hoppenstein (150) has advocated a new approach to the management of lumbar adhesive arachnoiditis and has reported a 72% success rate at short-term follow-up (9-30 months) in 26 patients. He screened patients with multiple selective spinal nerve blocks to identify the levels responsible for symptoms. If fewer than three nerves were implicated in the production of symptoms, he proceeded to microsurgical dorsal-root rhizotomies in which not more than two consecutive roots were severed. Although this approach is a positive contribution towards the management of an intractable condition, the conservatives and sceptics will await longer-term evaluation and satisfaction that deafferentation pains do not follow such rhizotomies.

Prevention of lumbar arachnoiditis is probably the most rewarding option at present and several papers have dealt with this aspect. In both animal (151, 152) and clinical (152) trials free fat grafts covering the lumbar nerve roots were found to be superior than other barriers in preventing postlaminectomy adhesions. Another group (153) has advocated a silicone implant called the lumbar shield.

Cervical Pain

Research activities into cervical pain have been few in the past year. A study of acute cervical pain (154) confirmed the general opinion that such pains generally subside within 1 to 2 weeks with the use of a collar and rest. TNS significantly reduced pain and hastened the restoration of cervical mobility. Patients treated by neck mobilization also had a higher mean improvement of both pain and mobility, but the results in these patients were not statistically better than those treated with a collar and rest alone.

Injections of steroids into the offending intervertebral disk have been reported to be of benefit for neck pain (155), but only 4 out of 18 patients studied sustained good results lasting at least 3 months. About 50% of the patients sustained limited and temporary improvement of their pain. Although considered by the authors to offer an additional therapeutic modality, the success rate of this technique is probably insufficiently impressive to induce its widespread adoption.

Given the popularity of radio-frequency facet denervation for low-back pain (1, 135), one could have expected the eventual adaptation of similar techniques for cervical pain. Indeed such has occurred. Sluijter and Koetsveld-Baart (156) have described their experience with radio-frequency neurotomy in the treatment of cervical pain syndromes. Clinically, they identified an upper syndrome constituting neck pain radiating into the occipital and frontal regions and a lower syndrome of neck pain radiating into the shoulders and upper limbs. They believed the etiology of these syndromes to be either nerve-root compression or disorders of the facetal joints. To confirm this, they used either paravertebral blocks of spinal nerves or local anesthetic blocks of cervical dorsal rami. If the blocks indicated that the patient's pain was mediated by a single nerve, then radio-frequency neurotomy was carried out: selective dorsal-root ganglionolysis in the case of segmental nerves and facet denervation in the case of dorsal ramus involvement. Despite the fact that all patients treated had been relieved by the appropriate nerve block, only about 40% of patients with either upper or lower syndromes sustained good results following neurotomy. Among other possible explanations for their failures, the authors considered incomplete denervation, which is most plausible. Their techniques were not prefaced by a review of the relevant anatomy. Whether their electrodes were accurately and appropriately located is open to question, particularly at upper cervical levels. Perhaps this is due to the lack of previous detailed anatomical descriptions of the relevant nerves. However, such descriptions have now been made available (157, 158) and perhaps future therapeutic trials based on accurate surgical anatomy can produce results more impressive to the critics and more satisfying to the patients.

Neck-tongue syndrome is a disorder typically affecting young adolescents. Sudden rotatory movements of the head precipitate attacks of pain in the occipital region associated with a sensation of numbness in the ipsilateral half of the tongue and sometimes in the occipital region (159). Recent anatomical studies have demonstrated the probable mechanism of this syndrome (160). The C_2 ventral ramus, which carries proprioceptive fibers from the tongue, is intimately related to the dorsal aspect of the lateral atlantoaxial joint and supplies articular branches to it. The symptoms of neck-tongue syndrome can be explained on the basis that an abnormal rotatory movement of the head causes a temporary subluxation of an atlantoaxial joint which produces local pain by straining the joint capsule. This also produces sensory changes in the tongue and upper neck or occipital region by stretching the C_2 ventral ramus over one or the other of the subluxated articular processes.

HEADACHE AND FACIAL PAIN

Headache may be considered as symptomatic when there is an identifiable organic cause and idiopathic or essential when no underlying structural change can be demonstrated. In the essential group, certain entities such as classic migraine and cluster headache can be clearly separated on clinical grounds when their presentation is typical, even though their pathophysiology is incompletely understood. The lines of demarcation between common migraine, tension-vascular headache, tension headache, and ordinary headache are less clear, and there has been considerable discussion as to whether these conditions are separable on grounds other than arbitrary clinical definition. The problem of definition is compounded when some migrainous patients develop a cyclical pattern (161) or other features usually associated with cluster headache, or who experience attacks that on some occasions would be considered as classic migraine and on other occasions as common migraine.

This review expands and brings up to date previous articles by one or both authors (1, 162). Recent observations on headaches of organic origin are discussed first before an attempt is made to discuss idiopathic headaches. For the background to headache problems not discussed here, the reader is referred to recent monographs (163-165).

Disease of the Extracranial Arteries

Temporal arteritis affects women, mostly 55 years or older, four times as frequently as men and is associated with polymyalgia rheumatica in about 25% of cases. In 50% of patients with polymyalgia, temporal artery biopsy shows evidence of arteritis (166). Autopsy studies of patients dying in the acute phase of temporal arteritis have shown that the superficial temporal, vertebral, ophthalmic, and posterior ciliary arteries are those most severely affected (167). Patterns of immunoglobulin deposition which were not present in the arteries of control subjects have been demonstrated in temporal arteries, although it is not clear whether they originated from circulating immune complexes or were antibodies to degenerating elastin in the arterial wall (168). The temporal artery is usually involved throughout its length but unaffected segments (skip lesions) were found in 17 of 60 patients reported by Klein and coworkers (169) and can account for false-negative biopsy reports. In such cases, the temporal arteries were normal to palpation in 65% compared with only 23% of those with continuous involvement.

Impairment of vision is said to occur in 50% of untreated cases (166, 169) but with early diagnosis and corticosteroid therapy, the figure is reduced to 13% (169). Claudication of the jaw muscles was a symptom in 28 of 42 patients studied over a period of 25 years (170). In this series, patients required corticosteroid therapy from 1-77 months (mean 7 months). Perhaps the most common reason for the diagnosis being missed is that a normal erythrocyte sedimentation rate (ESR) is mistakenly considered to exclude the diagnosis of temporal arteritis. Approximately 30% of biopsy-confirmed patients have an ESR of 40 mm/hour or less (171). Death may be caused early in the course of the disease from brain-stem infarction (172). Visual loss and the need for continuation of a high maintenance dose of steroids is associated with a shortened life span. Of surviving patients, the disease remitted in approximately one-third after a period of 6 months to 7 years, while one-third remained stable on steroid medication and one-third relapsed in spite of steroid therapy (172).

Carotidynia is a descriptive term rather than an entity. Carotid pain and tenderness may occur in migraine, viral infections, temporal arteritis, and other conditions. It has also been reported as a symptom of long intraluminal clots in the internal carotid artery (173) and of dissecting aneurysm involving the arterial wall (174). An elongated styloid process may sometimes give rise to pain in the cheek, chin, or neck along the distribution of the carotid artery [Eagle's syndrome] (175).

Pain from the Cranial Nerves

Excessive stimulation of the trigeminal nerve by diving into cold water, for example, or of the glossopharyngeal nerve by swallowing a bolus of ice cream can cause headache. A vascular mechanism could be responsible for some cases of ice-cream headache since frontal pain may take 25 seconds or more to develop after swallowing ice water or ice cream and is associated with a drop in forehead temperature of 1°C (176). Vascular involvement may account for the fact that ice-cream headache had been experienced by 93% of migrainous patients, compared with 31% of the members of a control group (177).

Peripheral receptors or affected cranial nerves may be distended by tumor, aneurysm, or granuloma. The first division of the trigeminal nerve can be compromised by orbital granuloma [Tolasa-Hunt syndrome] (178), pericarotid lesions (Raeder's para-trigeminal neuralgia), and by osteomyelitis or neoplasm affecting the apex of the petrous temporal bone (Gradenigo's syndrome).

The etiology of trigeminal neuralgia remains controversial despite mounting evidence that the majority of cases are caused by compression of the trigeminal root by aberrant vessels in the posterior fossa. Haines and coworkers (179) examined the trigeminal nerves in 20 cadavers of patients known to have been free of trigeminal neuralgia. Of the 40 nerves, 14 were in contact with an artery but only 4 of these were distorted by it. An additional four nerves were compressed by veins. In contrast, of 40 trigeminal nerves surgically exposed for the treatment of trigeminal neuralgia, 31 were compressed by adjacent arteries and 8 by veins. Kerr (180) pointed out that there is somatotopic

representation of the three divisions in the trigeminal ganglion but not in the root. This suggests that the former is more likely to be the site of origin of trigeminal neuralgia, since trigger points are usually found around the nose and mouth. This does not seem to be sufficient reason to postulate compression of the ganglion by the internal carotid artery, for example, because trigger points are situated in the central facial area which is innervated solely by the trigeminal nerve. The more peripheral parts of the face receive overlapping innervation from cervical roots (181).

Experimental demyelination of the trigeminal root in cats and monkeys happens about 3 weeks after the insertion of sutures through the root. At this time, the nerve was found to be hyperexcitable (182). Multiple discharges were evoked by a single stimulus and after-discharges by afferent volleys. Action potentials, which were generated at the site of the lesion, were enhanced by hyperventilation and suppressed by diphenyl-hydantoin. Such lesions could be caused in the peripheral or central trigeminal pathways of man by vascular or other compression or by primary demyelination as in multiple sclerosis.

Clinical reports of trigeminal neuralgia include an extraordinary case in which the trigger point was located not in the face but in the right index finger (183). A possible explanation lies in the convergent inputs to the nucleus caudalis of the descending or spinal nucleus of the trigeminal nerve from the upper limb (17). Trigeminal neuralgia may be secondary to trigeminal neuropathy. An instance recently reported was associated with vascular headaches, both apparently caused by sickle cell disease (184). The surgical management of trigeminal neuralgia includes decompression of the nerve by a posterior fossa approach and thermocoagulation of the trigeminal ganglion (1). Medical management has recently been improved by the addition of baclofen to the list of agents which suppress trigeminal neuralgia (186).

Intracranial Causes of Headache

A recent onset of headache or increasing severity of headache always arouses the suspicion of a space-occupying lesion, but there are occasional reports of the diagnosis being missed when events move swiftly, particularly with an acute extradural or subdural hematoma or when the cerebrospinal fluid pathways are blocked by a lesion such as colloid cyst of the third ventricle. In this case a headache history of only a few weeks' duration may precede coning and sudden death unless the condition is recognized and treated promptly (185).

Cough headache is caused by a transient increase in intracranial pressure. Normally intrathoracic and intra-abdominal pressure increases during coughing, thus causing a pressure wave to be transmitted from spinal to cranial CSF and back again. If there is intermittent obstruction in the CSF pathways, the rebound of the pressure wave may be prevented by a valve effect, causing a craniospinal dissociation of pressure. Cough headache may be symptomatic of a cerebral tumor or may be caused by a type I Arnold-Chiari malformation (187). Other causes prove to be benign in the sense that they do not require surgical intervention.

The incidence of post-lumbar puncture headache is thought to be reduced by using a small gauge needle and resting the patient prone or with the head tilted downwards after the procedure. Suggestion may play some part since headache was reported 24 hours after lumbar puncture by 7 out of 15 patients who were told to expect a headache compared with 1 out of 13 who were not warned (188). This study would not include those patients who develop headache more than 24 hours afterwards from continued CSF leakage. A low pressure headache and syncope has been reported in a patient with a pseudomeningocele which filled with 500 ml of fluid on standing (189).

Benign intracranial hypertension (BIH) appears to be caused by increased resistance to CSF absorption through the arachnoid villi, although the volume of the lateral and third ventricles is less than that of normal controls, indicating that the brain is swollen by edema or engorgement (190). Intracranial pressure builds up in waves followed by a sudden fall, suggesting that increased pressure periodically forces fluid through the arachnoid villi (191). Twenty-four hour monitoring of CSF pressure has shown pressure waves of 298-540 mm CSF with baseline pressures of less than 200 mm CSF (192). BIH may follow head injuries, nonspecific infections, medication with tetracycline and nalidixic acid, excessive vitamin A intake, and the cessation of corticosteroid therapy. It has been reported during low-dosage tetracycline therapy for acne and may be more likely to occur if vitamin A is prescribed at the same time (193). Obese young women are particularly susceptible to the condition. Papilledema is present in most patients when they are first examined. Sixth nerve palsy is found in 10%-40% of patients, and third nerve palsy has also been reported (194, 195). The condition usually responds to salt restriction and the use of diuretics, monitored by repeated lumbar puncture. The place of steroids in treatment is not established. Rarely, surgical decompression of the optic nerve in the orbit is undertaken to preserve vision if persistent papilledema threatens to cause optic atrophy.

Cerebral vascular disease may be responsible for headache, although the mechanism is uncertain since there is no correlation with the extent of collateral circulation (196). Headache is a symptom in about one-third of patients with internal carotid artery occlusion and one-quarter of patients with transient ischemic attacks. Severe unilateral headache may recur for up to 6 months after carotid endarterectomy (197) or be associated with dissecting aneurysm of the carotid arterial wall (174). Headache and pain in the neck over the carotid artery (carotodynia) may signal the presence of a long intraluminal clot, particularly if accompanied by symptoms of vascular insufficiency (173).

Rebound vasodilatation is presumably the cause of caffeine-withdrawal headache. Affected subjects are accustomed to consume 500 mg of caffeine (approximately 5 cups of coffee) or more daily and experience diffuse headache about 18 hours after ceasing their habitual intake. One survey of 205 hospitalized patients found that 25% had noticed headaches under these circumstances (198) and reported more symptoms of anxiety and depression than nonheadache subjects.

Headaches associated with sexual activity include a dull tension sensation building up as sexual excitement mounts, a sudden explosive headache at the time of orgasm (attributed to a surge of hypertension) and the rare disaster of subarachnoid hemorrhage. With the latter exception, most sex headaches are considered to be benign, although the onset of stroke (probably brain-stem infarction) at the time of orgasm has been reported in two young males, one aged 24 (199) and one aged 25 (200).

Episodic Vascular Headache

Migraine

Types. There are many variations on the theme of migraine. The following grouping of symptoms is presented (201) in an attempt to separate various components, which may turn out to have a different pathophysiology, although more than one component may comprise part of an attack in a patient at the same or different times.

In *premonitory migraine* episodes of mood changes occur. There is commonly a feeling of elation and hyperactivity. Thirst, increased appetite, craving for sweet foods or drowsiness precede a migraine headache by up to 24 hours. These symptoms may reflect central monoamine changes particularly in the hypothalamus. It could be relevant that the serotonin antagonist pizotifen often causes drowsiness and a craving for sweets (202).

Among the types of *prodromal migraine,* classical migraine has episodes in which visual disturbances or other focal neurological symptoms precede a migraine headache by 10-60 minutes. Retinal migraine appears to be a subgroup of classical migraine in which vasoconstriction is limited to the branches of one ophthalmic artery. Protracted prodromal migraine produces episodes in which focal neurological symptoms persist into the headache phase. This group includes most cases of vertebrobasilar migraine, migraine stupor, confusional states of childhood, and hemiplegic migraine.

Migraine equivalent has a gradual onset and subsidence of focal neurological symp-

toms in the manner of a migrainous prodrome without headache ensuing. An interesting subgroup in the middle-aged or older patient has been described by Fisher (203) as transient migrainous accompaniments (TMAs) to distinguish them from thromboembolic transient ischemic attacks (TIAs).

Nonprodromal migrane includes common and interposed migranes. *Common migraine* is an episodic headache, most commonly unilateral and associated with nausea, vomiting, and photophobia. There are no overt neurological symptoms or signs. Subgroups include most cases of premenstrual migraine and facial migraine (lower-half headache).

The interposed migraine has episodes of migraine headache during which focal neurological symptoms or signs develop as the headache intensifies. Ophthalmoplegic migraine appears to be a subgroup of interposed migraine.

In the final type, *complicated migraine,* retinal or neurological deficits persist after the usual duration of migraine headache or migraine equivalent (204).

In addition to the characteristic vascular pain of migraine, 42% of patients experience sudden jabbing (icepick-like) pains in the head. This can be experienced with or without the usual headache (205).

Clinical Observations. Discussion about the migraine personality has been animated and prolonged. Recent studies using standard personality inventories have not been able to demonstrate unequivocal deviation from normal in migrainous or cluster-headache patients (206, 207) and have not been able to confirm the traditional view of the perfectionistic, rigid, nature of the migraineur (208). By way of contrast, indices of depression, hypochondriasis, and neurosis were more common in patients with tension and post-traumatic headaches than in normal or migrainous subjects (208).

Migraine may be regarded as a neurovascular reaction occurring spontaneously or in response to specific trigger factors. Trigger factors may act through a neural mechanism (e.g., sunlight reflected from rippling water producing visual disturbance as a prodrome), through a vascular mechanism (e.g., exercise or alcohol causing vasodilatation), or a complex interaction of neurohumoral mechanisms (e.g., stress or relaxation after stress precipitating a typical migraine attack). Whether allergy to certain foods provokes migraine remains controversial although a recent study of elimination diets over a period of 2 years (209) supports this view. In this study, removal of certain foods from the diet benefited 23 of the 33 patients, and a good correlation was found with the results of radioallergosorbent (RAST) tests, but not with serum IgE levels. Pretreatment with oral sodium cromoglycate 200-400 mg 4 times daily protected patients from migraine when they were challenged with the offending foods. The question requires further investigation in view of a previous report of less favorable results from elimination diets (210).

Quite apart from the problem of food allergy, there is the question of the involvement of immune mechanisms in the precipitation of migraine attacks. Lord and Duckworth (211) reported that complement components C1s C1(I) and C4 were reduced early in migraine headache. Breakdown products of the third complement component were detected in the plasma of 3 headache-free patients, each of whom developed a migraine attack 3-24 hours after the sample was taken, while none of the 28 patients without detectable breakdown products had a headache within 24 hours. They deduced that complement activation played a part in the initiation of some migraine headaches as a type III immune response. In further studies (212) they detected circulating immune complexes only in the sera of those migraineurs without prodromal symptoms. Subsequent studies have not shown any difference between headache-free and headache periods in levels of complement components (213, 214), immune complexes (213) or C1 inhibitor levels (215). In none of these studies was it stated that samples were taken immediately before or after the onset of headache, so that the possibility of a transient immune reaction initiating migraine headache has not yet been excluded.

It has long been recognized that migraine can be induced by a minor blow to the head,

more often in children. Confirmation of this comes from a study of members of a football team in whom the symptoms of classical migraine following an injury gave rise to concern about the possibility of intracranial damage (216). The focal neurological symptoms of classical migraine may also suggest a viral meningoencephalitis at times, particularly if the episode is accompanied by a fever. Lumbar puncture may indeed disclose a mononuclear pleocytosis in the CSF, up to 300 white cells/mm^3, at the height of such a migraine attack (217, 218). It remains uncertain in these instances whether the migrainous symptoms were precipated by a viral infection or whether the CSF changes were simply a reaction to the migrainous process. When patients hyperventilate during a migraine attack, the resulting symptoms of circumoral and limb paresthesia or even carpopedal spasm may cause confusion with the symptoms of vertebrobasilar migraine (219). The low P_{CO_2} during hyperventilation may also aggravate cerebral vasoconstriction and worsen migrainous symptoms.

Seizures are liable to occur in association with migrainous focal neurological symptoms although no statistical link has been found between migraine and epilepsy. Some children and adolescents subject to both vertebrobasilar migraine and epilepsy have had interictal electroencephalograms (EEGs) showing slow spike-wave complexes in the occipital region, blocking on visual attention (220). This presumably means that the occipital cortex is in a constant state of hyperexcitability, although the relationship of this to migrainous symptoms is uncertain. The grossly abnormal EEG distinguishes the syndrome, which appears to have a good prognosis, from other forms of vertebrobasilar migraine in which the EEG is usually normal between attacks, even in those cases which progress to migraine stupor. A syndrome of recurrent headaches with dysphasia associated with a left temporal spike focus in the EEG has recently been reported as responding to phenytoin therapy (221), but its relation to migraine is uncertain.

Vertigo is a common accompaniment of migraine, presumably caused by ischemia of the brain stem. Of 20 children with basilar artery migraine, 16 were found to have abnormalities in their caloric responses on electronystagmography (222). Five children developed complex partial seizures thought to be caused by ischemic damage to the medial temporal lobe from diminished perfusion of the posterior cerebral-artery circulation. Attacks of spontaneous vertigo not precipitated by movement and not accompanied by cochlear or neurological symptoms in young or middle-aged adults were called benign recurrent vertigo by Slater (223). This disorder shows some features in common with migraine including female preponderance, positive family histories, and precipitation by alcohol, lack of sleep, and emotional stress. Moretti and coworkers (224) presented 5 additional patients, all of whom had a family history of migraine. Three of these patients were subject to migraine headache, although the episodes of vertigo were followed by headache in only one of them.

The literature on ophthalmoplegic migraine has been reviewed by Vijayan (225). Of 18 patients who fulfilled stringent criteria for the diagnosis, the third cranial nerve was the only one affected in 15. Because the pupillary reaction to light was completely or partially spared in two-thirds of the patients, Vijayan argues that the most common cause is an ischemic neuropathy rather than compression by an enlarged vessel.

There have been a number of reports in the literature of familial hemiplegic migraine associated with a cerebellar disturbance, which appears to be an hereditary cerebellar degenerative disorder rather than the result of ischemia from reported migraine attacks. The most recent report (226) describes a mother and son with hemiplegic migraine, essential tremor, and nystagmus. Other families have been described previously in which hemiplegic migraine has occurred with retinal degeneration, deafness, and ataxia.

The neurological symptoms of migraine may outlast the migraine attack, or permanent deficit can develop because of retinal, cerebral or brain-stem infarction. A recent report of 7 cases of such complicated migraine (204) discusses the possible role of edema of the arterial wall, platelet aggregation, and increased coagulability of the blood in causing infarction. Arterial occlusion was demonstrated in 5 of the 6 patients in this series investigated by cerebral angiography, in contrast to the negative findings of most angiographic studies performed during the prodromal phase of migraine in the past. The tendency to thrombosis of cerebral or retinal arteries in migraine seems to be the result of diminished cerebral blood flow and increased platelet aggregability rather than active constriction of the vessels which become occluded.

Computerized axial tomography of the brain (CAT scanning) in 94 patients subject to recurrent migrainous headache disclosed cortical infarcts in 4 patients with complicated migraine and in 2 patients with no obvious neurological deficit (227). Eleven patients were found to have a degree of cortical atrophy in excess of that expected for their age, 6 patients had some edema of the periventricular white matter, and 2 had an unsuspected glioma of the brain. Before too much importance is placed on reports of CAT scanning in migraine, controlled studies are required as most patients are selected for scanning because the patient's apparently migrainous headaches are atypical. Certainly routine CAT scanning of headache patients is unjustified in the absence of a sinister pattern of headache on history-taking or of neurological signs on physical examination (228).

Pathophysiology. Since the pioneering studies of Wolff and his colleagues (163), it has been assumed that the main cause of migraine headache is dilatation of extracranial vessels which have been rendered sensitive by the local accumulation of chemical pain-producing substances. Blau and Dexter (229) have assessed the contribution of extracranial arteries to migraine headache by systematically compressing the superficial temporal arteries and by inflating a modified sphygmomanometer cuff around the patient's head. These maneuvers relieved the headache in 14 of 39 patients and 19 of 37 patients, respectively. Intracranial sources of headache were assessed by the response to head jolting, coughing, and breath holding, which aggravated the headache in most cases.

They concluded that the majority of patients had some intracranial contribution to their pain and extracranial factors played no part at all in the pain of 18 patients. A similar conclusion was reached by Drummond and Lance (230) who compared the pulse amplitude of the superficial temporal arteries and their branches with the intensity of headache felt in the temple while the common carotid and temporal arteries were compressed alternately. It appears that migraine headache is accentuated by arterial pulsation (intracranial, extracranial, or both), but arterial pulsation is not essential for migraine headache, which may persist in one temple while the common carotid or temporal arteries are compressed.

Tfelt-Hansen and coworkers (231) infiltrated tender areas of muscle with lidocaine 1.5% or normal saline during migraine headache with relief of pain within 70 minutes in 28 of 48 patients. Whether lidocaine or saline was used did not affect the results. This study opens up the important question of the contribution made by direct or referred muscle pain to headache. It has become clear that dilatation of the extracranial vessels is not the primary source of headache in most instances, even though increased extracranial blood flow in migraine has been documented by radioactive xenon inhalation studies (232).

Earlier work had suggested that the extracranial pulses were greater on the habitually migrainous side even between headaches, but Drummond and Lance (233) were unable to confirm this. Temporal pulses of migrainous patients did not differ from normal at rest or on standing, but on exercise the temporal arterial pulse on the side most commonly affected by headache did increase in amplitude significantly more than its fellow on the headache-free side. This may represent a primary unilateral defect in vascular control or be secondary to the increases in extracranial blood flow that recur with each migraine attack. It has been shown that the responses of cerebral blood flow to the inhalation of 5% carbon dioxide in air is greater on the side of a recent migraine headache (234). Blockade of α-adrenergic receptors or stimulation of β-receptors increases cerebral blood flow more on the side

of headache or the side recently affected by headache (235). Conversely α-stimulation diminishes cerebral perfusion more on the affected side. On the basis of these results, Yamamoto and Meyer (235) postulate a primary sympathetic denervation hypersensitivity, but this could not account for those patients in whom hemicrania affects each side on different occasions.

The headache of migraine is usually associated with increased cerebral and extracranial blood flow but this is not invariable. Headache does not depend upon cerebral blood flow since it may be relieved by the injection of ergotamine tartrate or codeine (232) while cerebral perfusion is still increased. The cranial arteries of migrainous patients are more susceptible to the intravenous infusion of histamine than those of control subjects as shown by the incidence and severity of the headache produced (236). In summary, the headache of migraine is not necessarily associated with dilatation of extracranial arteries or increased intracerebral perfusion although it is aggravated by vascular pulsation. It appears to be of intracranial origin at least as often as of extracranial origin and may be related to increased sensitivity of vessels or perivascular structures. The reason for the headache of migraine being commonly unilateral remains obscure.

The prodromes of migraine are usually accompanied by diminution of cerebral blood flow. It is uncertain, though, whether the primary event is cortical ischemia or whether blood flow diminishes as a consequence of depressed cortical function. The most recent report, by Olesen and coworkers (237), comprises sequential studies in 8 patients with regional cerebral blood flow recorded by 254 sensors after the intracarotid injection of ^{113}xenon. This technique enables the pattern of change in different cortical areas to be established in relation to the developing symptoms of migraine. The correlation between symptoms and blood flow measurements lacked precision, though, because the changes in blood flow were unexpected, and the conclusion that they were part of a migraine attack was made retrospectively. One of the 8 patients studied suffered a right-sided headache without migrainous features while left-hemisphere measurements showed a triphasic pattern of increase, then diminution, then increase in parieto-occipital blood flow. Another patient developed a right-sided headache with nausea and metamorphopsia, which was associated with right parietal hyperemia. The headache was then followed by migraine stupor, which was accompanied by global reduction in cerebral blood flow and was particularly severe in the occipital area.

The remaining 6 patients were followed through a migraine attack, with prodromal symptoms in 5 and interposed visual disturbance at the height of the headache in the sixth patient. The characteristic feature in these 6 cases was occipito-parietal oligemia, starting posteriorly and spreading forwards over 15-45 minutes preceded in two instances by occipital hyperemia. Only in 1 case did perfusion drop to levels critical for normal metabolism, although this technique measures flow in a cone of cerebral tissue and could miss or minimize changes restricted to superficial layers of cortex. In 4 patients, severe headache was present at a time when cerebral blood flow was reduced. During a migraine attack, the increase in regional cerebral blood flow usually seen with activation procedures (such as reading and hand-clenching) was impaired or absent. This observation, together with the fact that autoregulation is also impaired in migraine (232), indicates paralysis of normal vaso-motor mechanisms. The fact that focal cerebral symptoms preceded overt oligemia, and appeared in some instances during hyperemia, casts doubt on the assumption that cortical vasoconstriction is the primary change, unless vasoconstriction was limited to the superficial layer of cortex in the early stages of the migraine attack.

As knowledge of neurogenic control of the circulation (particularly the cortical micro-circulation) increases, the number of chemical transmitter agents known to be involved has expanded to include acetylcholine (238), noradrenalin (239-242), serotonin (243), substance P (244), neurotensin (244), vasoactive intestinal polypeptide [VIP] (245), adenosine, and adenosine triphosphate [ATP]

(238). Therefore, almost any theory linking central neurotransmission, humoral changes, and vascular reactivity to the mechanism of migraine has become tenable. It is tempting to assume that sympathetic overactivity may initiate cortical vasoconstriction as the first phase of the migraine attack (246), but the failure of sympathectomy to prevent migraine is a forceful argument against this possibility. Perhaps direct connections from the brain stem to the small vessels in the parenchyma of the cortex may induce spreading depression of cortical function reducing the metabolic requirements of the cortex and thus reducing regional cerebral blood flow.

There is evidence of platelet aggregation (247-249) and a platelet release reaction (250) in migraine. Anthony and his colleagues (251) first reported that a serotonin-releasing factor was present in the blood during migraine headache, and this has been confirmed by others (252-253). Platelet serotonin content increases before a migrainous headache and then falls during the headache phase in most patients. It is possible that the released serotonin is absorbed to vessel walls since the combination of serotonin and bradykinin is known to produce vascular pain. Recently Fozard (254) has produced a succinct review of the relationship of serotonin to migraine, concluding that serotonin release from platelets may have its counterpart in the microvasculature of the circulation or in those areas of the central nervous system concerned with the perception or processing of pain.

The inhibition of transmission in pain pathways by enkephalins is known to be regulated by serotonergic neurons originating in the brain-stem raphe nuclei, which may well prove to be of relevance to the pathogenesis of migraine. Sicuteri (255) considers that migraine and tension headache are the result of defective monoaminergic activity in the central and peripheral nervous system, resulting in hypersensitivity of partially denervated vascular receptors and overactivity of central pathways involved in the perception of pain. It has been questioned that changes in plasma serotonin and catecholamines reflect changes taking place in the central nervous system. Certainly the premonitory symptoms of elation, hunger, craving for sweet foods, and drowsiness encountered in some patients indicate a hypothlamic disturbance. The fact that nausea may precede headache points to changes in dopaminergic transmission in the brain stem, and hypersensitivity to light, sound, and smells accompanying headache suggest a temporary suppression of central inhibitory mechanisms.

Interest has quickened in the study of prolactin as an indicator of hypothalamopituitary activity and, indirectly, of dopaminergic mechanisms. Prolactin secretion is inhibited by tuberoinfundibular neurons using dopamine as a transmitter and increased by serotonin, probably via prolactin-releasing factor. Nappi and his colleagues (256) reported that the dopamine agonist lisuride induced headache, nausea, vomiting, and weakness in patients prone to headache more than in normal controls. They administered sulpiride, which blocks dopamine receptors in the median eminence, to women during the follicular phase of the menstrual cycle. It produced a threefold greater increase in prolactin levels in those subject to menstrual headaches than in normal controls. These authors postulated a hypersensitivity of dopamine receptors in patients prone to headache. Giacovazzo and coworkers (257) associated headache with increasing prolactin levels from various causes, including drugs such as metoclopramide, sulpiride, and tricyclic antidepressants. The problem is complicated by the fact that migraine is uncommon during pregnancy when prolactin levels are high (258). The administration of levodopa during an attack of common migraine reduced the prolactin level while the same levodopa loading test increased the plasma level during those attacks of migraine that were accompanied by neurological symptoms or signs (259). It was suggested by the authors that this paradoxical effect could result from the effect of prostaglandin $F_{2\alpha}$ overcoming the levodopa effect in some patients by stimulating the production of prolactin. The concept of dopamine receptors being hypersensitive in migrainous subjects was supported by Fanciullacci and his colleagues (260) who found that the oral administration of 2.5 mg bromocriptine, a dopamine agonist, produced postural hypotension in migrainous patients but not in normal controls. They postulated that this could result from a chronic deficiency of endogenous opioids. CSF enkephalin is reduced during a migraine attack but not in headache-free periods (261), while no change was observed in serum β-endorphin in migrainous patients before, during, or after the attack (262). It is not possible at the moment to speculate beyond the statement that dopamine appears to share in the disturbance of monoamine metabolism which accompanies the migraine attack and that endogenous opioid systems may be secondarily implicated.

The mechanism of migraine thus appears to involve changes in monoamine transmission in the central nervous system associated with, or followed by, a platelet release reaction. The resulting neural and humoral changes are associated with depression of cortical function which spreads over both hemispheres from the occipital area forward, together with diminished regional cerebral blood flow, thus producing the classical neurological symptoms of migraine. Trigger factors all represent a change, usually sudden, in the internal or external environment which could be considered as a threat to the organism, of which the brain is the most precious and vulnerable part. The neurovascular reaction of migraine can thus be regarded as a quasiprotective mechanism to guard the brain by reducing its metabolic requirements or by shunting blood away from the cerebral cortex (201). The headache may be a side effect of this reaction which nevertheless, like any pain, alerts the organism to potential danger.

Treatment. If there proves to be a final common pathway for migraine, then it may be susceptible to pharmacological blockade. There is some hope for this concept in that individual patients are completely relieved of headache by the regular continued administration of propranolol or methysergide. There may well be ways of separating migrainous patients into groups on clinical grounds so that the result of drug therapy may become more predictable. Until that time arrives, migraine can be considered as an excessive neurovascular reaction in a vulnerable subject, a reaction to be regulated rather than a disease to be cured.

Behavioral Therapy. In the last few years much attention has been devoted to psychological and behavioral management of migraine, with particular emphasis on relaxation training assisted by biofeedback methods. Electromyographic studies have shown that migrainous patients have greater activity in the frontalis and neck muscles than normal controls (263), and that muscle activity increases during headache (264). Relaxation training assisted by biofeedback from frontalis muscles is associated with reduction in the frequency and severity of migraine headache (263, 265-266). The acquisition of voluntary control over the amplitude of pulsation of the frontal branch of the temporal artery was found to be superior to feedback from the frontal muscles (266) and to voluntary hand cooling (267) in reducing migraine headache. Relaxation training alone gave better results than learning to increase warmth in the hands by biofeedback of fingertip temperature (268). Patients trained to warm their hands had a slight edge over those trained to cool their hands in one study (269), although both groups improved. In another trial (270), those who were trained to lower finger temperature produced as good results as those who were trained to raise finger temperature, and neither group improved more than those patients who were unable to acquire these skills or those who simply kept a diary of their headaches as a control group. Mathew and coworkers (271) have demonstrated a mean increase in regional cerebral blood flow of 8.9% in the left hemisphere and 4.5% in the right hemisphere while hand-warming biofeedback was in progress. The comparable changes during hand cooling were +1.4% for the left hemisphere and –5.4% for the right hemisphere.

It thus appears that control of hand temperature is reflected by changes in cerebral blood flow, but there is some doubt as to whether the technique has a specific vascular effect in migraine or whether temperature control, like EMG feedback, acts as an aid to total body relaxation and reduced autonomic drive (272-274). It must be borne in mind that migraine tends to improve whenever a patient is under supervision in a clinical trial. In our own clinic, placebo results in controlled trials of drug therapy have varied from 20%-60% improvement, the latter figure being achieved when psychological counseling and relaxation training were part of general management. Parker and coworkers (275) found that migraine attacks were reduced by 28% in all groups during a trial of manipulative therapy and had diminished by a further 19% at a 20-month follow-up, which they attribute to the natural history of the disorder.

Pharmacotherapy. The usual management of the acute attack of migraine by ergotamine preparations, antiemetics, and analgesics is well known (163-165). A good therapeutic effect with ergotamine is associated with plasma levels of 0.2-0.5 ng/ml, with the mean maximum concentration being achieved within 1 hour (276). It is of interest that both ergotamine (277) and isometheptene (278), a sympathomimetic agent which is reported to be useful in aborting migraine headache, reduce carotid flow in the cat and increase capillary perfusion by reducing shunting through arteriovenous anastomoses.

The administration of metoclopramide 10 mg by intramuscular injection or 20 mg as a suppository at the onset of symptoms helps to promote gastric absorption and prevent nausea (279). This can be followed by one of the preparations containing ergotamine tartrate 1-2 mg, with or without aspirin or other analgesics. Tolfenamic acid, an anti-inflammatory agent which is said to block prostaglandin receptors, given in doses of 200 mg proved to be as effective in relieving migraine as ergotamine tartrate in a comparative trial (280). Both drugs were superior to aspirin, which in turn was superior to placebo.

Substances which have proven effective in reducing the frequency and severity of migraine headache when given as a prophylactic daily dosage include propranolol, pizotifen, methysergide, amitriptyline, and the monoamine oxidase inhibitor phenelzine. The new antidepressant agent zimelidene, which blocks serotonin uptake, may worsen migraine in the early stages of treatment, but improvement may occur later (281). Zimelidene reduces the whole blood serotonin concentration, though. Drugs which are not effective in preventing migraine include clonidine (282) and cimetidine (283, 284). The use of clonidine in migraine therapy is now invalid since acute or chronic administration has no demonstrable direct effect on vascular reactions (285).

Pizotifen, a drug with both antihistamine and antiserotonin actions, has recently been shown not only to diminish spontaneous platelet aggregation in migrainous patients but also to improve migraine headache (286). Masel and coworkers (287) also worked with reducing platelet hyperaggregability in migraine. They conducted a controlled crossover trial of aspirin 325 mg twice daily combined with dipyridamole 25 mg 3 times daily, finding that the frequency and severity of migraine attacks was significantly reduced compared with the placebo period. Of 22 patients in whom platelets were studied, excessive aggregation was demonstrated in 7, all of whom responded well to treatment.

Other controlled trials recently published have shown significant improvement of migraine with the β_1-adrenergic blocking agent, atenolol, 50 mg twice daily (288), the nonsteroid anti-inflammatory drug, naproxen, 250 mg twice daily (289), and a nonsedative barbiturate, proxibarbital, 100 mg-300 mg daily (290). Propranolol proved to be as effective as methysergide in reducing the frequency and severity of migraine attacks in a crossover trial of two 3-month periods (291). Side effects were fewer and milder in those patients treated with propranolol 40 mg three times daily. Drowsiness and feeling of weakness were the most common. Three patients had to be withdrawn from the trial because of vasoconstrictive side effects on methysergide 1 mg three times daily. Raskin and Schwartz (292) compared the progress of 146 patients treated by a variety of interval medications with 85 age-matched patients who declined drug therapy. Both groups were followed for a mean of 35 months. After 1 year substantial improvement was recorded in 55% of the drug-treated patients and 36% of the controls, falling to 31% and 12%, respectively, at the end of 2 years. At the present time, the successful management of migraine depends on a judicious blend of behavioral and drug therapy.

Cluster Headache

Since the summary of cluster headache in the last edition of this book (1), a comprehensive monograph by Kudrow (293) has been published which covers clinical aspects, pathophysiology, and management of this condition. When this type of headache recurs regularly in the manner of migraine rather than the characteristic bouts or clusters of pain, it is known as chronic cluster headache or chronic migrainous neuralgia (294). A third variety of cluster headache, in which the pain is typical but recurs more than 6 times daily and usually responds to the oral administration of indomethacin 50-75 mg daily, has been termed chronic paroxysmal hemicrania (295).

Patients with cluster headache do not have personality traits which are significantly different from migraine sufferers, or indeed from the normal population (293, 296). Between and during attacks of cluster headache, blood flow in the ipsilateral frontal region, which is supplied by terminal branches of the ophthalmic artery arising from the internal carotid artery, is diminished as estimated by Doppler studies (293) and thermography (164). Reports on cerebral blood flow in cluster headache are not consistent. Sakai and Meyer (232) found that cortical blood flow, estimated by the inhaled ^{113}xenon method, increases by 44.5% during the headache phase, while extracranial blood flow increases by as much as 250%. On the other hand, no change in cerebral blood flow could be demonstrated during headaches in 3 patients by Henry and coworkers (297) and, of 4 patients studied during spontaneous attacks by Nelson and coworkers (298), cerebral blood flow fell in 3 and rose in 1.

In a series of in vitro experiments by Hardebo and coworkers (299), short segments of the superficial temporal artery removed from patients with cluster headache have been compared with control specimens taken during craniotomy. They found no difference in the reactivity of arteries from cluster patients from normal controls to all vasoactive agents except histamine. The arteries of patients with chronic cluster headache dilated much more readily to histamine than those from patients with episodic cluster headache or from headache-free subjects. The reaction to histamine was reduced by cimetidine, a histamine-2 blocking agent. This is of particular interest since the dilator effect of histamine has been shown to depend mainly on histamine-2 receptors in the extracranial circulation of the monkey (300) and blood histamine levels increase during cluster headache (283). Unfortunately, cimetidine has not proven to be beneficial in preventing the usual episodic form of cluster headache (283). We are not aware of any trial of its use in chronic cluster headache, for which lithium carbonate is now a generally accepted method of treatment (293). Blood samples from patients who responded to lithium or to other forms of therapy, such as methysergide, were found to have lowered blood serotonin and histamine levels which remained stable as long as the headache was controlled but returned to pre-treatment levels if the headache recurred (301). It thus appears that the cause of cluster headache is related to blood levels of vasoactive amines, but the mechanism of pain production and the usual occurrence is still unknown.

Since the fluctuation of estrogen levels predisposes migraine to women, the level of testosterone has been investigated in cluster headache, a predominantly male disorder. Plasma testosterone was shown to be lower in patients during the active phase than in those enjoying a remission (293). The fact that luteinizing hormone, not other anterior pituitary hormones, was also decreased in the acute phase suggests a periodic disturbance of hypothalamic function. At the moment, it is not possible to link changes in hormones, vasoactive substances, and cranial blood flow in any satisfying hypothesis of the pathogenesis of cluster headache.

There are additions to the accepted treatment of cluster headache with ergotamine, methysergide, and prednisone (293). They are the use of chlorpromazine in doses ranging from 75-700 mg daily (302) in suppressing a bout and the inhalation of 100% oxygen in abbreviating the headache (303).

Tension Headache

Headache may be caused by emotional stress, fatigue, or exposure to glare or noise in most of the general population. When it recurs almost daily in frequency as a constant tight, pressing, or band-like sensation in frontal, temporal, or occipital areas it is known as chronic tension headache. The mechanism remains uncertain. Constant overcontraction of scalp muscles has long been thought to be an important etiological factor, and recently there has been speculation about a constitutional deficiency in the normal central mechanism for suppressing pain perception (255). Neither of these theories were supported by Martin and Matthews (304) who could find no consistent difference in the EMG of the forehead or neck muscles, or in the pain threshold to graded thermal stimuli, between tension headache patients and control subjects. They reported that the inhalation of amyl nitrite increased headache severity on 43% of occasions and did not alter the intensity on 48% of occasions, while no patient reported any increase after the inhalation of placebo. This suggests that the pain of tension headache is associated with vasodilatation rather than vasoconstriction, a point of interest in view of conflicting reports in the earlier literature. In another study (305) the intravenous infusion of histamine produced a pulsating headache in 24 of 25 migrainous patients, 5 out of 10 tension headache patients, and none of 13 normal controls. In spite of this apparent susceptibility to vascular pain in tension headache patients, no significant change in cortical or extracranial blood flow has been demonstrated during tension headache (232). Platelet serotonin was found to be consistently and significantly ($P = 0.001$) lower in patients with tension headache than in normal controls and headache-free migrainous patients (306). Since platelet serotonin falls and remains low during migraine headache, it is possible that tension headache also involves a defective serotoninergic mechanism which is chronically sustained rather than paroxysmal as in migraine. Patients who suffer from both forms of headache usually distinguish between them on the grounds of severity and associated symptoms, much in the same way as a clinician taking a case history (307). However, this does not answer the question as to whether they share the same basic pathophysiology. Tension headaches occur as often in migrainous and nonmigrainous subjects, indicating that they may be independent phenomena (308).

While excessive muscle contraction may not be essential for the development of tension headache, it is possible that it affects the intensity and duration of the headache (308). A logical extension of this thought is that EMG biofeedback would be most effective in reducing pain in those patients who do have consistent overcontraction of muscles. The relation of muscle contraction to headache has been investigated by measuring the resting levels of EMG in frontal or temporal muscles, the changes in EMG amplitude in response to problem solving or other forms of stress, and the changes in EMG with increasing or diminishing intensity of headache (309). The lack of consistency in results reported by different authors shows that there is no simple direct relationship between contraction of scalp muscles and headache. In spite of this, controlled trials of EMG biofeedback have found that it is effective in relieving tension headache (310-314), possibly by reducing the general level of anxiety and associated vascular changes (309). Behavioral management may be supplemented by the use of relaxing agents, antidepressant drugs, and analgesics although the ideal outcome is to free the patient from the necessity of using any form of drug therapy.

SUMMARY

The principal developments in the scientific understanding of pain have been the consolidation of the anatomy of the substantia gelatinosa and a start to the resolution of the complex connections of this center, which is critically involved in nociception. The neurophysiological analysis of the substantia gelatinosa has begun with the identification of a variety of neurons with different properties.

The role of various thalamic nuclei in pain perception has been reviewed and a new nociceptive nucleus has been identified. Various aspects of descending pain inhibitory pathways have been elaborated and new systems have been described. The role of serotonin in descending pain inhibitory systems has been challenged, as has their involvement in opiate analgesia.

Circumstantial evidence still favors the concept that substance P is the transmitter released by nociceptive afferents and that its release is inhibited by enkephalinergic neurons. Certain aspects of this concept have been questioned, however.

The efficacy of TNS has been reaffirmed but so too has its limited application and diminishing duration of effect. Similar conclusions have been reached about the therapeutic use of epidural morphine. Clinical and experimental studies have continued to elaborate the neurophysiology of deafferentation pain, causalgia, and reflex sympathetic dystrophy.

The classification of the cause of low-back pain has been refined, and provocation radiology promises to be a means of objectively diagnosing these causes. Postoperative lumbar adhesive arachnoiditis still remains a major problem in management. Radio-frequency neurotomy has been used for various cervical pain syndromes with limited success, but new anatomical data may possibly improve the success rates obtained with these procedures.

Anatomical and neurophysiological studies have provided data supporting the concept that demyelination of trigeminal roots by vascular anomalies is the cause of trigeminal neuralgia. There are still reservations about this concept, though.

Among intracranial causes of headache, benign intracranial hypertension following the use of tetracycline and vitamin A in the treatment of acne is worthy of note. Comments are also made on headache from other intracranial causes such as cough headache and headaches resulting from low intracranial pressure, cerebral vascular disease, and caffeine withdrawal and extracranial causes such as temporal arteritis.

The relationship between the various forms of migraine and tension headaches is explored. There is evidence that dilatation of the extracranial arteries is not the primary source of migraine in most cases and that excessive muscle contraction is not the cause of tension headache. Migraine is accompanied by reduction in cortical perfusion spreading forwards from the occipital poles, although it is uncertain whether this is caused by constriction of vessels supplying the cortex or is secondary to reduced metabolic require-ments. The roles played in migraine by central depletion of monoamines, neural discharge, platelet aggregation, and humoral changes remain to be determined.

There has been an upsurge in behavioral therapy for the management of both migraine and tension headache, although biofeedback techniques appear to confer no greater benefit than relaxation training alone. Agents which reduce platelet aggregation, a nonsteroid inflammatory drug, and a barbiturate have been advocated for the interval therapy of migraine while further studies of serotonin antagonists and β-noradrenergic blockers have been reported. Chlorpromazine has been added to the list of drugs such as prednisone, ergotamine, methysergide, indomethacin, and lithium, which benefit various forms of cluster headache.

REFERENCES

1. Bogduk N, Lance JW: Pain and pain syndromes including headache. In *Current Neurology*, vol 3. Edited by Appel S. Boston, Houghton Mifflin, 1981, pp 377-419

2. Bishop B: Pain: Its physiology and rationale for management. *Phys Ther* 60:13-37, 1980

3. Mendelson G: Pain. I. Basic mechanisms. *Med J Aust* 1:106-109, 1981

4. Mendelson G: Pain. II. Clinical aspects. *Med J Aust* 1:213-218, 1981

5. Mendelson G: Pain. III. Psychological aspects. *Med J Aust* 1:285-288, 1981

6. Wilson PR, Yaksh TL: Pharmacology of pain and analgesia. *Anaesth Intensive Care* 8:248-256, 1980

7. Zimmerman M: Peripheral and central nervous mechanisms of nociception, pain, and pain therapy: facts and hypotheses. *Advances in Pain Research and Therapy*, vol 3. Edited by Bonica JJ, Liebeskind JC, Albe-Fessard DG. New York, Raven Press, 1979, pp 3-32

8. Perl ER: Afferent basis of nociception and pain: evidence from the characteristics of sensory receptors and their projections to the spinal dorsal horn. In *Pain*. Edited by Bonica JJ. New York, Raven Press, 1980, pp 19-45

9. Kerr FWL, Fukushima T: New observations on the nociceptive pathways in the central nervous system. In *Pain*. Edited by Bonica JJ. New York, Raven Press, 1980, pp 47-61

10. Coggeshall RE, Maynard CW, Langford LA: Unmyelinated sensory and preganglionic fibers in rat L6 and S1 ventral spinal roots. *J Comp Neurol* 193:41-47, 1980

11. Hosobuchi Y: The majority of unmyelinated afferent axons in human ventral roots probably conduct pain. *Pain* 8:167-180, 1980

12. Cervero F, Iggo A: The substantia gelatinosa of the spinal cord. A critical review. *Brain* 103:717-772, 1980

13. Coggeshall RE, Chung K, Chung JM, et al: Primary afferent axons in the tract of Lissauer in the monkey. *J Comp Neurol* 196:431-442, 1981

14. Wall PD: The role of substantia gelatinosa as a gate control. In *Pain*. Edited by Bonica JJ. New York, Raven Press, 1980, pp 205-231

15. Ralston HJ, Ralston DD: The distribution of dorsal root axons in laminae I, II and III of the Macaque spinal cord: a quantitative electron microscope study. *J Comp Neurol* 184:643-684, 1979

16. Hu JW, Dostrovsky JO, Sessle BJ: Functional properties of neurons in cat trigeminal subnucleus caudalis (medullary dorsal horn). I. Responses to oral-facial noxious and non-noxious stimuli and projections to thalamus and subnucleus oralis. *J Neurophysiol* 45:173-192, 1981

17. Sessle BJ, Hu JW, Dubner R, et al: Functional properties of neurons in cat trigeminal subnucleus

caudalis (medullary dorsal horn). II. Modulation of responses to noxious and non-noxious stimuli by periaqueductal gray, nucleus raphe magnus, cerebral cortex, and afferent influences, and effect of naloxone. *J Neurophysiol* 45:193-207, 1981

18. Willis WD: Neurophysiology of nociception and pain in the spinal cord. In *Pain*. Edited by Bonica JJ. New York, Raven Press, 1980, pp 77-92

19. Wall PD: The substantia gelatinosa. A gate control mechanism set across a sensory pathway. *Trends Neurosc* 3:221-224, 1980

20. Abdelmoumene M, Bennett GJ, Hayashi H, et al: Functional and morphological features of layer I neurons in the cat spinal dorsal horn (abstract). *Neurosc Let* 5 (Suppl):S107, 1980

21. Price DD, Hayashi H, Dubner R, et al: Functional relationships between neurons of marginal and substantia gelatinosa layers of primate dorsal horn. *J Neurophysiol* 42:1590-1608, 1979

22. Gobel S, Falls WM, Bennett GJ, et al: An EM analysis of the synaptic connections of horseradish peroxidase-filled stalked cells and islet cells in the substantia gelatinosa of adult cat spinal cord. *J Comp Neurol* 194:781-807, 1980

23. Bennett GJ, Abdelmoumene M, Hayashi H, et al: Physiology and morphology of substantia gelatinosa neurons intracellularly stained with horseradish peroxidase. *J Comp Neurol* 194:809-827, 1980

24. Cervero F, Iggo A, Molony V: An electrophysiological study of neurons in the substantia gelatinosa Rolandi of the cat's spinal cord. *Q J Exp Physiol* 64:297-314, 1979

25. Cervero F, Iggo A, Molony V: Segmental and intersegmental organization of neurones in the substantia gelatinosa Rolandi of the cat's spinal cord. *Q J Exp Physiol* 64:315-326, 1979

26. Cervero F, Molony V, Iggo A: Functional characteristics of neurons in the substantia gelatinosa Rolandi of the cat. *Advances in Pain Research and Therapy*, vol 3. Edited by Bonica JJ, Liebeskind JC, Albe-Fessard DG. New York, Raven Press, 1979, pp 877-882

27. Craig AD, Burton H: Spinal and medullary lamina I projection to nucleus submedius in medial thalamus: a possible pain centre. *J Neurophysiol* 45:443-466, 1981

28. Carmon A, Friedman Y, Coger R, et al: Single trial analysis of evoked potentials to noxious thermal stimulation in man. *Pain* 8:21-32, 1980

29. Shah Y, Dostrovsky JO: Electrophysiological evidence for a projection of the periaqueductal gray matter to nucleus raphe magnus in cat and rat. *Brain Res* 193:534-538, 1980

30. Sanders KH, Klein CE, Mayer TE, et al: Differential effects of noxious and non-noxious input on neurones according to location in ventral periaqueductal grey or dorsal raphe nucleus. *Brain Res* 186:83-97, 1980

31. Carstens E, Klumpp D, Zimmermann M: Time course and effective sites for inhibition from midbrain periaqueductal gray of spinal dorsal horn neuronal responses to cutaneous stimuli in the cat. *Exp Brain Res* 38:425-430, 1980

32. Hammond DL, Levy RA, Proudfit HK: Hypoalgesia induced by microinjection of a norepinephrine antagonist in the raphe magnus; reversal by intrathecal administration of a serotonin antagonist. *Brain Res* 201:475-479, 1980

33. Hammond DL, Levy RA, Proudfit HK: Hypoalgesia following microinjection of noradrenergic antagonists in the nucleus raphe magnus. *Pain* 9:85-101, 1980

34. Gerhart KD, Wilcox TK, Chung JM, et al: Inhibition of nociceptive and non-nociceptive responses of primate spinothalamic cells by stimulation in medial brain stem. *J Neurophysiol* 45:121-136, 1981

35. Dostrovsky JO: Raphe and periaqueductal gray induced suppression of non-nociceptive neuronal responses in the dorsal column nuclei and trigeminal sub-nucleus caudalis. *Brain Res* 200:184-189, 1980

36. Duggan AW, Griersmith BT, North RA: Morphine and supraspinal inhibition of spinal neurones: evidence that morphine decreases tonic descending inhibition in the anaesthetized cat. *Br J Pharmacol* 69:461-466, 1980

37. Jurna I: Effect of stimulation in the periaqueductal grey matter on activity in ascending axons of the rat spinal cord: selective inhibition of activity evoked by afferent Aδ and C fibre stimulation and failure of naloxone to reduce inhibition. *Brain Res* 196:33-42, 1980

38. Le Bars D, Dickenson AH, Besson JM: Microinjection of morphine within nucleus raphe magnus and dorsal horn neurone activities related to nociception in the rat. *Brain Res* 189:467-481, 1980

39. Proudfit HK: Reversible inactivation of raphe magnus neurons: effects on nociceptive threshold and morphine-induced analgesia. *Brain Res* 201:459-464, 1980

40. Carstens E, Fraunhoffer M, Zimmermann M: Serotonergic mediation of descending inhibition from midbrain periaqueductal gray but not reticular formation of spinal nociceptive transmission in the cat. *Pain* 10:149-167, 1981

41. Berge OG, Hole K: Morphine analgesia measured by the tail flick (TF) test is not reduced by 5-hydroxytryptamine (5-HT) blockers (abstract). *Neurosci Let* 5(Suppl): S106, 1980

42. Barton C, Basbaum AI, Fields HL: Dissociation of supraspinal and spinal actions of morphine: a quantitative evaluation. *Brain Res* 188:487-498, 1980

43. Griersmith BT, Duggan AW, North RA: Methysergide and supraspinal inhibition of the spinal transmission of nociceptive information in the anaesthetized cat. *Brain Res* 204:147-158, 1981

44. Rivot JP, Calvino B, Besson JM: Effects of 5-HT antagonists (cinanserin and methysergide) on the C fiber response of dorsal horn convergent units of the rat (abstract). *Neurosci Let* 5 (Suppl):S106, 1980

45. Griersmith BT, Duggan AW: Prolonged depression of spinal transmission of nociceptive information by 5-HT administered in the substantia gelatinosa: antagonism by methysergide. *Brain Res* 187:231-236, 1980

46. Le Bars D, Rivot JP, Dickenson AH, et al: Rôle de la sérotonine dans les controlês inhibiteurs diffus induits par des stimulations nociceptives. *C R Acad Sci (Paris) 290:379-382, 1980*

47. Reddy SVR, Yaksh TL: Spinal noradrenergic terminal system mediates antinociception. *Brain Res* 189:381-401, 1980

48. Kuraishi Y, Harada Y, Takagi H: Antinociceptive effects of intrathecal catecholamines and opiates in the rat (abstract). *Neurosci Let* 4 (Suppl):S74, 1980

49. Hodge CJ, Woods CI, Delatizky J: Noradrenaline, serotonin, and the dorsal horn. *J Neurosurg* 52:674-685, 1980

50. Zemlan FP, Corrigan SA, Pfaff DW: Noradrenergic and serotonergic mediation of spinal analgesia mechanisms. *Eur J Pharmacol* 61:111-124, 1980

51. Hammond DL, Proudfit HK: Effects of locus coeruleus lesions on morphine-induced antinociception. *Brain Res* 188:79-91, 1980

52. Watkins LR, Griffin G, Leichnetz GR, et al: The somatotopic organization of the nucleus raphe magnus and surrounding brain stem structures as revealed by HRP slow-release gels. *Brain Res* 181:1-15, 1980

53. Satoh M, Akaike A, Nakazawa T, et al: Evidence for involvement of separate mechanisms in the production of analgesia by electrical stimulation of the nucleus reticularis paragigantocellularis and nucleus raphe magnus in the rat. *Brain Res* 194:525-529, 1980

54. Takagi H: The nucleus reticularis paragigantocellularis as a site of analgesic action of morphine and enkephalin. *Trends Pharmacol Sci* 1:182-184, 1980

55. Skagergerg G, Björklund A: Monoaminergic and non-aminergic projection to the spinal cord from the catecholamine and indolamine cell groups in the rat brainstem as revealed by transmitter specific fluorescent retrograde tracing (abstract). *Neurosci Let* 5(Suppl):S105, 1980

56. Carstens E, Klumpp D, Zimmermann M: Differential inhibitory effects of medial and lateral midbrain stimulation on spinal neuronal discharges to noxious skin heating in the cat. *J Neurophysiol* 43:332-342, 1980

57. Carstens E, Zimmermann M: The opiate antagonist naloxone does not consistently block inhibition of spinal nociceptive transmission produced by stimulation in lateral midbrain reticular formation of the cat. *Neurosci Let* 20:335-339, 1980

58. Dickenson AH, Le Bars D, Besson JM: Diffuse noxious inhibitory controls (DNIC). Effects on trigeminal nucleus caudalis neurones in the rat. *Brain Res* 200:293-305, 1980

59. Le Bars D, Guilbaud G, Chitour D, et al: Does systemic morphine increase descending inhibitory controls of dorsal horn neurones involved in nociception? *Brain Res* 202:223-228, 1980

60. Johnson SM, Duggan AW: Evidence that the opiate receptors of the substantia gelatinosa contribute to the depression, by intravenous morphine, of the spinal transmission of impulses in unmyelinated primary afferents. *Brain Res* 207:223-228, 1981

61. Davies J, Dray A: Depression and facilitation of synaptic responses in cat dorsal horn by substance P administered into substantia gelatinosa. *Life Sci* 27:2037-2042, 1980

62. Maruyama Y, Shimoji K, Shimizu H, et al: Effects of morphine on human spinal cord and peripheral nervous activities. *Pain* 8:63-74, 1980

63. Willer JC, Bussel B: Possible explanation for analgesia mediated by direct spinal effect of morphine. *Lancet* 1:158-159, 1980

64. Willer JC, Bussel B: Evidence for a direct spinal mechanism in morphine-induced inhibition of nociceptive reflexes in humans. *Brain Res* 187:212-215, 1980

65. Zieglgänsberger W: An enkephalinergic gating system involved in nociception? In *Neural Peptides and Neuronal Communication*. Edited by Costa E, Trabucchi M. New York, Raven Press, 1980, pp 425-434

66. Hunt SP, Kelly JS, Emson PC: The electron microscopic localization of methionine-enkephalin within the superficial layers (I and II) of the spinal cord. *Neuroscience* 5:1871-1890, 1980

67. Nicoll RA, Schenker C, Leeman SE: Substance P as a transmitter candidate. *Annu Rev Neurosci* 3:227-268, 1980

68. Yaksh TL, Jessel TM, Gamse R, et al: Intrathecal morphine inhibits substance P release from mammalian spinal cord in vivo. *Nature* 286:155-157, 1980

69. Glazer EJ, Basbaum AI: Immunohistochemical localization of leucine-enkephalin in the spinal cord of the cat: enkephalin-containing marginal neurons and pain modulation. *J Comp Neurol* 196:377-389, 1981

70. Henry JL: Substance P and pain: an updating. *Trends Neurosci* 3:95-97, 1980

71. Hayes AG, Tyers MB: Effects of capsaicin on nociceptive heat, pressures and chemical thresholds and on substance P levels in the rat. *Brain Res* 189:561-564, 1980

72. Wright DM, Roberts MHT: Responses of spinal neurones to a substance P analogue, noxious pinch and bradykinin. *Eur J Pharmacol* 64:165-167, 1980

73. Henry JL, Sessle BJ, Lucier GE, et al: Effects of

substance P on nociceptive and non-nociceptive trigeminal brain stem neurons. *Pain* 8:33-45, 1980

74. Duggan AW, Griersmith BT, Headley PM, et al: Lack of effect by substance P at sites in the substantia gelatinosa where met-enkephalin reduces the transmission of nociceptive impulses. *Neurosci Let* 12:313-317, 1979

75. Hökfelt T, Johansson O, Ljungdahl A, et al: Peptidergic neurones. *Nature* 284:515-521, 1980

76. Snyder SH: Peptide neurotransmitters with possible involvements in pain perception. In *Pain*. Edited by Bonica JJ. New York, Raven Press, 1980, pp 233-243

77. Jeftinija S, Miletic V, Randic M: Cholecystokinin octapeptide excites dorsal horn neurones both in vivo and in vitro. *Brain Res* 213:231-236, 1981

78. Baker SBC, Wong CC, Wong PC, et al: Transcutaneous electrostimulation in the management of postoperative pain: initial report. *Can Anaesth Soc J* 27:150-155, 1980

79. Fields HL: Pain. II. New approaches to management. *Ann Neurol* 9:101-106, 1981

80. Schuster GD, Infante MC: Pain relief after low back surgery: the efficacy of transcutaneous electrical nerve stimulation. *Pain* 8:299-302, 1980

81. Richardson RR, Siqueira EB: Transcutaneous electrical neurostimulation in postlaminectomy pain. *Spine* 5:361-365, 1980

82. Sodipo JOA, Adadeji SA, Olumide O: Postoperative pain relief by transcutaneous electrical nerve stimulation. *Am J Chin Med* 8:190-194, 1980

83. Richardson RR, Meyer PR, Cerullo LJ: Transcutaneous electrical neurostimulation in muskuloskeletal pain of acute spinal cord injuries. *Spine* 5:42-45, 1980

84. Johansson F, Almay BGL, Von Knorring L, et al: Predictors for the outcome of treatment with high frequency transcutaneous electrical nerve stimulation in patients with chronic pain. *Pain* 9:55-61, 1980

85. Bates JAV, Nathan PW: Transcutaneous electrical nerve stimulation for chronic pain. *Anaesthesia* 35:817-822, 1980

86. Ignelzi RJ, Nyquist JK: Excitability changes in peripheral nerve fibers after repetitive electrical stimulation. *J Neurosurg* 51:824-833, 1979

87. Janko M, Trontel JV: Transcutaneous electrical nerve stimulation: a microneurographic and perceptual study. *Pain* 9:219-230, 1980

88. Woolf CJ, Mitchell D, Barrett GD: Antinociceptive effect of peripheral segmental electrical stimulation in the rat. *Pain* 8:237-252, 1980

89. Salar G, Job I, Mingrino S, et al: Effect of transcutaneous electrotherapy on CSF β-endorphin content in patients without pain problems. *Pain* 10:169-172, 1981

90. Krainick JU, Thoden U, Riechert T: Pain reduction in amputees by long-term spinal cord stimulation. *J Neurosurg* 52:346-350, 1980

91. Richardson RR, Meyer PR, Cerullo LJ: Neurostimulation in the modulation of intractable paraplegic and traumatic neuroma pains. *Pain* 8:75-84, 1980

92. Tasker RR, Organ LW, Hawrylyshyn P: Deafferentation and causalgia. In *Pain*. Edited by Bonica JJ. New York, Raven Press, 1980, pp 305-329

93. Sweet WH: Central mechanisms of chronic pain (neuralgias and certain other neurogenic pain). In *Pain*. Edited by Bonica JJ. New York, Raven Press, 1980, pp 287-303

94. Chung SH, Dickenson A: Pain, enkephalin and acupuncture. *Nature* 283:243-244, 1980

95. Takeshige C, Luo CP, Murai M, et al: Afferent pathway of acupuncture analgesia to limbic system and its correlation with morphine analgesia (abstract). *Neurosci Let* 4 (Suppl):S76, 1980

96. Anzhong Z, Xiaoping P, Shaofen X, et al: Endorphins and acupuncture analgesia. *Chin Med J* 93:673-680, 1980

97. Wall PD, Woolf CJ: What we don't know about pain. *Nature* 287:185-186, 1980

98. Kosterlitz HW: Possible functions of the enkephalins. In *Neural Peptides and Neuronal Communication*. Edited by Costa E, Trabucchi M. New York, Raven Press, 1980, pp 633-642

99. Chapman CR, Colpitts YM, Benedetti C, et al: Evoked potential assessment of acupuncture analgesia: attempted reversal with naloxone. *Pain* 9:183-197, 1980

100. Coan RM, Wong G, Ku SL, et al: The acupuncture treatment of low back pain: a randomized controlled study. *Am J Chin Med* 8:181-189, 1980

101. Johnston JR, McCaughey W: Epidural morphine. A method of management of multiple fractured ribs. *Anaesthesia* 35:155-157, 1980

102. Layfield DJ, Lemberger RJ, Hopkinson BR, et al: Epidural morphine for ischemic rest pain. *Br Med J* 282:697-698, 1981

103. Dirksen R, Nijhuis GMM: Epidural opiate perioperative analgesia. *Acta Anaesthesiol Scand* 24:367-374, 1980

104. Graham JL, King R, McCaughey W: Postoperative pain relief using epidural morphine. *Anaesthesia* 35:158-160, 1980

105. Ebert J, Varner PD: The effective use of epidural morphine sulfate for postoperative orthopaedic pain. *Anaesthesiology* 53:257-258, 1980

106. Boskovski N, Lewinski A, Xuereb, J, et al: Caudal epidural morphine for postoperative pain relief (letter). *Anaesthesia* 36:67-68, 1981

107. Baraka A, Noueihid R, Hajj S: Intrathecal injection of morphine for obstetric analgesia. *Anaesthesiology* 54:136-140, 1981

108. Francis DM, Justins D, Reynolds FJM: Obstetric pain relief using epidural narcotic agents (letter). *Anaesthesia* 36:69, 1981

109. Husemeyer RP, O'Connor MC, Davenport HT: Failure of epidural morphine to relieve pain in labour. *Anaesthesia* 35:161-163, 1980

110. Crawford JS: Experience with epidural morphine in obstetrics. *Anaesthesia* 36:207-209, 1981

111. McClure JH, Chambers WA, Moore E, et al: Epidural morphine for postoperative pain. *Lancet* 1:975-976, 1980

112. Howard RP, Milne LA, Williams NE: Epidural morphine in terminal care. *Anaesthesia* 36:51-53, 1981

113. Magora F, Olshwang D, Eimerl D, et al: Observations on extradural morphine analgesia in various pain conditions. *Br J Anaesth* 52:247-252, 1980

114. Torda TA: Epidural analgesia with morphine. A preliminary communication. *Anaesth Intensive Care* 7:367-370, 1979

115. Torda TA, Pybus DA, Liberman H, et al: Experimental comparison of extradural and I.M. morphine. *Br J Anaesth* 52:939-943, 1980

116. Boas RA: Hazards of epidural morphine (letter). *Anaesth Intensive Care* 8:377-378, 1980

117. Collier CB: Epidural morphine (letter). *Anaesthesia* 36:67, 1981

118. Duffy BL: Itching as a side effect of epidural morphine (letter). *Anaesthesia* 36:67, 1981

119. Hirlekar G: Is itching after caudal epidural morphine dose related? (letter) *Anaesthesia* 36:68, 1981

120. Wynn Parry CB: Pain in avulsion lesions of the brachial plexus. *Pain* 9:41-53, 1980

121. Levitt M, Levitt JH: The deafferentation syndrome in monkeys: dysethesias of spinal origin. *Pain* 10:129-147, 1981

122. Bonica JJ: The need of a taxonomy. *Pain* 6:247-252, 1979

123. Loh L, Nathan PW, Schott GD, et al: Effects of regional guanethidine infusion in certain pain states. *J Neurol Neurosurg Psychiatry* 43:446-451, 1980

124. Tahmoush AJ: Causalgia: redefinition as a clinical pain syndrome. *Pain* 10:187-197, 1981

125. Bentley JB, Hameroff SR: Diffuse reflex sympathetic dystrophy. *Anaesthesiology* 53:256-257, 1980

126. Fager CA, Freidberg SR: Analysis of failures and poor results of lumbar spine surgery. *Spine* 5:87-94, 1980

127. Anderson JAD: Occupational aspects of low back pain. *Clin Rheum Dis* 6:17-35, 1980

128. Frymoyer JW, Pope MH, Costanza MC, et al: Epidemiologic studies of low-back pain. *Spine* 5:419-423, 1980

129. Loeser JD: Low back pain: In *Pain*. Edited by Bonica JJ. New York, Raven Press, 1980, pp 363-377

130. Hamblen DL: The role of surgery in low back pain. *Clin Rheum Dis* 6:191-216, 1980

131. Spengler DM, Freeman C, Miller JW, et al: Low-back pain following multiple spine procedures: failure of initial selection? *Spine* 5:356-360, 1980

132. Weir BKA, Jacobs GA: Reoperation rate following lumbar discectomy. An analysis of 662 lumbar discectomies. *Spine* 5:366-370, 1980

133. Bogduk N: The anatomy and pathology of lumbar back disability. *Bull Postgrad Committee Med Univ Sydney* 36:2-17, 1980

134. Bogduk N, Tynan W, Wilson AS: The nerve supply of the human lumbar intervertebral discs. *J Anat* 132:39-56, 1981

135. Bogduk N: Lumbar dorsal ramus syndrome. *Med J Aust* 2:537-541, 1980

136. Park WM: The place of radiology in the investigation of low back pain. *Clin Rheum Dis* 6:93-132, 1980

137. Howe JF: A neurophysiological basis for the radicular pain of nerve root compression. *Advances in Pain Research and Therapy*, vol 3. Edited by Bonica JJ, Liebeskind JC, Albe-Fessard DG. New York, Raven Press, 1979, pp 647-657

138. Farfan H: The pathological anatomy of degenerative spondylolisthesis: a cadaver study. *Spine* 5:412-418, 1980

139. Cole JP, Gossman D: Ultrasonic stimulation of low lumbar nerve roots as a diagnostic procedure: a preliminary report. *Clin Orthop* 153:126-131, 1980

140. Gunn CC, Milbrandt WE, Little AS, et al: Dry needling of muscle motor points for chronic low-back pain: a randomized clinical trial with long-term follow-up. *Spine* 5:279-291, 1980

141. Garfin SR, Pye SA: Bed design and its effect on chronic low back pain—a limited controlled trial. *Pain* 10:87-91, 1981

142. Bogduk N, Long DM: Percutaneous lumbar medial branch neurotomy. A modification of facet denervation. *Spine* 5:193-200, 1980

143. Ignelzi RJ, Cummings TW: A statistical analysis of percutaneous radiofrequency lesions in the treatment of chronic low back pain and sciatica. *Pain* 8:181-187, 1980

144. Graham CE: Chemonucleolysis. *Clin Rheum Dis* 6:179--189, 1980

145. Ravichandran G, Mulholland RC: Chymopapain chemonucleolysis. A preliminary report. *Spine* 5:380-384, 1980

146. Javid MJ: Treatment of herniated lumbar disk syndrome with chymopapain. *JAMA* 243:2043-2048, 1980

147. Brena SF, Wolf SL, Chapman SL, et al: Chronic back pain; electromyographic, motion and behavioural assessments following sympathetic nerve blocks and placebos. *Pain* 8:1-10, 1980

148. White AH, Derby R, Wynne G: Epidural injections for the diagnosis and treatment of low-back pain. *Spine* 5:78-86, 1980

149. Benoist M, Ficat C, Baraf P, et al: Postoperative

lumbar epiduro-arachnoiditis: diagnostic and therapeutic aspects. *Spine* 5:432-436, 1980

150. Hoppenstein R: A new approach to the failed, back syndrome. *Spine* 5:37-379, 1980

151. Yong-Hing K, Reilly J, de Korompay V, et al: Prevention of nerve root adhesions after laminectomy. *Spine* 5:59-64, 1980

152. Jacobs RR, McClain O, Neff J: Control of postlaminectomy scar formation: an experimental and clinical study. *Spine* 5:223-229, 1980

153. Feild JR, McHenry H: The lumbar shield: a progress report. *Spine* 5:264-278, 1980

154. Nordemar R, Thorner C: Treatment of acute cervical pain—a comparative group study. *Pain* 10:93-101, 1981

155. Wilkinson HA, Schuman N: Intradiscal corticosteroids in the treatment of lumbar and cervical disc problems. *Spine* 5:385-389, 1980

156. Sluijter ME, Koetsveld-Baart CC: Interruption of pain pathways in the treatment of the cervical syndrome. *Anaesthesia* 35:302-307, 1980

157. Bogduk N: The clinical anatomy of the cervical dorsal rami. *Spine*. In press, 1982

158. Bogduk N: Local anaesthetic blocks of the second cervical ganglion cephalalgia 1. In press, 1982

159. Lance JW, Anthony M: Neck-tongue syndrome on sudden turning of the head. *J Neurol Neurosurg Psychiatry* 43:97-101, 1980

160. Bogduk N: An anatomical basis for the neck tongue syndrome. *J Neurol Neurosurg Psychiatry* 44:202-208, 1981

161. Diamond S, Medina LJ: Cyclical migraine (abstract). Third International Symposium, London, The Migraine Trust, 1980, pp 11-12

162. Lance JW: Headache. *Ann Neurol* 10:1-10, 1981

163. Dalessio DJ: Wolff's *Headache and Other Head Pain,* 4th ed. New York, Oxford University Press, 1980

164. Lance JW: *The Mechanism and Management of Headache,* 3rd ed. London, Butterworths, 1978

165. Raskin NH, Appenzeller O: Headache. In *Major Problems in Internal Medicine,* vol 14. Edited by Smith LH. Philadelphia, Saunders, 1980

166. Murray TJ: Temporal arteritis. *J Am Geriatr Soc* 25:450-453, 1977

167. Wilkinson IMS, Russell RWF: Arteries of the head and neck in giant cell arteritis. *Arch Neurol* 27:378-391, 1972

168. Liang GC, Simkin PA, Mannik M: Immunoglobulins in temporal arteritis. An immunofluorescent study. *Ann Intern Med* 81:19-24, 1974

169. Klein RG, Campbell RJ, Hunder GG, et al: Skip lesions in temporal arteritis. *Mayo Clin Proc* 51:504-510, 1976

170. Huston KA, Hunder GG, Lie JT, et al: A 25 year epidemiologic, clinical and pathologic study in temporal arteritis. *Ann Intern Med* 88:162-167, 1978

171. Kansut, Corbett JJ, Savino P, et al: Giant cell arteritis with normal sedimentation rate. *Arch Neurol* 34:624-625, 1977

172. Graham E, Holland H, Avery A, et al: Prognosis in giant-cell arteritis. *Br Med J* 282:269-271, 1981

173. Donnan GA, Bladin PF: The stroke syndrome of long intraluminal clot with incomplete vessel obstruction. *Clin Exp Neurol* 16:41-47, 1979

174. West TET, Davies RJ, Kelly RE: Horner's syndrome and headache due to carotid artery disease. *Br Med J* 1:818-820, 1976

175. Massey EW, Massey J: Elongated styloid process (Eagle's syndrome) causing hemicrania. *Headache* 19:339-344, 1979

176. Mumford JM: Thermography and ice cream headache. *Acta Thermograph* 4:33-37, 1979

177. Raskin NH, Knittle SC: Ice cream headache and orthostatic symptoms in patients with migraine. *Headache* 16:222-225, 1976

178. Vallet JM, Vallet M, Julien J, et al: Painful ophthalmoplegia (Tolosa Hunt) accompanied by peripheral facial paralysis. *Ann Neurol* 8:645, 1980

179. Haines SJ, Janetta PJ, Zorub DS: Microvascular relations of the trigeminal nerve. An anatomical study with clinical correlation. *J Neurosurg* 52:381-386, 1980

180. Kerr FWL: Craniofacial neuralgias. In *Advances in Pain Research and Therapy,* vol 3. Edited by Bonica JJ, Liebeskind JC, Albe-Fessard DG. New York, Raven Press, 1979, pp 283-295

181. Denny-Brown D, Yanigisawa N: The function of the descending root of the fifth nerve. *Brain* 96:783-814, 1973

182. Burchiel KJ: Abnormal impulse generation in focally demyelinated trigeminal roots. *J Neurosurg* 53:674-683, 1980

183. Ruskin AP: Facial neuralgia with trigger point on finger. One case suggesting a cortically mediated response. *Arch Neurol* 37:672, 1980

184. Asher SW: Multiple cranial neuropathies, trigeminal neuralgia, and vascular headaches in sickle cell disease, a possible common mechanism. *Neurology* 30:210-211, 1980

185. Fromm GH, Terrence CF, Chattha AS: Treatment of face pain with baclofen (abstract). *Ann Neurol* 8:130-131, 1980

186. Harper CG: A rare cause of sudden death. *Med J Aust* 1:562-565, 1981

187. Williams B: Cough headache due to craniospinal pressure dissociation. *Arch Neurol* 37:226-230, 1980

188. Daniels AM, Sallie R: Headache, lumbar puncture, and expectation. *Lancet* 1:1003, 1980

189. Marlin AE, Epstein F, Rouit R: Positional headache and syncope associated with a pseudo-meningocele. *Arch Neurol* 37:736-737, 1980

190. Reid AC, Matheson MS, Teasdale G: Volume of the ventricles in benign intracranial hypertension. *Lancet* 2:7-8, 1980

191. Johnson I, Paterson A: Benign Intracranial Hypertension. II. CSF pressure and circulation. *Brain* 97:301-312, 1974

192. Spence JD, Amacher AL, Willis NR: Cerebrospinal fluid (CSF) pressure monitoring in the management of benign intracranial hypertension without papilledema. *Neurology* 29:551, 1979

193. Walters BNJ, Gubbay SS: Tetracycline and benign intracranial hypertension: report of five cases. *Br Med J* 282:19-20, 1981

194. Snyder DA, Frenkel M: An unusual presentation of pseudotumor cerebri. *Ann Ophthalmol* 11:1823-1827, 1979

195. McCammon A, Kaufman HH, Sears ES: Transient oculomoter paralysis in pseudotumor cerebri. *Neurology* 31:182-184, 1981

196. Edmeads J: The headaches of ischemic cerebrovascular disease. *Headache* 19:345-349, 1979

197. Pearce J: Headache after carotid endarterectomy. *Br Med J* 3:85-86, 1979

198. Greden JF, Victor BS, Fontaine P, Lubetsky M: Caffeine-withdrawal headache: a clinical profile. *Psychosomatics* 21:411-418, 1980

199. Levy RL: Strokes and orgasmic cephalgia. *Headache* 21:12-13, 1981

200. Lance JW: Headaches related to sexual activity. *J Neurol Neurosurg Psychiatry* 39:1226-1230, 1976

201. Lance JW: What is migraine? In *Headache '80*. Edited by Sicuteri F. Proceedings of International Headache Symposium, Florence, March 1980, New York, Raven Press. In press, 1981

202. Doleček R: Experimental and clinical results with pizotifen in the treatment of underweight patients. *Pharmatherapeutica* 2:363-371, 1980

203. Fisher CM: Late-life migraine accompaniments as a cause of unexplained transient ischemic attacks. *Can J Neurol Sci* 7:9-17, 1980

204. Rascol A, Cambier J, Guiraud B, Manelfe C, et al: Accidents ischémiques cérébraux au cours de crises migraineuses. *Rev Neurol (Paris)* 135:867-884, 1979

205. Raskin NH, Schwartz RK: Icepick-like pain. *Neurology* 30:203-205, 1980

206. Cuypers J, Altenkirch H, Bunge S: Personality profiles in cluster headache and migraine. *Headache* 21:21-24, 1981

207. Sternbach RA, Dalessio DJ, Kunzel M, et al: MMPI patterns in common headache disorders. *Headache* 20:311-315, 1980

208. Kudrow L, Sutkus BJ: MMPI pattern specificity in primary headache disorders. *Headache* 19:18-24, 1979

209. Monro J, Brostoff J, Carini C, et al: Food allergy in migraine: study of dietary exclusion and RAST. *Lancet* 2:1-4, 1980

210. Medina JL, Diamond S: The role of diet in migraine. *Headache* 18:31-34, 1978

211. Lord GDA, Duckworth JW: Immunoglobulin and complement studies in migraine. *Headache* 17:163-168, 1977

212. Lord GDA, Duckworth JW: Complement and immune complex studies in migraine. *Headache* 18:355-360, 1978

213. Moore TL, Ryan RE Jr, Pohl DA, et al: Immunoglobulin, complement and immune complex levels during a migraine attack. *Headache* 20:9-12, 1980

214. Behan WMH, Behan PO, Durward WF: Complement studies in migraine. *Headache* 21:55-57, 1981

215. Sovak M, Kunzel M, Dalessio DJ, et al: C_{-1} inhibitor levels in migraineurs and normals. *Headache* 20:132-133, 1980

216. Bennett DR, Fuenning SI, Sullivan G, et al: Migraine precipitated by head trauma in athletes. *Am J Sports Med* 8:202-205, 1980

217. Schraeder PL, Burns RA: Hemiplegic migraine associated with an aseptic meningeal reaction. *Arch Neurol* 37:377-379, 1980

218. Swanson JW, Bartleson JD, Whisnant JP: A migrainous syndrome with CSF pleocytosis (abstract). *Neurology* 30:418, 1980

219. Blau JN, Dexter SL: Hyperventilation during migraine attacks. *Br Med J* 280:1254, 1980

220. Panayiotopoulos CP: Basilar migraine? Seizures, and severe epileptic EEG abnormalities. *Neurology* 30:1122-1125, 1980

221. Riley TL, Massey EW: The syndrome of aphasia, headaches and left temporal spikes. *Headache* 20:90-92, 1980

222. Eviatar L: Vestibular testing in basilar artery migraine. *Ann Neurol* 9:126-130, 1981

223. Slater R: Benign recurrent vertigo. *J Neurol Neurosurg Psychiatry* 42:363-367, 1979

224. Moretti G, Manzoni GC, Caffarra P, et al: 'Benign recurrent vertigo' and its connection with migraine. *Headache* 20:344-346, 1980

225. Vijayan N: Ophthalmoplegic migraine: ischemic or compressive neuropathy? *Headache* 20:300-304, 1980

226. Zifkin B, Andermann E, Andermann F, et al: An autosomal dominant syndrome of hemiplegic migraine, nystagmus, and tremor. *Ann Neurol* 8:329-332, 1980

227. Cala LA, Mastaglia FL: Computerized axial tomography in the detection of brain damage. II. Epilepsy, migraine and general medical disorders. *Med J Aust* 2:616-620, 1980

228. Larson EB, Omenn GS, Lewis H: Diagnostic evaluation of headache: impact of computerized tomography and cost-effectiveness. *JAMA* 243:359-362, 1980

229. Blau JN, Dexter SL: The site of pain origin during migraine headaches (abstract). Third International Symposium, London, The Migraine Trust, 1980, p 31

230. Drummond PD, Lance JW: Temporal artery pulsation in migraine headache. Unpublished data

231. Tfelt-Hansen P, Lous I, Olesen J: Prevalance and significance of muscle tenderness during common migraine attacks. *Headache* 21:49-54, 1981

232. Sakai F, Meyer JS: Regional cerebral hemodynamics during migraine and cluster headache measured by the ^{113}Xe inhalation method. *Headache* 18:122-132, 1978

233. Drummond PD, Lance JW: Extracranial vascular reactivity in migraine and tension headache. *Cephalalgia* 1:149-155, 1981

234. Sakai F, Meyer JS: Abnormal cerebrovascular reactivity in patients with migraine and cluster headache. *Headache* 19:357-366, 1979

235. Yamamoto M, Meyer JS: Hemicranial disorder of vasomotor adrenoceptors in migraine and cluster headache. *Headache* 20:321-335, 1980

236. Krabbe AA, Olesen J: Headache provocation by continuous intravenous infusion of histamine. Clinical results and receptor mechanisms. *Pain* 8:253-259, 1980

237. Oleson J, Larsen B, Lauritzen M: Focal hyperemia followed by spreading oligemia and impaired activation of rCBF in classical migraine. *Ann Neurol* 9:344-352, 1981

238. Burnstock G: Cholinergic and purinergic regulation of blood vessels. In *Handbook of Physiology*, vol 2. Edited by Bohr DF, Somlyo AD, Sparks HW, et al. Baltimore, Waverly Press, 1980, pp 567-612

239. Raichle ME, Hartman BK, Eichling JO, et al: Central noradrenergic regulation of cerebral blood flow and vascular permeability. *Proc Natl Acad Sci USA* 72:3726-3730, 1975

240. Bates D, Weinshilboum RM, Campbell RJ, et al: The effects of lesions in the locus ceruleus on the physiological responses of the cerebral vessels in cats. *Brain Res* 136:431-443, 1977

241. Kogure K, Scheinberg P, Kishikawa H, et al: Adrenergic control of cerebral blood flow and energy metabolism in the rat. *Stroke* 10:179-184, 1979

242. Harik SI, Sharma VK, Wetherbee JR, et al: Adrenergic receptors of cerebral microvessels. *Eur J Pharmacol* 61:207-208, 1980

243. Reinhard JF Jr, Liebmann JE, Schlosberg AJ, et al: Serotonin neurons project to small blood vessels in the brain. *Science* 206:85-87, 1979

244. Chan-Palay V: Innervation of cerebral blood vessels by norepinephrine, indoleamine, substance P and neurotensin fibers and the leptomeningeal axons: their role in vasomotor activity and local alterations of brain blood composition. In *Neurogenic Control of the Brain Circulation.* Wenner-Gren Center International Symposium Series, vol 30. Edited by Owman C, Edvinsson L. New York, Pergamon Press, 1977, pp 39-53

245. Larsson L-I, Edvinsson L, Fahrenkrug J, et al: Immunohistochemical localization of a vasodilatory polypeptide (VIP) in cerebrovascular nerves. *Brain Res* 113:400-404, 1976

246. Johnson ES: A basis for migraine therapy—the autonomic theory reappraised. *Postgrad Med J* 54:231-242, 1978

247. Kalendowsky Z, Austin JH: 'Complicated migraine.' Its association with increased platelet aggregability and abnormal plasma coagulation factors. *Headache* 15:18-35, 1975

248. Couch JR, Hassanein RS: Platelet aggregability in migraine. *Neurology* 27:843-848, 1977

249. Deshmukh SV, Meyer JS: Cyclic changes in platelet dynamics and the pathogenesis and prophylaxis of migraine. *Headache* 17:101-108, 1977

250. Gawal M, Burkitt M, Rose FC: The platelet release reaction during migraine attacks. *Headache* 19:323-327, 1979

251. Anthony M, Hinterberger H, Lance JW: The possible relation of serotonin to the migraine syndrome. *Res Clin Stud Headache* 2:29-59, 1968

252. Dvilansky A, Rishpon S, Nathan I, et al: Release of platelet 5-hydroxytryptoamine by plasma taken from platelets during and between migraine attacks. *Pain* 2:315-318, 1976

253. Mück-Šeler D, Deanović Ž, Dupelj M: Platelet serotonin (5-HT) and 5-HT releasing factor in plasma of migrainous patients. *Headache* 19:14-17, 1979

254. Fozard JR: Serotonin, migraine and platelets. In *Progress in Pharmacology*, vol 4. Edited by Van Zwieten PA, Schonbaum E. Stuttgart, Gustav Fischer. In press, 1982

255. Sicuteri F: The nature of pain in headache and central panalgesia. In *Mechanism of Pain and Analgesic Compounds.* Edited by Beers RF Jr, Bassett EG. New York, Raven Press, 1979, pp 295-307

256. Nappi G, Martignoni E, Bono G, et al: Mammotrophs receptors sensitivity changes in headache patients, (abstract). Third International Symposium, London, The Migraine Trust, 1980, pp 37-39

257. Giacovazzo M, Romiti A, Martelletti P: Headache and prolactin: clinical findings, In *Headache, Pavia 1979.* IV. *Meeting of the Italian Headache Society.* Edited by Savoldi F, Nappi G. Padua, Fidia Research Laboratories, 1979, pp 149-151

258. Nattero G. Menstrual migraine (recent statistical, clinical, haemodynamic and hormonal data). In *Headache, Pavia 1979.* IV. *Meeting of the Italian Headache Society.* Edited by Savoldi F, Nappi G. Padua, Fidia Research Laboratories, 1979, pp 161-167

259. Vardi J, Flechter S, Ayalon D, et al: L-dopa effect on prolactin plasma levels in complicated and common migrainous patients. *Headache* 21:14-20, 1981

260. Fanciullacci M, Michelacci S, Curradi C, et al: Hyper-responsiveness of migraine patients to the hypotensive action of bromocriptine. *Headache* 20:99-102, 1980

261. Anselmi B, Baldi E, Casacci F, et al: Endogenous opioids in cerebrospinal fluid and blood in idiopathic headache sufferers. *Headache* 20:294-299, 1980

262. Appenzeller O, Standefer J, Atkinson R: Endogenous opioid peptides and vascular headache (abstract). Third International Symposium, London, The Migraine Trust, 1980, p 36

263. Bakal DA, Kaganov JA: Muscle contraction and migraine headache: psychophysiologic comparison. *Headache* 17:208-215, 1977

264. McArthur DL, Cohen MJ: Measures of forehead and finger temperature, frontalis EMG, heart rate and finger pulse amplitude during and between migraine headaches. *Headache* 20:134-136, 1980

265. Lake A, Rainey J, Papsdorf JD: Biofeedback and rational-emotive therapy in the management of migraine headache. *J Appl Behav Anal* 12:127-140, 1979

266. Bild R, Adams HE: Modification of migraine headaches by cephalic blood volume pulse and EMG biofeedback. *J Consult Clin Psychol* 48:51-57, 1980

267. Friar LR, Beatty J: Migraine: management by trained control of vasoconstriction. *J Consult Clin Psychol* 44:46-53, 1976

268. Blanchard EB, Theobald DE, Williamson DA, et al: Temperature biofeedback in the treatment of migraine headaches. *Arch Gen Psychiatry* 35:581-588, 1978

269. Largen JW, Mathew RJ, Dobbins K, et al: Specific and non-specific effects of skin temperature control in migraine management. *Headache* 21:36-44, 1981

270. Kewman D, Roberts AH: Skin temperature biofeedback and migraine headaches. *Biofeedback Self Regul* 5:327-345, 1980

271. Mathew RJ, Largen JW, Dobbins K, et al: Biofeedback control of skin temperature and cerebral blood flow in migraine. *Headache* 20:19-28, 1980

272. Diamond S, Diamond-Falk J, De Veno T: Biofeedback in the treatment of vascular headache. *Biofeedback Self Regul* 3:385-408, 1978

273. Adams HE, Feuerstein M, Fowler JL: Migraine headache review of parameters, etiology and intervention. *Psychol Bull* 87:217-237, 1980

274. Cohen MJ, McArthur DL, Rickles WH: Comparison of four biofeedback treatments for migraine headache: physiological and headache variables. *Psychosom Med* 42:463-481, 1980

275. Parker GB, Pryor DS, Tupling H: Why does migraine improve during a clinical trial? Further results from a trial of cervical manipulation for migraine. *Aust NZ J Med* 10:192-198, 1980

276. Ala-Hurula V, Myllylä VV, Hokkanen E: Ergotamine plasma levels in relation to its clinical efficacy (abstract). Third International Symposium, London, The Migraine Trust, 1980, pp 51-52

277. Spierings ELH, Saxena PR: The action of ergotamine on the distribution of carotid blood flow—the migraine shunt theory revisited. *Headache* 20:143-145, 1980

278. Spierings ELH, Saxena PR: Effect of isomeptene on the distribution and shunting of 15 μm microspheres throughout the cephalic circulation of the cat. *Headache* 20:103-106, 1980

279. Tfelt-Hansen P, Olesen J, Aebelholt-Krabbe A, et al: A double blind study of metoclopramide in the treatment of migraine attacks. *J Neurol Neurosurg Psychiatry* 43:369-371, 1980

280. Hakkarainen H, Vapaatolo H, Gothoni G, et al: Tolfenamic acid is as effective as ergotamine during migraine attacks. *Lancet* 2:326-328, 1979

281. Syvalahti E, Kangasniemi P, Ross SB: Migraine headache and blood serotonin levels after administration of zimelidine, a selective inhibitor of serotonin uptake. *Curr Ther Res* 25:299-310, 1979

282. Ryan RE, Ryan RE Jr: Clonidine—its use in migraine therapy. *Headache* 14:190-192, 1975

283. Anthony M, Lord GDA, Lance JW: Controlled trials of cimetidine in migraine and cluster headache. *Headache* 18:261-264, 1978

284. Nanda RN, Arthur GP, Johnson RH, et al: Cimetidine in the prophylaxis of migraine. *Acta Neurol Scand* 62:90-95, 1980

285. Mylecharane EJ, Duckworth JW, Lord GDA, et al: Effects of low doses of clonidine in the monkey cranial circulation. *Eur J Pharmacol* 68:163-173, 1980

286. Mazal S, Rachmilewitz EA: The effect of an antiserotonin agent pizotifen on platelet aggregability in migraine patients. *J Neurol Neurosurg Psychiatry* 43:1137-1140, 1980

287. Masel BE, Chesson AL, Peters BH, et al: Platelet antagonists in migraine prophylaxis. A clinical trial using aspirin and dipyridamole. *Headache* 20:13-18, 1980

288. Stensrud P, Sjaastad O: Comparative trial of Tenormin (atenolol) and Inderal (propranolol) in migraine. *Headache* 20:204-207, 1980

289. Lindegaard K-F, Ovrelid L, Sjaastad O: Naproxen in the prevention of migraine attacks. A double-blind placebo-controlled cross-over study. *Headache* 20:96-98, 1980

290. Sulman FG, Pfeifer Y, Superstine E: Preventive treatment of migraine with enzyme induction by Proxibarbital in a 'double-blind' trial. *Headache* 20:269-273, 1980

291. Behan PO, Reid M: Propranolol in the treatment of migraine. *Practitioner* 224:201-204, 1980

292. Raskin NH, Schwartz RK: Interval therapy of migraine: long-term results. *Headache* 20:336-340, 1980

293. Kudrow L: *Cluster Headache: Mechanisms and Management.* Oxford, Oxford University Press, 1980

294. Pearce JMS: Chronic migrainous neuralgia: a variant of cluster headache. *Brain* 103:149-159, 1980

295. Sjaastad O, Apfelbaum R, Caskey W, et al: Chronic paroxysmal hemicrania (CPH). The clinical manifestations. A review. *Ups J Med Sci* 31 (Suppl):27-33, 1980

296. Cuypers J, Altenkirch H, Bunge S: Personality profiles in cluster headache and migraine. *Headache* 21:21-24, 1980

297. Henry PY, Vernhiet J, Orgogozo JM, et al: Cerebral blood flow in migraine and cluster headache. *Res Clin Stud Headache* 6:81-88, 1978

298. Nelson RF, du Boulay GH, Marshall J, et al: Cerebral blood flow studies in patients with cluster headache. *Headache* 20:184-189, 1980

299. Hardebo JE, Krabbe AA, Gjerris F: Enhanced dilatory response to histamine in large extracranial vessels in chronic cluster headache. *Headache* 20:316-320, 1980

300. Lord GDA, Mylecharane EJ, Duckworth JW, et al: Effects of histamine H_1- and H_2- receptor antagonists in the cranial circulation of the monkey. *Clin Exp Pharmacol Physiol* 8:89-100, 1980

301. Medina JL, Fareed J, Diamond S: Lithium carbonate therapy for cluster headache. Changes in number of platelets and serotonin and histamine levels. *Arch Neurol* 37:559-563, 1980

302. Caviness VS, O'Brien P: Cluster headache: response to chlorpromazine. *Headache* 20:128-131, 1980

303. Kudrow L: Response of cluster headache attacks to oxygen inhalation. *Headache* 21:1-4, 1981

304. Martin PR, Mathews AM: Tension headaches: psychophysiological investigation and treatment. *J Psychosom Res* 22:389-399, 1978

305. Krabbe AA, Olesen J: Headache provocation by continuous intravenous infusion of histamine. Clinical results and receptor mechanisms. *Pain* 8:253-259, 1980

306. Rolf LH, Wiele G, Brune GG: 5-hydroxytryptamine in platelets of patients with muscle contraction headache. *Headache* 21:10-11, 1981

307. Cohen MJ, McArthur DL: Classification of migraine and tension headache from a survey of 10,000 headache diaries. *Headache* 21:25-29, 1981

308. Philips C: Tension headache: theoretical problems. *Behav Res Ther* 16:249-261, 1978

309. Martin PR: Behavioral management of headaches: a review of the evidence. *Int J Ment Health* 9:88-110, 1980

310. Bruhn P, Olesen J, Melgaard B: Controlled trial of EMG feedback in muscle contraction headache. *Ann Neurol* 6:34-36, 1979

311. Nuechterlein KM, Holroyd JC: Biofeedback in the treatment of tension headache—current status. *Arch Gen Psychiatry* 37:866-873, 1980

312. Jessup BA, Neufeld RWJ, Merskey H: Biofeedback therapy for headache and other pain: an evaluative review. *Pain* 7:225-270, 1979

313. Blanchard EB, Andrasik F, Ahles TA, et al: Migraine and tension headache: a meta-analytic review. *Behav Ther* 11:613-631, 1980

314. Sturgis ET, Tollison CD, Adams HE: Modification of combined migraine-muscle contraction headaches using BVP and EMG feedback. *J Appl Behav Anal* 11:215-223, 1978

9

On Prions Causing Dementia: Molecular Studies of the Scrapie Agent

Stanley B. Prusiner

With increasing longevity, senile dementia has become a major disease. The cause of most cases of senile dementia is unknown. Laboratory investigations of senile dementia have been greatly hampered by the lack of good animal models. The dementias accompanying two human degenerative disorders, kuru and Creutzfeldt-Jakob disease (CJD), possess features that are similar to those found in senile dementia of the Alzheimer's type. Dementia occurs early in the course of CJD and late in kuru. Both kuru and CJD are caused by slow transmissible agents that appear to be similar to the infectious agent causing scrapie in sheep and goats many months or years after exposure or inoculation. Six lines of evidence, including sensitivity to proteases, demonstrate that the scrapie agent contains a protein which is required for infectivity. Although the scrapie agent is irreversibly inactivated by alkali, five procedures with more specificity for modifying nucleic acids failed to cause inactivation. The apparent heterogeneity of the scrapie agent with respect to size appears to result from its hydrophobicity; the smallest form of the agent may have a molecular weight of 50,000 or less. Nonpolar side chains of amino acid residues within a protein may be responsible for its hydrophobic properties. Because the novel properties of the scrapie agent appear to distinguish it from viruses, plasmids, and viroids, a new term *"prion"* is proposed to denote a small *pro*teinaceous *in*fectious particle which resists inactivation by most procedures that modify nucleic acids. Current knowledge does not allow exclusion of a small nucleic acid buried inside of a protein shell. However, it is unlikely that this hypothetical nucleic acid is of sufficient size to code for the protein coat. Although many features of Alzheimer's senile dementia resemble facets of scrapie, kuru, and CJD, the role of prions in the causation of senile dementia is unknown. The study of prions may also have significance for understanding the causes of many other degenerative diseases, the etiologies of which remain elusive.

INTRODUCTION

Diseases that diminish intellect, memory, and judgment are perhaps the most demeaning and cruel of all illnesses. It is these very functions—the hallmarks of the human species—that are lost in dementia. The patient with dementia progressively loses those intellectual qualities that have distinguished him as an individual. In many cases the patient observes, with great frustration and sadness, his slow but progressive deterioration of intellectual function. His family, friends, colleagues, and physicians must watch helplessly.

This study was supported by research grants from the National Institutes of Health (NS14069) and the National Science Foundation (PCM77-24076).

The problem of dementia is growing, particularly among the elderly. As longevity increases, the number of individuals with dementia increases. Most patients with dementia appear to have Alzheimer's disease, which is thought to have two forms: presenile and senile. The senile form is the most common. It is estimated that 3 million individuals currently suffer from dementia in the United States (1). One million who are unable to care for themselves comprise the majority of nursing home patients. While the statistics are overwhelming, the cost to society is staggering. At present 10 billion dollars are spent annually to care for these demented patients. With more and more people living into old age the problem is expected to grow to enormous proportions over the next 3 decades. By the year 2010 we could be spending 50-100 billion dollars annually for the care of demented patients.

Because the incidence of senile dementia rises with increasing age, any person reaching the age of 80 has nearly a one in three chance of becoming senile (2). For many years senility or senile dementia was thought to be a normal accompaniment of the aging process; however, this is no longer thought to be the case. It is believed that senile dementia is caused by a group of disorders, the most common of which is Alzheimer's disease. These disorders are subject to investigation as well as eventual treatment and prevention. So little is known about the causes of these disorders, especially Alzheimer's disease, in part because there are no ideal animal models for investigative studies (3). Until such models become available, investigators must continue to use human specimens and imperfect animal models.

Over the past 2 decades, two human degenerative neurological diseases in which dementia is a prominent feature have been shown to be caused by unusual slow virus-like agents (4). These diseases are Creutzfeldt-Jakob disease (CJD) and kuru. Dementia is an early feature of CJD while it does not occur until late in kuru (5, 6). In kuru and CJD as well as Alzheimer's disease only the central nervous system is affected. Curiously, many other aspects of these three human diseases are similar including: (1) afebrile courses, (2) no pleocytosis or abnormal proteins in cerebrospinal fluid, (3) numerous amyloid or senile plaques, (4) prominent loss of dendritic spines, and (5) widespread proliferation of astrocytes.

Although kuru and CJD are primarily transmissible to primates, an analogous disease of sheep and goats, scrapie, is readily transmitted to laboratory rodents. The chemical structure of the infectious agent causing scrapie was completely unknown until recently (7). Studies on the kuru and CJD agents suggest that their structures will probably be similar to the agent causing scrapie (8, 9).

The scrapie agent—like viruses, plasmids, and viroids—passes through filters that retain bacteria and other large pathogens. All of these filterable microbes replicate inside of living cells using cellular synthetic machinery (10). They are all intracellular parasites, and their lack of cellular organization clearly distinguishes them from other intracellular parasites such as the Rickettsiae and Chlamydiaceae, which reproduce by division.

SMALL INFECTIOUS AGENTS

Recognition of a new class of infectious particles seems imminent from studies of the scrapie agent. These particles clearly extend the virus concept and may force revision of some of the dogmatic tenets that are the current foundations of modern molecular biology (11). While recent studies have shown that the scrapie agent contains a hydrophobic protein, which is required for infectivity, no nucleic acid has been identified (7, 12-14). The scrapie agent appears to be a prototype for a novel class of *prot*einaceous *inf*ectious particles (*prions*). The molecular properties of the scrapie agent reflect this proteinaceous structure. Similar small infectious agents may not only cause kuru and CJD but might also exist in *Naegleria amoeba* (4, 15). The scrapie agent is readily distinguished from regulatory proteins, including repressors, toxins, and hormones, because the agent triggers its own replication.

Table 1 lists the macromolecular compo-

Table 1. Classification and Molecular Structure of Small Infectious Agents

Agents	Nucleic Acid	Protein	Lipid
Virions	+	+	+/−
Plasmids and viroids	+	−	−
Prions	( )*	+	+/−

*( ) denotes resistance of the scrapie agent to inactivation by procedures that modify nucleic acids.

nents of viruses, viroids, plasmids, and prions. Viruses contain nucleic acid genomes, which replicate intracellularly and which possess all of the information needed for their multiplication (10). These genomes are either RNA or DNA. No virus containing an RNA-DNA hybrid has been identified to date. The viral genome codes for proteins that generate a shell or capsid within which the viral nucleic acid is enclosed. In some viruses, spikes or even tails are added to the capsid structure; in other viruses, lipid bilayers containing viral specific proteins form envelopes around the capsid. In addition, many viral proteins are glycosylated. Thousands of viruses have been isolated from bacteria, fungi, plants, insects, animals, and humans in contrast to viroids and prions. Viruses produce a broad spectrum of diseases ranging from acute, brief illnesses to prolonged, chronic disorders. Both slow and latent viruses may persist for many years undetected and then become activated.

Viroids are small "naked" nucleic acids which infect plants (16). To date, viroids have been found only in plants, with one possible exception (17). Eleven different viroid diseases of plants have been identified. Viroids are single-stranded covalently closely circular RNAs (18, 19). Viroids contain no protein or lipid (Table 1).

Plasmids, like viroids, are also "naked" nucleic acids (20). Both RNA and DNA plasmids have been identified. Plasmids possess many of the attributes of other filterable infectious agents, although these episomal elements generally enjoy a symbiotic relationship with their hosts. Plasmids express their pathogenicity in several fascinating ways. DNA plasmids confer drug resistance on bacteria that may be pathogenic. In some cases, these plasmids cause disease by conferring upon nonpathogenic bacteria the ability to produce an enterotoxin (20). Plasmids may code for the production of bacteriocins, the most well-studied of which are the colicins. Recent studies have shown that a portion of the Ti plasmid of *Agrobacterium tumefaciens* becomes integrated into the host plant DNA and is the cause of crown gall tumors (21). Double-stranded RNA plasmids of yeast are known to code for a killer protein toxin (22, 23).

Prions contain proteins, and no nucleic acid has been identified to date. The scrapie agent contains a hydrophobic protein, which presumably binds lipid [Table 1] (7, 12, 13). The slow infectious processes of scrapie, kuru, and CJD proceed without any sign of an inflammatory process such as fever, cerebrospinal fluid pleocytosis, or perivascular accumulation of mononuclear cells. How these slow infections are able to evade recognition by the immune system remains a fascinating question (24). An encephalopathy of mink appears to be caused by an agent quite similar or identical to the one causing scrapie [Table 2] (25).

Table 2. Classification of *Prions*

Diseases of Prions	Natural Hosts
Scrapie	Sheep and goats
Mink encephalopathy	Mink
Kuru	Humans (Fore)*
Creutzfeldt-Jakob disease	Humans

*A tribal population in Papua New Guinea.

KURU AND CREUTZFELDT-JAKOB DISEASE

A fascinating saga surrounds the discovery of kuru and its subsequent impact on medical science. As early as 1952 Australian patrol officers (kiaps) charged with bringing order to stone age societies as well as anthropologists studying the organization of these societies commented on a strange trembling disorder, which was common among the Fore people in New Guinea (26, 27). Early observers thought that the disorder was hysterical, and not until 1956 was this common trembling disorder appreciated as an unusual neurological disease. These observations were made by Vincent Zigas, the first medical officer to enter the area (4). Carleton Gajdusek joined Zigas to begin an intensive investigation of the disease (28-30). Gajdusek and coworkers (31) eventually demonstrated that kuru was caused by a slow transmissible agent. These studies were prompted by Hadlow (32) who called attention to the neuropathological similarities between scrapie and kuru.

Likewise, the neuropathological similarities between kuru and CJD were so striking that subsequent studies were undertaken to search for a transmissible agent in CJD (33). For nearly half a century CJD had been classified as a degenerative nervous system disorder of unknown etiology much like Alzheimer's disease is still described. In 1968 Gibbs and Gajdusek (34) demonstrated the transmission of CJD to nonhuman primates (34). One and a half years after intracerebral inoculation with crude suspensions of brain tissue from patients dying of CJD, these experimental primate hosts developed a central nervous system disorder. Subsequently more than 100 cases of CJD have been transmitted to monkeys or chimpanzees (35). Only a few cases of CJD have been transmitted to nonprimate hosts (36).

A recent study has brought scrapie and CJD more closely together than was previously imagined (37). Goats inoculated with brain tissue from demented patients dying of CJD developed a neurological disorder 3-5 years after inoculation (Fig. 1). This disorder was indistinguishable both clinically and neuropathologically from natural scrapie. Monkeys have been used as a common experimental host for scrapie and CJD; curiously, chimpanzees are susceptible to CJD but not scrapie (38, 39). Numerous attempts to link scrapie epidemiologically to

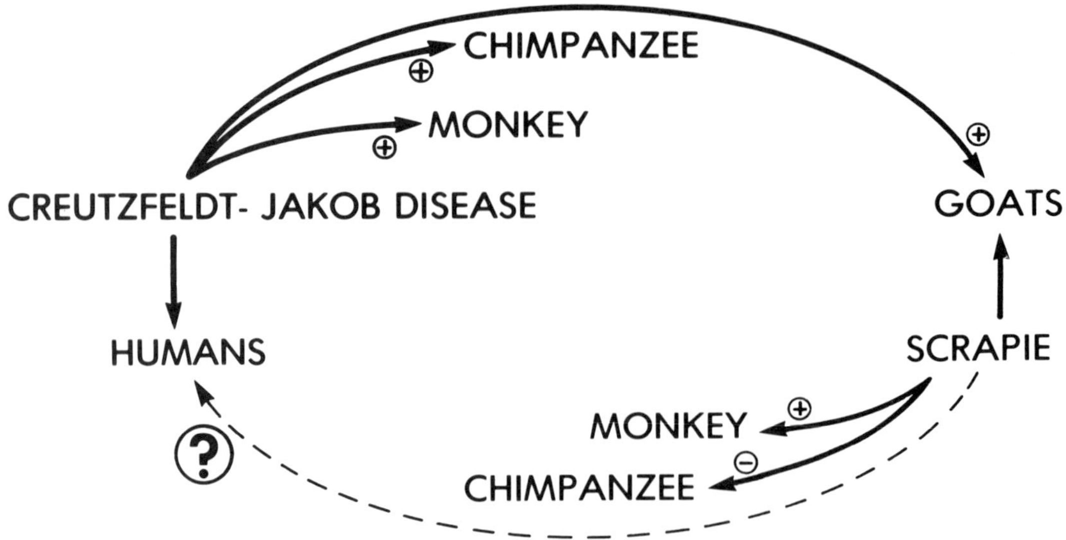

Figure 1. Relationship of Creutzfeldt-Jakob disease of humans and scrapie of goats and sheep.

CJD have been unsuccessful (35). At present there is no evidence that the scrapie agent is a cause of human disease.

In contrast to CJD which occurs worldwide, kuru is found only in a small mountainous region of Papua New Guinea. Epidemiological studies of kuru provide evidence for incubation periods of 20-30 years (4, 40). With the cessation of ritualistic cannibalism in the Fore region, the age of the youngest patients with kuru has progressively increased with each passing year. Studies on the prototypic scrapie agent suggest that current kuru patients may have been exposed to extremely small doses of the kuru agent more than 2 decades ago (6). Studies of familial cases of CJD suggest the possibility of incubation periods of similar length.

Although considerable evidence implicates cannibalism in the spread of kuru, no direct observations of cannibalistic acts among the Fore have been recorded. Attempts to transmit kuru by feeding infected brain tissue to chimpanzees have been unsuccessful, although one monkey developed a kuru-like illness 36 months after oral ingestion of the kuru agent (41). In contrast, goats fed scrapie-infected tissue frequently develop disease (42, 43). Recently, we have taken advantage of the natural cannibalistic activities of hamsters and developed an experimental model of scrapie transmitted by cannibalism (44). When scrapie-infected hamsters died, they were cannibalized by their uninfected cage mates. The cannibals developed scrapie 110-130 days later. Although the clinical signs and progression of scrapie transmitted by cannibalism were identical to those observed after intracerebral inoculation, the efficiency of infection was reduced by a factor of 10^9. These results provide compelling evidence for transmission of the prototypic scrapie agent during cannibalism and may offer new insights into the spread of kuru among the Fore people and their neighboring tribes.

ALZHEIMER'S DISEASE

Alzheimer's disease is at least 5000 times more common than CJD in the United States [Table 3] (1). Two forms of Alzheimer's disease have been proposed: presenile and senile. No clear distinctions exist between the two forms of Alzheimer's disease except for age of onset (3). The senile form is far more common. The incidence of Alzheimer's disease at age 80 is 400 times greater than that between the ages of 30 and 60. The incidence of CJD reaches a maximum around age 60. Neither CJD nor Alzheimer's disease are seen in childhood and rarely do these diseases afflict young adults. The sex ratios of both diseases are near unity. In both CJD and Alzheimer's disease 10%-20% of all cases are familial, exhibiting an autosomal dominant pattern of inheritance (45). Some families with multiple cases of both CJD and Alzheimer's disease have been reported. The origin of these familial cases is unknown. Are these cases due to vertical transmission or horizontal spread within the family? Epidemiological studies in the kuru region clearly support the absence of vertical transmission (4, 40). Similarly, no firm evidence exists for vertical transmission of either natural or experimental scrapie.

Dementia is the primary symptom in both CJD and Alzheimer's disease (3, 5). Multifocal myoclonus is frequently found in CJD but rarely in Alzheimer's disease. There is a distinct absence of focal neurological signs in both disorders. Only those neurological signs associated with bilateral cortical hemispheric disease such as grasps, suck, snout, and root are frequently found. Although spasticity is rare, bilateral extensor plantar responses are not uncommon. Neither fever nor leukocytosis are found in either disease, and examination of the cerebrospinal fluid is always normal. Computerized tomography (CT scan) shows varying degrees of cortical atrophy and ventricular enlargement in both disorders. Patients with CJD frequently die within a year after the onset of illness, but prolonged clinical courses up to 5 years have been recorded. Prolonged clinical courses lasting up to 10 years are frequently seen in Alzheimer's disease.

The pathology of both CJD and Alzheimer's disease is confined to the central nervous system (46, 47). Neuronal vacuolation is frequently prominent in CJD but is not

Table 3. Comparison of Alzheimer's and Creutzfeldt-Jakob Diseases

Parameter	*Creutzfeldt-Jakob Disease*	*Alzheimer's Disease*
Incidence/10^6	1	5×10^3
Age of onset	55-65 years	Presenile: 55-65 years Senile: 75-85 years
Female to male ratio	1:1	3:1
Familial cases	10%-20%	10%-20%
Pattern of inheritance	Autosomal dominant	Autosomal dominant
Duration of illness	0.5-5 years	1-10 years
Fever, or leukocytosis, or both	None	None
Symptoms	Dementia and myoclonus	Dementia
Cerebrospinal fluid	Normal	Normal
CT scan	Cortical atrophy Enlarged ventricles	Cortical atrophy Enlarged ventricles
Neuronal vacuolation	Frequently prominent	Minimal
Astrogliosis	Frequently severe	Moderate
Senile or amyloid plaques	Sometimes numerous	Numerous
Neurofibrillary tangles	None	Numerous
Dendritic spine loss	Severe	Severe
Cause	Slow prions	Unknown

always present. In natural scrapie of sheep neuronal vacuolation is rarely detectable (48). Neuronal vacuolation is not a prominent feature of Alzheimer's disease. Astrogliosis is frequently severe in CJD and somewhat less prominent in Alzheimer's disease. In some cases of CJD, amyloid or senile plaques abound (49, 50). These cases usually present with ataxia rapidly followed by dementia. Amyloid or senile plaques are frequently seen in kuru and have been reported with a specific strain of the scrapie agent inoculated into mice (51). Senile plaques are one of two neuropathological hallmarks in Alzheimer's disease. The other hallmark is the neurofibrillary tangle, which is not found in CJD, kuru, or scrapie. In both CJD and Alzheimer's disease a marked loss of dendritic spines has been observed (52, 53). Similar reductions in dendritic spines have also been recorded in scrapie (54).

While the cause of CJD is clearly a slow prion, the cause of Alzheimer's disease is unknown. The proposed causes of Alzheimer's disease are similar to those listed for kuru and CJD prior to demonstration of their transmissibility. These postulated causes for Alzheimer's disease include: (1) genetic disorder, (2) aluminum intoxication, (3) slow virus or prion, (4) abiotrophy, and (5) nutritional deficiency (3). Attempts to transmit Alzheimer's disease to nonhuman primates have not been successful (55). Two familial cases of Alzheimer's disease may have been transmitted to monkeys, but these transmissions could not be reproduced. Certainly the general lack of transmissibility of Alzheimer's disease to monkeys and chimpanzees does not eliminate the possibility that Alzheimer's disease is caused by prions. While CJD is readily transmissible to apes, it is only occasionally transmissible to rodents (36). The host range of CJD in nonprimates has been used as evidence of multiple strains of the CJD agent.

The similarities between CJD and Alzheimer's disease are impressive (Table 3). They make a good case for continuing to consider a possible role for prions in the etiology of Alzheimer's disease (56).

THE SCRAPIE AGENT

Bioassays

Studies on the scrapie, kuru, and CJD agents have been greatly limited by the extremely slow, tedious, and costly bioassays used to detect these agents. Since tissue culture systems are not available for the replication and assay of these agents, and they appear to be nonantigenic in their native forms, animal bioassays must be employed. Until recently, virtually all studies on the scrapie agent were performed with end-point titrations in laboratory rodents. Indeed, the assay is heroic, for quantitation of a single sample requires eight to ten serial tenfold dilutions and injection of each dilution into six mice (57). Then 50 to 60 mice must be held for 1 year and examined weekly for signs of scrapie. The number of animals at each dilution developing scrapie is used to calculate an end point. The time period required for titration of a sample was reduced to 200 days when a more rapid form of the disease in hamsters was discovered (25, 58).

Recently, studies on the scrapie agent have been dramatically accelerated by the development of a new bioassay based on measurements of incubation time intervals (13, 59). It is now possible to quantitate samples with high titers of the scrapie agent using four animals in 60-70 days. As shown in Fig. 2*A*, the time interval from inoculation to onset of illness (y) was found to be inversely proportional to the dose injected intracerebrally into random bred weanling Syrian hamsters. The logarithm of the mean interval ($\bar{y}$) in days minus a time factor of 40 is a linear function of the logarithm of the dose over a wide range. The time factor was determined by maximizing the linear relationship between the time interval and dose. With a

factor of 40, the regression coefficient of the line is 0.87. A similar analysis was performed for the time interval from inoculation to death ($\bar{z}$). With a time factor of 61, the regression coefficient of the line is 0.86. Equations were written to describe these linear functions which relate the titer of the inoculum to the time intervals both from inoculation to onset of illness (equation I) and from inoculation to death (equation II):

$$\text{Log } T_y = 26.66 - (12.99) \log (\bar{y} - 40) - \log D \quad (I)$$
$$\text{Log } T_z = 25.33 - (12.47) \log (\bar{z} - 61) - \log D \quad (II)$$

where T is the titer expressed in ID_{50} units/ml, D is the dilution defined as the fractional concentration of the diluted sample, $\bar{y}$ is the mean interval from inoculation to onset of clinical illness in days, and $\bar{z}$ is the mean interval from inoculation to death in days. The most precise estimate of titer is obtained by calculating a weighted average for T_y and T_z.

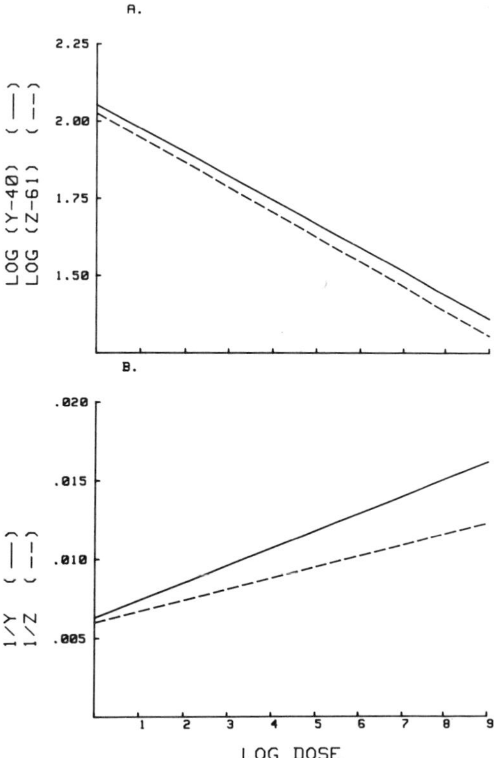

Figure 2. Assay of the scrapie agent by incubation time interval measurements. Linear relationships were obtained by plotting (*A*) logarithm of time intervals minus a time factor as function of logarithm of dose and (*B*) reciprocal of time intervals as a function of logarithm of dose.

Similar linear relationships were obtained when the reciprocals of the time intervals were plotted as a function of the logarithm of the dose (Fig. 2*B*). Regression coefficients of 0.87 and 0.88 were obtained for lines relating $1/y$ and $1/z$ to the logarithm of the dose, respectively. Equations describing these functions gave similar results to those obtained with equations I and II.

While the new bioassay is still greatly prolonged compared to most assays of biological activities, the economies with respect to time and resources represent a highly significant methodological advance.

Replication

Replication of the scrapie agent in the brains of hamsters inoculated intracerebrally with 10^7 ID_{50} units shows a progressive increase in the titer of the agent with time (60). Maximum titers of $10^{9.5}$ ID_{50} units/g are found in the brain about 50 days after inoculation. At this time the agent is widely distributed throughout the brain, and no regional differences can be discerned (61). Light microscopic pathology is minimal, and the animals still exhibit no signs of neurological dysfunction. During the next 10-15 days the animals develop a neurological illness characterized by ataxia, difficulty righting themselves from a supine position, generalized tremor, and head bobbing. By 60-70 days, vacuolation of neurons and astrogliosis are found throughout the brain, even though the titer of the agent has remained constant. Thus, the "pathological hallmarks" of this spongiform encephalopathy do not correlate with the extent of agent replication. The clinical phase of scrapie is characterized by progressive neurological dysfunction, and death follows within 2-3 weeks.

A few cases of CJD have been transmitted to rodents and the extent of agent replication measured (36, 62-64). Titers of $>10^6$ ID_{50} units/g of brain have been found in both guinea pigs and mice (62-64). The incubation periods of these rodent adapted CJD agent strains range from 3-24 months.

Purification and Hydrophobicity

Over the past 20 years several laboratories have been actively engaged in purification studies of the scrapie agent. Hunter (65) and Kimberlin (66) suggested that the scrapie agent was distributed throughout virtually all subcellular fractions. The interpretation of those observations was complicated by the imprecision of the end-point titration assay. Nevertheless, the scrapie agent was reported to be intimately associated with cellular membranes and from this association the "membrane hypothesis" evolved. When a variety of extraction procedures failed to release the agent from membrane fractions, it was concluded that the agent is a replicating membrane fragment that cannot be separated from cellular membranes. It was in this setting that Diener proposed that the scrapie agent might be a viroid (67). While we now know that the scrapie agent is not a "naked" nucleic acid, the hypothesis was useful because it stimulated investigation.

From a synaptosomal fraction of scrapie-infected murine brain, Hunter and coworkers (65, 68) isolated a small DNA molecule of molecular weight 60,000. No similar molecule was found in control fractions. Unfortunately isolation of this DNA molecule required phenol extraction so that no infectivity was recovered with the molecule. Subsequently, these investigators have been unable to reproduce their own findings.

Difficulty with confirmation of experimental findings in scrapie research have also plagued other investigators (69). Marsh and coworkers (70) reported that digestion with DNase of a fraction containing less than 0.01% of the initial scrapie infectivity from an hydroxyapatite column diminished scrapie agent titer by $10^{1.5}$ ID_{50} units. In addition, infectivity of a fraction eluted from a sodium dodecyl sulfate (SDS) electrophoretic gel was diminished nearly 10^3 ID_{50} units by DNase digestion (70, 71). These results are puzzling since the residual SDS in the gel eluates was probably sufficient to inactivate the DNase (72).

Siakotos and coworkers (73) attempted to purify the scrapie agent from murine brain using equilibrium sucrose/sodium chloride density gradients. These authors suggested that there was a peak of infectivity at a sucrose density of 1.19 g/cm³. However, multiple peaks of infectivity were found throughout the gradients, demonstrating considerable heterogeneity of the agent with respect to density and showing that the technique when applied to crude suspensions of membranous material from brain is probably not useful in isolating the scrapie agent. Other studies from the laboratory of Gajdusek have shown considerable heterogeneity of the agent in metrizamide and cesium chloride density gradients (74).

Since the initial purification of most biological macromolecules involves a series of differential centrifugations (75), we began our studies on the scrapie agent by defining its sedimentation properties in fixed-angle rotors to develop a preparative protocol (76). These studies showed that the sedimentation profile of the agent in both murine spleen and brain extracts was unchanged upon the addition of 0.5% sodium deoxycholate and that the agent sedimented over a range of particle sizes from 60S to 1000S (57).

Using the information derived from these sedimentation profiles, a partial purification scheme for the murine scrapie agent from spleen was derived (12). The preparation was devoid of cellular membranes and enriched for the scrapie agent 20- to 30-fold with respect to protein and DNA. Rate-zonal sucrose gradient centrifugation studies gave sedimentation coefficients for the agent ranging from 40S to > 500S. Sucrose density gradient centrifugation showed the agent to have a density ranging from 1.08 g/cm³ to >1.30 g/cm³, indicating that some forms of the agent might be associated with lipids. Further sedimentation studies showed that the agent aggregated with cellular elements on heating in the partially purified fraction (77). The agent in this fraction was stable in nonionic and nondenaturing anionic detergents but was destroyed by the denaturing detergent SDS at a detergent:protein ratio of 1.5 g SDS/g protein. Free-flow electrophoresis of the agent showed that most of the agent has a net negative charge, but significant charge heterogeneity was found.

The remarkable heterogeneity of the scrapie agent with respect to size, density, and charge seemed to be best explained by hydrophobic domains on the surface of agent. The most likely structure responsible for this hydrophobicity is a protein composed of amino acid residues with juxtaposed non-polar side chains (12, 78, 79).

From these initial studies on the murine agent from spleen, the complexities of scrapie agent purification became clear. The possibility of proceeding without a greatly improved assay for the agent seemed remote. Thus, a considerable effort was devoted to developing the incubation time interval assay described above. With this new bioassay system, we developed a purification scheme for the agent from hamster brain where the titers were highest (58). The initial steps of the purification protocol were similar to those employed for the murine agent (12). Deoxycholate extracts (P_4) were digested sequentially with micrococcal nuclease and proteinase K. The digestions were performed at 4°C to prevent aggregation of the agent observed at elevated temperatures (78). The digested preparations were then subjected to cholate-sarkosyl extraction followed by $(NH_4)_2SO_4$ precipitation (P_5). Most of the remaining digested proteins and nucleic acids were separated from the scrapie agent by sarkosyl agarose gel electrophoresis at 4°C (7). Such preparations of the eluted scrapie agent (E_6) were 100- to 1000-fold purified with respect to cellular protein (7). The availability of these enriched preparations has allowed us to identify a protein within the agent which is required for infectivity (7). Fraction E_6 is optically clear and contains $10^{6.5} - 10^{8.5}$ ID$_{50}$ units/ml of the scrapie agent, 20-50 μg/ml of protein and < 1 μg/ml of DNA.

The hydrophobicity of the agent in fraction E_6 was reflected by diminished titers when detergent was removed (7). Presumably this decrease in infectivity was due to aggregation. Further evidence for the hydrophobicity of the scrapie agent comes from its binding to phenyl-Sepharose (7). The agent could not be eluted in 8.5 M ethylene glycol; however, addition of 4% Nonidet P40 and 2% sarkosyl to the ethylene glycol eluate resulted in the almost quantitative recovery of the agent from phenyl-Sepharose.

Not only is the hydrophobic nature of the scrapie agent important with respect to purification, it may also explain some of its enigmatic properties. That hydrophobic interactions increase with elevated temperature may be reflected in the extreme heat stability of the agent (79). Our unsuccessful attempts to detect antibodies against the native scrapie agent in fraction E_6 might be explained by its hydrophobicity (80). Hydrophobic proteins in their native state are poor antigens in some cases (81). An alternative explanation for the apparent lack of immunogenicity of the scrapie agent evolves from the possibility that the agent may be closely related to a normal cellular protein to which the host is tolerant.

Protein Required for Infectivity

Five separate and distinct lines of evidence now clearly show that the scrapie agent contains a protein that is required for infectivity: (1) inactivation by proteinase K digestion, (2) inactivation by chemical modification with diethylpyrocarbonate (DEP), (3) inactivation by the denaturing detergent SDS, (4) inactivation by chaotropic salts such as guanidinium SCN, and (5) inactivation by the denaturing organic solvent, phenol (7). The cumulative evidence for a protein within the scrapie agent is compelling (Table 4).

Digestion with crystalline proteinase K inactivated the scrapie agent purified from hamster brain (7). The decrease in scrapie agent titer was a function of proteinase K concentration as well as the temperature and time of digestion. Prior treatment of proteinase K with the protease inhibitor, phenylmethylsulfonylfluoride (PMSF), completely abolished the protease catalyzed degradation of the agent. Preliminary studies indicate that the scrapie agent is also destroyed by trypsin digestion. It is important to note that the protease sensitivity of the scrapie agent was revealed only after considerable purification (fraction E_6). Chemical modification by DEP also inactivated the scrapie agent in these purified preparations (7). Addition of protein or histidine prevented chemical modification of the scrapie agent by DEP (82). The carbethoxylated, inactive agent was restored to its original level of infectivity upon decarbethoxylation by treatment with hydroxylamine. This reversibility of the inactive, chemically modified agent provides a further argument for a protein target.

Table 4. Molecular Properties of the Scrapie Agent—Evidence That It Contains a Protein

Treatment	Stable	Labile
Protease digestion	. . .	Proteinase K Trypsin
Chemical modification	. . .	DEP
Detergents	TX-100, OGS SB 3-14, and ET-12H	SDS and LiDS
Inorganic ions	Na^+, K^+, Cl^-, and SO_4^- EDTA	Gdn^+, SCN^-, and TCA^-
Organic solvents	Ethanol	Phenol

Note.—Abbreviations: diethylpyrocarbonate, DEP; Triton X–100, TX–100; octylglucoside, OGS; sulfobetaine 3–14, SB 3–14; 1–dodecyl propanediol–3–phosphorylcholine, ET–12H; sodium dodecyl sulfate, SDS; lithium dodecyl sulfate, LiDS; and guanidinium, Gdn.

Besides inactivation of the scrapie agent by protease digestion and chemical modification with DEP, three reagents commonly used to denature proteins and isolate biologically active nucleic acids (83) have been found to inactivate the agent. First, sodium dodecyl sulfate diminished scrapie agent titer when the ratio of detergent to protein exceeded 1.8 g SDS/g protein (13). In contrast, the agent was stable in a wide variety of nondenaturing ionic and nonionic detergents. Simultaneous addition of a nonionic detergent and SDS to a preparation containing the scrapie agent prevented the inactivation observed with SDS alone. Second, recent studies with a variety of chaotropic ions have shown that low concentrations of these ions readily inactivate the agent (13, 14). Irreversible inactivation of the agent was found upon exposure to 1 M guanidinium SCN at 4°C. Higher concentrations of less potent chaotropic salts were required to achieve irreversible inactivation. Studies with KSCN and CsTCA have identified three states of scrapie agent infectivity: (1) a native state, (2) an intermediate state from which infectivity may be recovered, and (3) a denatured state from which infectivity cannot be restored. Third, phenol, which has been widely used in nucleic acid isolation, readily inactivates the scrapie agent (84). In contrast, the agent is stable in ethanol but readily precipitates. Phenol is a particularly potent denaturant of protein. Phenol extractions, under a variety of salt and pH conditions, uniformly destroyed infectivity (13). In these studies partially purified preparations were first digested with proteinase K to prevent the formation of an interface in which the agent might be trapped. We have attempted to restore scrapie agent infectivity from phenol extracted preparations by incorporation into liposomes and by transfection into cultured cells. Using reverse phase liposome formation (85), no infectivity was recovered from the aqueous phase, dialyzed phenol phase or combination of these two phases. (86). Preparations of phenol extracted DNA and RNA from scrapie-infected murine spleen failed to produce infectious scrapie agent upon transfection of L cells (87). Ca^{2+}

phosphate and DEAE-dextran were used to promote the entry of the DNA and RNA, respectively. The conditions used were similar to those employed in transfection studies of visna virus nucleic acid (88). The cultured cells were passaged eight times. Aliquots were removed at each passage and stored at $-70°$C. Ten percent (w/v) homogenates were diluted tenfold and inoculated into six weanling mice. The mice were observed weekly for clinical signs of scrapie over the next 18 months; none of the mice developed a neurological disorder. Similar transfection experiments with murine fetal brain cells and embryonic fibroblasts also failed to produce infectious agent (89). From all of these studies with chemical reagents that denature proteins but permit isolation of biologically active nucleic acids, we conclude that denaturation of a protein within the scrapie agent leads to inactivation of the infectious particle. It is noteworthy that CJD agents adapted to guinea pigs and mice are also inactivated upon phenol extraction (90).

Of interest with respect to the proteinaceous structure of the scrapie agent is also the effect of pH on infectivity (14). At pH 3 no loss of infectivity was observed over a 16-hour period at 37°C. In contrast, at pH 10 the titer of the agent was reduced 1000-fold upon exposure for 1 hour at 4°C (86). Neutralization of the sample with acid did not restore infectivity. The lability of the scrapie agent in alkali is probably due to protein denaturation, but we cannot exclude RNA hydrolysis. Resistance of the agent to Zn^{2+} catalyzed hydrolysis of nucleic acids at neutral pH would tend to favor the former interpretation (86). Also of note are studies showing a large oxygen effect upon exposure of the scrapie agent to ionizing radiation (91). These results are consistent with a protein or lipoprotein target since nucleic acids characteristically show a small oxygen effect.

Nucleic Acid Content

Over the past 15 years, two lines of evidence have suggested that the scrapie agent might not contain a nucleic acid. The scrapie agent in crude preparations has been found to be resistant to nuclease digestion and to irradiation at 254 nm (8, 65, 66, 78, 92). The objection to the nuclease studies was that the nuclease failed to penetrate the protective coat of the scrapie agent, and thus it could not inactivate the agent. This is certainly the case for many viruses. The other objection raised was that shielding of the agent by a protein or carbohydrate coat might be responsible for its extreme resistance to ultraviolet (UV) irradiation.

At several different stages of purification we have searched for susceptibility of the agent to nuclease digestion (Table 5). No decrease in scrapie infectivity has been observed with micrococcal nuclease, nuclease P, DNase I, DNase II, RNase A, and RNase T_1 at 100 μg/ml for 2-3 hours at 37°C. Only one report has described nuclease sensitivity for the scrapie agent (70), but we as well as others have not been able to confirm the observation (69).

The complete lack of scrapie agent sensitivity to nucleases in the face of inactivation by proteases is of interest. Numerous viruses are resistant to nucleases; presumably, these enzymes do not penetrate the viral protein coats (93, 94). In contrast, 0.1 μg/ml of RNase A added to a crude nucleic acid extract containing potato spindle tuber viroid (PSTV) decreased the PSTV titer $>$ 10^6-fold in 1 hour at 25°C (95). In these extracts it is estimated that viroid RNA was $<$ 0.01% of the total RNA (96). Hydrolysis of a single phosphodiester bond within a viroid

probably inactivates it (16, 97). There are many examples of proteins that retain their biological activities after limited proteolysis (98). We do not know in the case of the scrapie agent how many peptide bonds must be cleaved to cause inactivation.

UV-inactivation studies with the optically clear fraction E_6 have confirmed the resistance of the scrapie agent to inactivation (8, 92). Fractions S_2, P_5, and E_6 were irradiated at 254 nm with increasing doses. Although no inactivation of the agent in fraction S_2 was observed, a minimal but probably significant decrease was found in fractions P_5 and E_6 as a function of dose (99). The kinetics of inactivation by 254 nm irradiation suggest a single hit process. The decreases in titer as a function of UV dose for fractions P_5 and E_6 give a D_{37} of 42,000 J/m². The resistance of the scrapie agent to irradiation at 254 nm is compared to that observed for viruses, viroids, and the *Naegleria* agent in Table 6. Clearly, the inactivation of the scrapie agent at these extreme energy levels indicates a photochemistry of a far different nature than that observed for virus inactivation through the formation of thymine or uracil dimers. Proteins are extremely resistant to irradiation at 254 nm (100) and are probably the target within the scrapie agent in these irradiation studies.

The resistance of the scrapie agent to procedures attacking nucleic acids has been extended using two other techniques (Table 5). The agent has been incubated at pH 7 in

Table 5. Resistance of Scrapie Agent to Procedures That Attack Nucleic Acids

Procedures	*Possible Cause of Resistance*
Nuclease digestion	Nucleic acid protected from enzymatic hydrolysis by protein shell
Ultraviolet irradiation (254 nm)	Nucleic acid small and no critical pyrimidine dimers formed
Zn^{2+} hydrolysis	Nucleic acid protected from Zn^{2+} catalyzed hydrolysis by protein shell
Psoralen photoreactoin	Nucleic acid single-stranded, and monoadditions do not inactivate

the presence of 2 mM $Zn(NO_3)_2$ at 65°C for periods as long as 24 hours without loss of infectivity (86). Under these conditions polymers of RNA are completely reduced to mononucleotides, and polymers of DNA, undergo considerable hydrolysis (101). Even more surprising are results with psoralens. Photochemical inactivation of the scrapie agent with psoralens has been attempted with samples at several levels of purification, both from murine spleen and hamster brain. Five different psoralens of varying degrees of hydrophobicity were employed (102). It is expected that the most hydrophobic psoralens readily partitioned into the scrapie agent. No inactivation of the scrapie agent was observed with any of these psoralens over a wide range of dosages (103). Psoralens have been found to inactivate numerous viruses (104, 105). Psoralens may form diadducts upon photoaddition within base-paired regions of nucleic acids and monoadducts within single-stranded regions. Psoralens have several advantages in searching for a nucleic acid genome: (1) low reactivity with proteins, (2) penetration of viral protein and lipid coats, and (3) stable covalent linkages formed upon photoactivation. Even with all of these negative results in our search for a nucleic acid polymer, the possibility that the genome of the scrapie agent is composed of a polymer with unusual base structure or that the genome is especially well-shielded, must be entertained.

Table 6. Inactivation of Small Infectious Agents by Ultraviolet Irradiation at 254 nm

Infectious Agents	D_{37} (J/m^2)
Bacteriophage T2	4
Bacteriophage S13	20
Bacteriophage ϕX174	20
Rous sarcoma virus	150
Polyoma virus	240
Friend leukemia virus	500
Murine leukemia virus	1400
Potato spindle tuber viroids	5000
Scrapie agent	42,000
Naegleria agent	50,000

Note.—Data were taken from references (8, 15, 16, 99).

Molecular Size

The extreme resistance of the scrapie agent to inactivation by ionizing radiation raised the possibility that the agent is quite small (106). Ignoring two potentially important factors, target size calculations gave a molecular weight of 150,000. First, the possibility that multiple copies of the agent might exist within a single infectious particle, as would occur with aggregation, was not considered. We have good evidence that the agent readily associates with cellular elements and probably aggregates with itself in purified preparations (12, 77, 79). Second, the efficiency of the cellular repair processes was not addressed. Polyoma virus dsDNA (3×10^6 daltons) has been found to be almost as resistant to ionizing radiation as either viroids or the scrapie agent (8). The extreme efficiency of the cellular repair processes for the polyoma virus dsDNA genome accounts for its apparent resistance to damage by ionizing radiation.

Studies on the scrapie agent in murine spleen have shown a continuum of sizes ranging from 40S or less to > 500S by rate-zonal sucrose gradients (12, 79). Parvoviruses are among the smallest viruses identified, and they have sedimentation coefficients of 100 to 110S (93, 94). The scrapie agent in detergent-extracted preparations associated with cellular elements when heated to form large infectious particles of > 10,000S (77, 79). Such particles are the size of mitochondria. Sedimentation studies of CJD agents adapted to both guinea pigs and mice suggest that the sizes of these agents are similar to that observed for the scrapie agent (90).

Gel electrophoresis studies have also shown that the scrapie agent exists as a succession of particles of varying size (69, 78). Sarkosyl agarose gel electrophoresis of partially purified fractions containing the agent showed that some forms of the agent migrated more slowly than DNA restriction fragments of 15×10^6 daltons. Some smaller forms of the agent migrated ahead of 3×10^5 dalton DNA fragments. Digestion of crude preparations with nucleases and proteases facilitated the entry of the agent into these gels. One report by other workers showed that the majority of the scrapie agent migrated with 5S RNA molecules in the presence of SDS (71). We have been unable to confirm these findings and, as noted above, SDS inactivates the agent (13, 69).

Until recently, gel filtration studies employing a variety of anionic detergents and chaotropic ions have given results similar to those described for rate-zonal sucrose gradients and gel electrophoresis. Typically a portion of the agent eluted in the void volume followed by a continuum of particles apparently of decreasing size (14, 78). In contrast, incubation of the scrapie agent overnight with 10% (w/v) sulfobetaine 3-14 (SB 3-14), a zwitterionic detergent, appears to have dissociated the agent [Fig. 3] (86). Under these conditions the scrapie agent eluted as a peak behind bovine serum albumin, but slightly ahead of ovalbumin. If the agent has a globular shape in SB 3-14, then it should have a molecular weight of 50,000 or less. How much detergent is bound to the agent under these conditions remains to be determined. While these studies are as yet preliminary, similar observations have been recorded with another detergent, 1-dodecyl propanediol-3-phosphorylcholine, which is a synthetic derivative of lysolecithin. Confirmation of these findings by rate-zonal sucrose gradient centrifugation is awaited. Thus, the monomeric form of the scrapie agent may

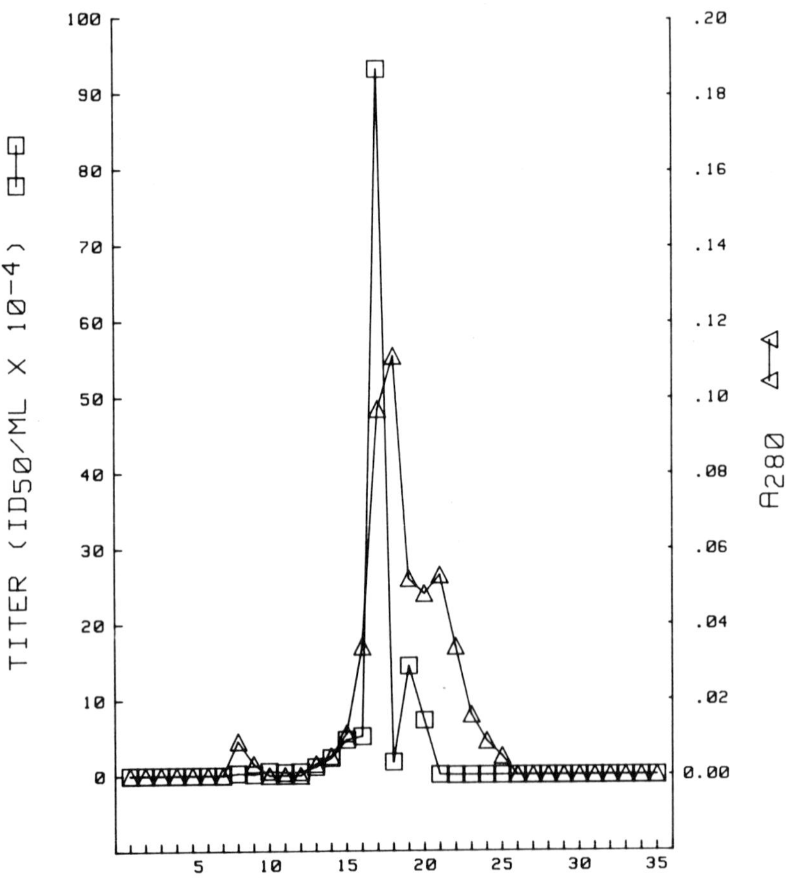

FRACTION NUMBER

Figure 3. High pressure liquid chromatography of the scrapie agent in sulfobetaine 3-14 (SB 3-14). Fraction P₅ was exposed to 10% (w/v) SB 3-14 for 16 hours at 4°C and then chromatographed in 60 mM Tris OAc pH 7.2 containing 1 mM EDTA and 0.024% SB 3-14 over a TSK 4000 column. One ml fractions were collected and assayed in hamsters by incubation time interval measurements. Blue dextran, bovine serum albumin, and tryptophan eluted in fractions 7, 15, and 22, respectively.

indeed be considerably smaller than that of a viroid, which until now has been the smallest infectious agent known.

If the scrapie agent does have a molecular weight of 50,000 or less, then a nucleic acid within such a globular structure will be too small to code for a protein. A spherical scrapie agent of molecular weight 50,000 would have a diameter of 4-6 nm. Let us assume that the agent has a protective protein which is 1 nm (10 Å) thick. The volume of the core will be 14.1 nm³. From measurements of DNA packing in crystals and bacteriophage (107), there is space for a 12 nucleotide polymer consisting of six base pairs. Dehydration of the polymer would permit 32 nucleotides to be encapsulated. Indeed, if such oligonucleotides exist within the agent, they must have a function other than that of a template directing the synthesis of scrapie coat proteins.

Novel Properties

The foregoing summary of experimental data indicates that the molecular properties of the scrapie agent differ from those of viruses, viroids, and plasmids. Its resistance to procedures that attack nucleic acids, its resistance to inactivation by heat, and its apparent small size all suggest that the scrapie agent is a novel infectious entity. Because the dominant characteristics of the scrapie agent resemble those of a protein, an acronym is introduced to emphasize this feature. In place of such terms as "unconventional virus" or "unusual slow virus-like agent," the term *"prion"* is suggested. Prions are small *pro*teinaceous *in*fectious particles which resist inactivation by most procedures that modify nucleic acids. The term prion underscores the requirement of a protein for infection; current knowledge does not allow exclusion of a small nucleic acid within the interior of the particle.

Our data and that of other investigators suggest two possible models for the scrapie agent: (1) a small nucleic acid surrounded by a tightly packed protein coat or (2) a protein devoid of nucleic acid—that is, an infectious protein. While the first model might seem the most plausible, there is no evidence for a nucleic acid within the agent. The second model is consistent with the experimental

data but is clearly heretical. Skepticism of the second model is certainly justified. Only purification of the scrapie agent to homogeneity and determination of its chemical structure will allow a rigorous conclusion as to which of these two models is correct.

There seems to be little advantage in championing one model over another; however, several previously postulated structures for the scrapie agent can now be discarded. The requirement of a protein for infectivity eliminates the possibilities that the scrapie agent is composed entirely of polysaccharide or nucleic acid. Thus, the replicating polysaccharide and naked nucleic acid-viroid hypotheses are no longer viable. The hypothetical nucleic acid surrounded by a polysaccharide coat can also be eliminated. Studies demonstrating the small size of the scrapie agent clearly distinguish it from conventional viruses, spiroplasma-like organisms and parasites such as sarcosporidia.

Rigid categorization of the scrapie agent at this time would be premature. Determination of its molecular structure will be required prior to deciding whether prions represent a distinct subgroup of extraordinarily small viruses or a completely different type of pathogen which lacks a nucleic acid genome.

NAEGLERIA AGENT

The similarities between the scrapie agent and an agent from *Naegleria amoeba* are striking (Table 7). Whether or not the *Naegleria* agent should be included within the classification of prions remains to be established. The agent has been called *Naegleria Amoeba* Cytopathic Material (NACM) because it causes a cytopathic process to occur in chicken embryo cells 4-6 days after exposure to the agent (15). The amount of the agent increases 10- to 20-fold in chicken embryo cells prior to the onset of cytopathology. This limited increase has raised the possibility that replication of the agent is not occurring in the chicken embryo cells and that the apparent increase is due to disaggregation or activation. If this is the case, then the *Naegleria* agent must be considered a toxin.

Like the scrapie agent, there is clear evidence for a protein within the *Naegleria* agent. The agent was destroyed by digestion

Table 7. Comparison of Molecular Properties of the Scrapie and *Naegleria* Agents

Properties	*Scrapie*	*Naegleria*
Molecular weight	~50,000	~50,000
Hydrophobic	+	−
Protein component	+	+
Nucleic acid component	−	−
Heat inactivation	$> 90°C$	$37°C$
Ultraviolet inactivation (D_{37})	42,000 J/m^2	50,000 J/m^2

with papain and pronase, and inactivated by SDS as well as urea (15). The *Naegleria* agent has been shown to be resistant to inactivation by both RNases and DNases as well as irradiation at 254 nm (15). A D_{37} of 50,000 J/m^2 for the *Naegleria* agent is of similar magnitude to that found for the scrapie agent (Table 6). Gel filtration of the *Naegleria* agent has shown a peak of infectivity which eluted in the region where globular proteins of molecular weight 50,000 chromatograph (15). Certainly, a variety of techniques must be employed to determine accurately whether the molecular weights of both the *Naegleria* and scrapie agents are similar.

PRION REPLICATION

One of the most fascinating questions about prions concerns their mode of replication. If, in fact, prions do not contain a nucleic acid genome, then studies on the replication of prions may reveal unprecedented mechanisms of reproduction.

The first possibility is that prions contain a protected nucleic acid which, like a viral genome, codes for the protein shell (Table 8). The hypothetical prion genome could derive its protection from the protein-lipid coat or from an unusual chemical structure. Such an unusual genomic structure might confer upon prions the characteristics of proteinaceous particles which are resistant to most procedures that attack nucleic acids. Alternatively, prions may contain an oligonucleotide that acts as a regulatory element instead of a coding template. This oligonucleotide might act as an inducer to promote the synthesis of prions. Small

nuclear RNAs are thought to be regulatory elements controlling the splicing of genes (109). If the postulated nucleic acid within the scrapie agent does not code for the protein in its coat, then this would be a major feature distinguishing prions from viruses.

The second possibility is that, in fact, prions are devoid of nucleic acid. If this is the case, then alternative modes of replication for these infectious proteins must exist (Table 8). The macromolecular information required for the synthesis of prions must be contained either in the host cell or in the prion itself.

If cellular genes coding for the scrapie prion do exist, then they are highly regulated, not readily activated, and present in a variety of mammalian cells ranging from mice to monkeys. It is pertinent that hundreds of mice and hamsters inoculated with homogenates from the brains of control animals have never developed a neurological disorder (11, 109). These animals have been observed for up to 1 year—a period of time sufficient to detect one infectious unit in the inoculum. An occasional activation of such cellular genes might explain the sporadic occurrence of CJD with an incidence of 1/10^6 (35). A few clusters of CJD with higher rates of incidence have been identified and 10% of CJD cases are familial. The molecular mechanism by which prions might activate cellular genes which code for their biosynthesis is unknown. The emerging story of oncogenes within retroviruses and their cellular counterparts provides an interesting analogy (110).

In addition, we must account for the evolutionary pressure that preserves such hypothetical cellular genes that code for prions. Perhaps these hypothetical genes code

Table 8. Possible Mechanisms of *Prion* Replication

I. Prions contain undetected nucleic acids
   A. Code for prion proteins
   B. Activate transcription of host genes coding
      for prion proteins
II. Prions are devoid of nucleic acids
   A. Activate transcription of host genes coding
      for prion proteins
   B. Code for their own replication
      1. Reverse translation
      2. Protein-directed protein synthesis

---

for some necessary, related protein when they are under normal regulation. It is interesting to speculate that tolerance to a normal, crossreacting gene product might allow the scrapie prion to replicate unnoticed by the immune system. Another explanation for tolerance toward the scrapie agent involves selective suppression of small populations of potentially reactive lymphocytes (111).

Alternatively, prions could code for their own biosynthesis. This hypothesis contradicts the "central dogma" of molecular biology (11, 112). Unorthodox mechanisms such as reverse translation or protein-directed protein synthesis would allow prions to replicate (113, 114). We have no precedents for either of these synthetic processes in biology. The possibility that prions are devoid of nucleic acid brings to mind early studies on crystalline tobacco mosaic virus (TMV) where no RNA was found, and Stanley suggested that the protein of TMV was auto-catalytic (115).

Relevant to the mechanism by which the scrapie agent replicates are two observations. First, multiple strains of the scrapie and CJD agents have been identified by repeated passage at limiting dilution and by their host range in experimental animals (36, 116). Second, adaptation of the agent has been observed upon repeated passage in the same host species as evidenced by a reduction in the length of the incubation period (58, 73, 117). A fascinating series of experiments on adaptation has been conducted by Hadlow (118, 119) who observed that the scrapie agent passaged in mink retains its ability to infect goats but loses its ability to infect mice. The

scrapie agent from sheep or goats is transmissible to both mice and hamsters (Fig. 4). The agent causing mink encephalopathy is transmissible to goats and hamsters but not mice. A disease identical to mink encephalopathy has been produced by feeding mink scrapie-infected sheep meat. Presumably this is how the disease arises. The above studies clearly indicate that the scrapie agent is modified during its passage in mink. While adaptation is most readily explained by modification of a nucleic acid genome within the agent, multiple host genes coding for a variety of agents could also explain these observations. The presence of multiple genes coding for different proteins with the same biological activities is underscored by the multitude of interferons (120, 121).

The genetic background of the host clearly influences the length of the incubation period in scrapie. Dickinson and colleagues (122, 123) have identified two genetic loci in mice that influence the length of the incubation period. In a survey of immunodeficient mice, we found that NZB and NZBxW F_1 mice inoculated intracerebrally have an incubation period of similar magnitude to that found in BALB/c and C57/Bl mice (124). In contrast, NZW mice have a significantly shorter incubation period. Further studies with F_2 backcrosses are required to determine if a single gene is responsible for these differences. From these studies and those on the murine CJD agent, we conclude that longer incubation time alleles are autosomal dominant. Murine CJD studies have show that the D subregion of the H-2 complex plays a central role in controlling the length of

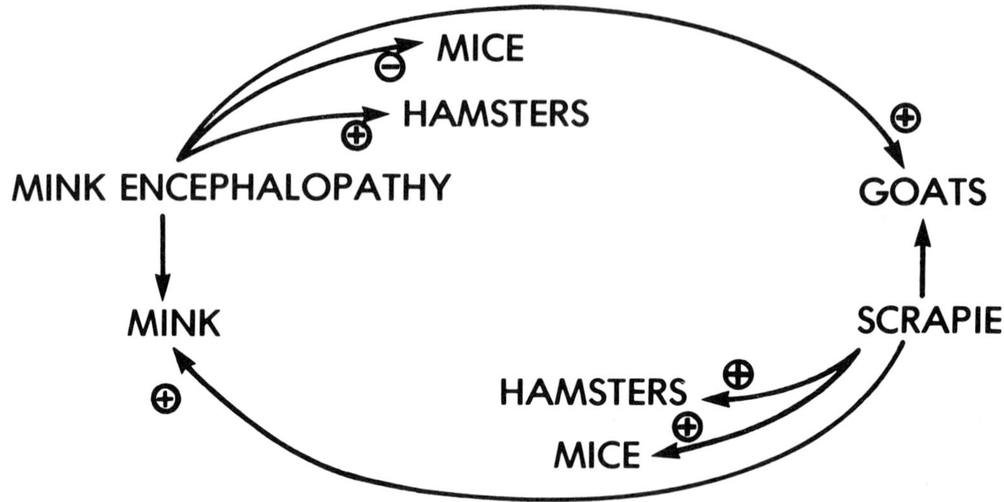

Figure 4. Relationship of scrapie and mink encephalopathy. Modification of the scrapie agent after passage in mink.

the incubation period (125). The q allele in this subregion resulted in shorter incubation times and the d allele in longer ones.

CONCLUSION

The consequences of understanding the structure, function, and replication of prions are significant. If prions do not contain a nucleic acid genome that codes for its proteins, then they will be unique among microorganisms. Novel mechanisms of replication and information transfer must then be entertained. Unraveling the chemistry of such functions will certainly be fascinating.

A knowledge of the molecular structure of prions may help identify the etiologies of some chronic degenerative diseases of humans. Development of sensitive probes for detecting prions in such diseases is clearly needed. It seems unlikely that kuru and CJD are the only human diseases caused by prions. Although transmission studies using non-human primates have failed to identify an etiological agent in Alzheimer's disease, we should not be dissuaded from continuing to consider the possibility that an infectious agent causes senile dementia. The virological literature contains numerous examples of viral diseases where the causative agent was

not readily identified by routine isolation procedures. In some cases the viruses could be rescued by cocultivation of infected tissue with permissive cells, coinfection with a helper virus, chemical or ultraviolet light induction, or fusion with susceptible cells. In all of these cases and in some others where viruses could not be isolated, radiolabeled complementary DNA probes were able to detect the virus genome by hybridization. The most reasonable approach would seem to necessitate first elucidating the structure of the prototypic scrapie agent followed by structural studies on the kuru and CJD agents. Once the molecular biology of these slow prions is understood, then we can construct molecular probes capable of detecting prions. At that time, investigations directed toward finding similar etiological agents in senile dementia of the Alzheimer's type can commence.

The importance of prion research in the potential elucidation of a wide variety of medical illnesses underscores the need for purification of the scrapie agent to homogeneity and the subsequent identification of its macromolecular components. Only then can we determine with certainty whether or not prions are devoid of nucleic acids. Indeed, recent progress in scrapie research has transformed an intriguing yet forbidding problem into an exciting and productive area of investigation.

ACKNOWLEDGEMENTS

This article is dedicated to Dr. William J. Hadlow on the occasion of his sixtieth birthday and in appreciation of both his enduring friendship and instructive collaboration. The author gratefully acknowledges the continuing help in these studies of F. Elvin, L. Gallagher, C. Boghosian, S. P. Cochran, D. F. Groth, M. P. McKinley, P. E. Bendheim, D. Bolton, F. R. Masiarz, K. Bowman, D. Downey, N. Mock, D. P. Stites, J. R. Baringer, R. N. Hogan, and K. Kasper. The author thanks Drs. R. C. Williams, R. C. Morris, Jr., A. Gordon, and H. Fields for critical discussions. The past support of the Howard Hughes Medical Institute during many phases of these studies is also gratefully acknowledged.

REFERENCES

1. Katzman R: Dementia. *Curr Neurol* 3:138-158, 1981

2. Gruenberg E: Epidemiology. In *Alzheimer's Disease: Senile Dementia and Related Disorders.* Edited by Katzman R, Terry RD, Bick KL. New York, Raven Press, 1978, pp 323-335

3. Katzman R, Terry RD, Bick KL (eds): *Alzheimer's Disease: Senile Dementia and Related Disorders.* New York, Raven Press, 1978, pp 1-595

4. Gajdusek DC: Unconventional viruses and the origin and disappearance of kuru. *Science* 197:943-960, 1977

5. Kirschbaum WR: *Jakob-Creutzfeldt Disease.* New York, American Elsevier, 1968, pp 1-251

6. Prusiner SB, Gajdusek DC, Alpers MP: Kuru with incubation periods exceeding two decades. *Ann Neurol.* In press, 1982

7. Prusiner SB, McKinley MP, Groth DF, et al: Scrapie agent contains a hydrophobic protein. *Proc Natl Acad Sci USA* 78:6675-6679, 1981

8. Latarjet R: Inactivation of the agents of scrapie, Creutzfeldt-Jakob disease, and kuru by radiations. In *Slow Transmissible Diseases of the Nervous System,* vol 2. Edited by Prusiner SB, Hadlow WJ. New York, Academic Press, 1979, pp 387-408

9. Gibbs CJ Jr, Gajdusek DC, Latarjet R: Unusual resistance to ionizing radiation of the viruses of kuru, Creutzfeldt-Jakob disease and scrapie. *Proc Natl Acad Sci USA* 75:6268-6270, 1978

10. Luria SE, Darnell JE Jr, Baltimore D, et al: *General Virology.* New York, John Wiley, 1978, pp 1-490

11. Crick F: Central dogma of molecular biology. *Nature* 227:561-563, 1970

12. Prusiner SB, Hadlow WJ, Garfin DE, et al: Partial purification and evidence for multiple molecular forms of the scrapie agent. *Biochemistry* 17:4993-4999, 1978

13. Prusiner SB, Groth DF, Cochran SP, et al: Molecular properties, partial purification and assay by incubation period measurements of the hamster scrapie agent. *Biochemistry* 19:4883-4891, 1980

14. Prusiner SB, Groth DF, McKinley MP, et al: Thiocyanate and hydroxyl ions inactivate the scrapie agent. *Proc Natl Acad Sci USA* 78:4606-4610, 1981

15. Dunnebacke TH, Schuster FL: The nature of a cytopathogenic material present in amebae of genus *Naegleria. Am J Trop Med Hyg* 26:412-421, 1977

16. Diener TO: *Viroids and Viroid Diseases.* New York, John Wiley, 1979, pp 1-252

17. Coggin JH Jr, Oakes JE, Huebner RJ, et al: Unusual filterable oncogenic agent isolated from horizontally transmitted Syrian hamster lymphomas. *Nature* 290:336-338, 1981

18. Diener TO: Potato spindle tuber "virus." IV. A replicating, low molecular weight RNA. *Virology* 45:411-428, 1971

19. Sänger HL, Klotz G, Riesner D, et al: Viroids are single-stranded covalently closed circular RNA molecules existing as highly base-paired rod-like structures. *Proc Natl Acad Sci USA* 73:3852-3856, 1976

20. Broda P: *Plasmids.* San Francisco, WH Freeman, 1979, pp 1-148

21. Depicker A, Van Montagu M, Schell J: Homologous DNA sequences in different Ti-plasmids are essential for oncogenicity. *Nature* 275:150-153, 1978

22. Vodkin MH, Fink GR: A nucleic acid associated with a killer strain of yeast. *Proc Natl Acad Sci USA* 70:1069-1072, 1973

23. Wicker RB: Plasmids controlling exclusion of the K$_2$ killer double-stranded RNA plasmid of yeast. *Cell* 21:217-226, 1980

24. Stites DP, Garfin DE, Prusiner SB: The immunology of scrapie. In *Slow Transmissible Diseases of the Nervous System*, vol 2. Edited by Prusiner SB, Hadlow WJ. New York, Academic Press, 1979, pp 211-224

25. Marsh RF, Kimberlin RH: Comparison of scrapie and transmissible mink encephalopathy in hamsters. II. Clinical signs, pathology and pathogenesis. *J Infect Dis* 131:104-110, 1975

26. Berndt RM: A "devastating disease syndrome"— kuru sorcery in the Eastern Central Highlands of New Guinea. *Sociologus* 8:4-28, 1958

27. Macarthur JR: Patrol Report. Territory of Papua and New Guinea, Department of Native Affairs, December, 1954

28. Gajdusek DC, Zigas V: Degenerative disease of the central nervous system in New Guinea. The endemic occurrence of "kuru" in the native population. *N Engl J Med* 257:974-978, 1957

29. Gajdusek DC: Observations on the early history of kuru investigations. In *Slow Transmissible Diseases of the Nervous System*, vol 1. Edited by Prusiner SB, Hadlow WJ. New York, Academic Press, 1979, pp 7-36

30. Farguhar J, Gajdusek DC (eds): *Kuru: Early Letters and Field-Notes from the Collection of D. Carleton Gajdusek*. New York, Raven Press, 1981, pp 1-338

31. Gajdusek DC, Gibbs CJ Jr, Alpers M: Experimental transmission of a kuru-like syndrome to chimpanzees. *Nature* 209:794-796, 1966

32. Hadlow WJ: Scrapie and kuru. *Lancet* 2:289-290, 1959

33. Klatzo I, Gajdusek DC, Zigas V: Pathology of kuru. *Lab Invest* 8:799-847, 1959

34. Gibbs CJ Jr, Gajdusek DC: Infection as the etiology of spongiform encephalopathy. *Science* 165:1023-1025, 1969

35. Masters CL, Harris JO, Gajdusek DC, et al: Creutzfeldt-Jakob disease: patterns of worldwide occurrence and the significance of familial and sporadic clustering. *Ann Neurol* 5:177-188, 1979

36. Gibbs CJ Jr, Gajdusek DC, Amyx H: Strain variation in the viruses of Creutzfeldt-Jakob disease and kuru. In *Slow Transmissible Diseases of the Nervous System*, vol 2. Edited by Prusiner SB, Hadlow WJ. New York, Academic Press, 1979, pp 87-110

37. Hadlow WJ, Prusiner SB, Kennedy RC, et al: Brain tissue from persons dying of Creutzfeldt-Jakob disease causes scrapie-like encephalopathy in goats. *Ann Neurol* 8:628-631, 1980

38. Gibbs, CJ Jr, Gajdusek DC: Transmission of scrapie to the cynomolgus monkey (*Macaca fasicularis*). *Nature* 236:73-74, 1972

39. Gibbs CJ Jr, Gajdusek DC: Experimental subacute spongiform virus encephalopathies in primates and other laboratory animals. *Science* 182:67-68, 1973

40. Alpers MP: Epidemiology and ecology of kuru. In *Slow Transmissible Diseases of the Nervous System*, vol 1. Edited by Prusiner SB, Hadlow WJ. New York, Academic Press, 1979, pp 67-92

41. Gibbs CJ Jr, Amyx HL, Bacote A, et al: Oral transmission of kuru, Creutzfeldt-Jakob disease, and scrapie to nonhuman primates. *J Infect Dis* 142:205-208, 1980

42. Pattison IH, Millson GC: Experimental transmission of scrapie to goats and sheep by the oral route. *J Comp Pathol Ther* 71:171-176, 1961

43. Pattison IH, Hoare MN, Jebbett JN, et al: Spread of scrapie to sheep and goats by oral dosing with foetal membranes from scrapie-affected sheep. *Vet Rec* 90:465-468, 1972

44. Prusiner SB, Cochran SP: In preparation, 1982

45. Masters CL, Gajdusek DC, Gibbs CJ Jr, et al: Familial Creutzfeldt-Jakob disease and other familial dementias: an inquiry into possible modes of virus-induced familial diseases. In *Slow Transmissible Diseases of the Nervous System*, vol 1. Edited by Prusiner SB, Hadlow WJ. New York, Academic Press, 1979, pp 143-194

46. Tomlinson BE: The pathology of dementia. In *Dementia*, 2nd ed. Edited by Wells CE. Philadelphia, FA Davis, 1977, pp 113-154

47. Beck, E, Daniel PM: Kuru and Creutzfeldt-Jakob disease: neuropathological lesions and their significance. In *Slow Transmissible Diseases of the Nervous System*, vol 1. Edited by Prusiner SB, Hadlow WJ. New York, Academic Press, 1979, pp 253-270

48. Hadlow WJ, Race RE, Kennedy RC, et al: Natural infection of sheep with scrapie virus. In *Slow Transmissible Diseases of the Nervous System*, vol 2. Edited by Prusiner SB, Hadlow WJ. New York, Academic Press, 1979, pp 3-12

49. Gomori AJ, Partnow MJ, Horoupian DS, et al: The ataxic form of Creutzfeldt-Jakob disease. *Arch Neurol* 29:318-323, 1973

50. Zarranz JJ, Rivera-Pomar JM, Salisachs P: Kuru plaques in the brain of two cases with Creutzfeldt-Jakob disease. *J Neurol Sci* 43:291-300, 1979

51. Wisniewski HM, Bruce ME, Fraser H: Infectious etiology of neuritic (senile) plaques in mice. *Science* 190:1108-1110, 1975

52. Landis DMD, Williams RS, Masters CL: Golgi and electromicroscopic studies of spongiform encephalopathy. *Neurology* 31:538-549, 1981

53. Scheibel AB: Dendritic changes in senile and presenile dementia. In *Congenital and Acquired Cognitive Disorders*. Edited by Katzman R. New York, Raven Press, 1979, pp 107-122

54. Hogan RN, Baringer JR, Prusiner SB: In preparation, 1982

55. Goudsmit J, Morrow CH, Asher DM, et al: Evidence for and against the transmissibility of Alzheimer's disease. *Neurology* 30:945-950, 1980

56. Gajdusek DC: Slow and latent viruses and the aging

nervous system. In *Survey Report on the Aging of the Nervous System.* Edited by Maletta GJ. Washington DC, USDHEW, PHS, NIH No 74-296, 1974, pp 149-168

57. Prusiner SB, Hadlow WJ, Eklund CM, et al: Sedimentation characteristics of the scrapie agent from murine spleen and brain. *Biochemistry* 17:4987-4992, 1978

58. Kimberlin R, Walker C: Characteristics of a short incubation model of scrapie in the golden hamster. *J Gen Virol* 34:295-304, 1977

59. Prusiner SB, Cochran SP, Groth DF, et al: Measurement of the scrapie agent using an incubation time interval assay. *Ann Neurol* 11:353-358, 1982

60. Hogan RN, Baringer JR, Prusiner SB: Progressive retinal degeneration in scrapie-infected hamsters. *Lab Invest* 44:34-42, 1981

61. Baringer JR, Bowman KA, Prusiner SB: Regional neuropathology and titers in hamster scrapie. *J Exp Neurol Neuropathol* 40:329, 1981

62. Manuelidis EE, Manuelidis L: Observations on Creutzfeldt-Jakob disease propagated in small rodents. In *Slow Transmissible Diseases of the Nervous System*, vol 2. Edited by Prusiner SB, Hadlow WJ. New York, Academic Press, 1979, pp 147-173

63. Tateishi J, Ohta M, Koga M, et al: Transmission of chronic spongiform encephalopathy with kuru plaques for humans to small rodents. *Ann Neurol* 5:581-584, 1979

64. Kingsbury DT, Smeltzer DA, Amyx HL, et al: Properties of a mouse adapted agent from a case of spongiform encephalopathy. In preparation, 1982

65. Hunter GD: The enigma of the scrapie agent: biochemical approaches and the involvement of membranes and nucleic acids. In *Slow Transmissible Diseases of the Nervous System*, vol 2, Edited by Prusiner SB, Hadlow WJ. New York, Academic Press, 1979, pp 365-385

66. Kimberlin RH: *Scrapie in the Mouse.* Durham, England, Meadowfield Press, 1976, pp 1-77

67. Diener TO: Is the scrapie agent a viroid? *Nature New Biol* 235:218-219, 1972

68. Somerville RA, Millson GC, Hunter GD: Changes in a protein-nucleic acid complex from synaptic plasma membrane of scrapie-infected mouse brain. *Biochem Soc Trans* 4:1112-1114, 1976

69. Prusiner SB, Groth DF, Bildstein C, et al: Electrophoretic properties of the scrapie agent in agarose gels *Proc Natl Acad Sci USA* 77:2984-2988, 1980

70. Marsh RF, Malone TG, Semancik JS, et al: Evidence for an essential DNA component in the scrapie agent. *Nature* 275:146-147, 1978

71. Malone TG, Marsh RF, Hanson RP, et al: Evidence for the low molecular weight nature of scrapie agent. *Nature* 278:575-576, 1979

72. Liao TH: Reversible inactivation of pancreatic deoxyribonuclease A by sodium dodecyl sulfate. *J Biol Chem* 250:3831-3836, 1975

73. Siakotos AN, Gajdusek DC, Gibbs CJ Jr, et al: Partial purification of the scrapie agent from mouse brain by pressure disruption and zonal centrifugation in sucrose-sodium chloride gradients. *Virology* 70:230-237, 1976

74. Brown P, Green EM, Gajdusek DC: Effect of different gradient solutions on the buoyant density of scrapie infectivity. *Proc Soc Exp Biol Med* 158:513-516, 1978

75. Prusiner SB: An approach to the isolation of biological particles using sedimentation analysis. *J Biol Chem* 253:916-921, 1978

76. Prusiner SB, Hadlow WJ, Eklund CM, et al: Sedimentation properties of the scrapie agent. *Proc Natl Acad Sci USA* 74:4656-4660, 1977

77. Prusiner SB, Garfin DE, Cochran SP, et al: Experimental scrapie in the mouse: electrophoretic and sedimentation properties of the partially purified agent. *J Neurochem* 35:574-582, 1980

78. Prusiner SB, Groth DF, Cochran SP, et al: Gel electrophoresis and glass permeation chromatography of the hamster scrapie agent after enzymatic digestion and detergent extraction. *Biochemistry* 19:4892-4898, 1980

79. Prusiner SB, Garfin DE, Baringer JR, et al: On the partial purification and apparent hydrophobicity of the scrapie agent. In *Slow Transmissible Diseases of the Nervous System*, vol 2, Edited by Prusiner SB, Hadlow WJ. New York, Academic Press, 1979, pp 425-464

80. Kasper K, Stites DP, Bowman KA, et al: In preparation, 1982

81. Scanu AM: Structural studies on serum lipoproteins. *Biochim Biophys Acta* 265:471-508, 1972

82. McKinley MP, Masiarz FR, Prusiner SB: Reversible chemical modification of the scrapie agent. *Science* 214:1259-1261, 1981

83. Chirgwin JM, Przybyla AE, MacDonald RJ, et al: Isolation of biologically active ribonucleic acid from sources enriched in ribonuclease. *Biochemistry* 24:5294-5299, 1979

84. Hunter GD, Millson GC: Attempts to release the scrapie agent from tissue debris. *J Comp Pathol* 77:301-307, 1967

85. Szoka F Jr, Papahadjopoulos D: Procedure for preparation of liposomes with large internal aqueous space and high capture by reverse-phase evaporation. *Proc Natl Acad Sci USA* 75:4194-4298, 1978

86. Prusiner SB, Groth DF: Unpublished observations, 1981

87. Haase A, Hadlow WJ, Prusiner SB: Unpublished observations, 1981

88. Haase AT, Traynor BL, Ventura PE: Infectivity of visna virus DNA. *Virology* 70:65-79, 1976

89. Borras MT, Kingsbury DT, Gajdusek DC, et al: Inability to transmit scrapie by transfection of mouse embryo cells *in vitro. J Gen Virol.* In press, 1982

90. Kingsbury DT: In preparation, 1982

91. Alper T, Haig DA, Clarke MC: The scrapie agent: evidence against its dependence for replication on intrinsic nucleic acid. *J Gen Virol* 41:503-516, 1978

92. Alper T, Cramp WA, Haig DA, et al: Does the agent of scrapie replicate without nucleic acid? *Nature* 214:764-766, 1967

93. Rose JA: Parvovirus reproduction. In *Comprehensive Virology*, vol 3. Edited by Fraenkel-Conrat H, Wagner RR. New York, Plenum Press, 1974, pp 1-61

94. Schaffer FL, Schwerdt CE: Purification and properties of poliovirus. *Adv Virus Res* 6:159-204, 1959

95. Diener TO, Raymer WB: Potato spindle tuber virus: a plant virus with properties of a free nucleic acid. II. Characterization and partial purification. *Virology* 37:351-366, 1969

96. Mulbach H-P, Camacho-Henriquez A, Sänger HL: Infection of tomato protoplasts by ribonucleic acid of tobacco mosaic virus and by viroids. *Phytopathol Z* 90:289-305, 1977

97. Sanger HL, Ramm K, Domdey H, et al: Conversion of circular viroid molecules to linear strands. *FEBS Lett* 99:117-122, 1979

98. Mihalyi E: *Application of Proteolytic Enzymes to Protein Structure Studies.* Cleveland, CRC Press, 1972, pp 1-364

99. Prusiner SB, Cleaver J, Groth DF: Unpublished observations, 1981

100. McLaren AD, Shugar D: *Photochemistry of Proteins and Nucleic Acids.* New York, Pergamon Press, 1964, pp 110-162

101. Butzow JJ, Eichhorn GL: Interactions of metal ions with polynucleotides and related compounds. IV. Degradation of polynucleotides by zinc and other divalent metal ions. *Biopolymers* 3:95-107, 1965

102. Issacs ST, Shen CJ, Hearst JE, et al: Synthesis and characterization of new psoralen derivatives with superior photoreactivity with DNA and RNA. *Biochemistry* 16:1058-1064, 1977

103. McKinley MP, Masiarz FR, Hearst J, et al: In preparation, 1982

104. Hearst JE, Thiry L: The photoinactivation of an RNA animal virus, vesicular stomatitis virus, with the aid of newly synthesized psoralen derivatives. *Nucl Acid Res* 4:1339-1348, 1977

105. Hanson CV, Riggs JL, Lennette EH: Photochemical inactivation by DNA and RNA viruses by psoralen derivatives. *J Gen Virol* 40:345-358, 1978

106. Alper T, Haig DA, Clarke MC: The exceptionally small size of the scrapie agent. *Biochem Biophys Res Commun* 22:278-284, 1966

107. Earnshaw WC, Casjens SR: DNA packaging by double-stranded DNA bacteriophages. *Cell* 21:319-331, 1980

108. Clarke MC: Infection of cell cultures with scrapie agent. In *Slow Transmissible Diseases of the Nervous System*, vol 2. Edited by Prusiner SB, Hadlow WJ. New York, Academic Press, 1979, pp 225-234

109. Yang VW, Lerner MR, Steitz JA, et al: A small nuclear ribonucleoprotein is required for splicing of adenoviral early RNA sequences. *Proc Natl Acad Sci USA* 78:1371-1375, 1981

110. Bishop JM: Enemies within: the genesis of retrovirus oncogenes. *Cell* 23:5-6, 1981

111. Weigle WO: Cellular events in experimental autoimmune thyroiditis, allergic encephalomyelitis and tolerance to self. In *Autoimmunity: Genetic, Immunologic, Virologic and Clinical Aspects.* New York, Academic Press, 1977, pp 141-170

112. Temin H: The DNA provirus hypothesis: the establishment and implications of RNA-directed DNA synthesis. *Science* 192:1075-1080, 1976

113. Craig R: The theoretical possibility of reverse translation of proteins into genes. *J Theor Biol* 88:757-760, 1981

114. Kleinkauf H, von Döhren H: Nucleic acid independent synthesis of peptides. *Curr Top Microbiol Immunol* 91:129-176, 1981

115. Stanley WM: Isolation of a crystalline protein possessing the properties of tobacco mosaic virus. *Science* 81:644-645, 1935

116. Kimberlin RH, Walker CA: Evidence that the transmission of one source of scrapie agent to hamsters involves separation of agent strains from a mixture. *J Gen Virol* 39:487-496, 1978

117. Prusiner SB, Cochran SP, Groth DF, et al: Aging of the nervous system and prolonged incubation periods of the spongiform encephalopathies. In *Aging of the Brain and Dementia.* Edited by Amaducci L, Davison AN, Antuono P. New York, Raven Press, 1980, pp 205-216

118. Hadlow WJ: Unpublished observations, 1981

119. Hanson RP, Eckroade RJ, Marsh RF, et al: Susceptibility of mink to sheep scrapie. *Science* 172:859-861, 1971

120. Allen G, Fantes KH: A family of structural genes for human lymphoblastoid (leukocyte-type) interferon. *Nature* 287:408-411, 1980

121. Nagata S, Mantei N, Weissmann C: The structure of one of the eight or more distinct chromosomal genes for human interferon-α. *Nature* 287:401-408, 1980

122. Dickinson AG, Meikle V, Fraser H: Identification of a gene which controls the incubation period of some strains of scrapie agent in mice. *J Comp Pathol* 78:293-299, 1968

123. Dickinson AG, Fraser H: An assessment of the genetics of scrapie in sheep and mice. In *Slow Transmissible Diseases of the Nervous System*, vol 1. Edited by Prusiner SB, Hadlow WJ. New York, Academic Press, 1979, pp 367-386

124. Stiets DP, Prusiner SB, Kasper KC, et al: Genetic control of scrapie in mice with immunodysfunction. *Fed Proc* 41:567, 1982

125. Kingsbury DT, Watson JD: Genetic control of the incubation time of mice infected with a human agent of spongiform encephalopathy. In preparation, 1982

10
Epilepsy: Changing Concepts and Approaches

Timothy A. Pedley and Eli S. Goldensohn

INTRODUCTION

The movement toward greater standardization in the treatment of seizures, which began with the widespread use of anticonvulsant blood levels, has accelerated. This has been achieved in part by the almost universal use of the International Classification of Seizures in neurological publications, and in part as the result of a number of recent well-structured clinical investigations on the use of anticonvulsant drugs. Of greatest impact are several widely disseminated reports that define conditions in which anticonvulsant medication may be discontinued with minimal risk in patients whose seizures are controlled, and situations in which the institution of chronic anticonvulsant treatment may not be clinically justified. This information takes on added significance in view of recent studies, also discussed in this chapter, in which toxic and teratogenic effects of both old and new anticonvulsants are assessed. Several worthwhile changes to the International Classification of Seizures have been offered.

Efforts toward expanding the pool of patients with uncontrolled seizures who can benefit by temporal lobectomy, and efforts toward improving the overall results of lobectomy are being made. In addition to conventional presurgical evaluation criteria, some centers now include closed circuit television recordings of clinical seizures and the electroencephalogram (EEG), intracerebral electrical depth recordings, and positron emisson tomography (PET).

At the cellular and molecular levels, studies on in vitro and in vivo preparations of mammalian neuronal networks continue to add to the understanding of basic processes involved in epileptogenesis. However, the premature application of experimental physiological phenomena such as kindling and the mirror focus to clinical decisions affecting the management of patients with seizures does not seem justified.

PATHOPHYSIOLOGY

Mirror Focus and Kindling

Bilateral, apparently independent epileptogenic foci are common in human focal epilepsy. Homotopic areas are most often involved. The question frequently arises, when surgical extirpation is being considered, whether one focus is dependent on the other or at least of secondary importance to the area of origin of the patient's habitual seizures. In this connection, the term "mirror focus" is often used to describe the contralateral activity deemed secondary in clinical cases.

Despite vigorous advocacy, mainly by Morrell and his coworkers, that the mirror focus represents a persistent new zone of epileptogenic tissue induced by but eventually independent of the primary focus (1-4), there is actually little experimental support for this concept, and most studies are subject to criticism. Practically the entire hypothesis is based on electroencephalographic or electrocorticographic evidence that paroxysmal activity on the two sides does not always occur synchronously or in obvious relationship. Cellular studies are few in number and have not reliably documented burst firing patterns in the secondary focus. One such chronic study we view as unconvincing because of technique and absence of controls (3). In an acute preparation, Ajmone-Marsan (5) found only projected phenomena in the homotopic area with "hardly any of the features characteristic of the epileptic neuronal pool." It might be argued that insufficient time had elapsed for independence of the secondary focus to have occurred. However, in a study of neuronal activities in the homotopic cortex of monkeys contralateral to an alumina-induced epileptogenic focus, Wyler (6) also was unable to find firing patterns typical of "epileptic" neurons. Use of surgical ablation of the primary focus as a means of establishing independence in the opposite hemisphere may be particularly misleading since it is often difficult to determine whether all the potentially epileptogenic brain tissue at or surrounding the primary focus has been removed. Lowrie and Ettlinger (7) have been unable to replicate their own earlier findings in monkeys that secondary, independent foci develop in homotopic cortex contralateral to the site of topical aluminum hydroxide application. And most recently, Harris and Lockard (8) have shown decisively in rhesus monkeys that total removal of a primary epileptogenic focus made by cortical injection of alumina invariably prevented further seizures or the development of contralateral "independent" epileptiform activity. Further, only projected (not independent) epileptiform discharges were seen contralateral to the focus prior to excision.

There is even less data regarding the relevance, or indeed the occurrence, of mirror foci in man. This is not altogether surprising as Wilder and coworkers (9) have reported that the ease with which secondary or mirror foci develop shows a strong phylogenetic hierarchy with such foci developing in amphibia within hours, but taking 2-10 days in rabbits, 1-2 months in cats, and up to 2 years in rhesus monkeys. Gupta and coworkers (10) have inferred the existence of mirror foci in some patients with temporal lobe epilepsy by demonstrating a longer duration of illness in patients with bilateral as opposed to unilateral spike foci. Their data are open to an alternative interpretation, however, as patients with bilateral epileptogenic lesions may have a more severe form of epilepsy which begins earlier than epilepsy in patients with unilateral lesions. To our knowledge, there is no documentation of persistent clinical or electrographic seizures, either in animals or man, that arise from foci attributed to secondary epileptogenesis after the primary focus is removed.

It is nevertheless reasonable to hypothesize that an epileptic focus acting as a site of neuronal hyperactivity might have both short- and long-term effects on neural circuits involved in the propagation of its abnormal activity. The practical questions that concern the clinican are twofold. First, does epilepsy under certain circumstances act as a progressive disease with each ictal and interictal discharge contributing to the creation of new substrates for additional seizures? Second, if long-term functional changes in neuronal processing of information occur, do they have implications for interictal interference with function distinct from seizure activity per se? Penfield (11) concluded long ago that "continuous conduction of spontaneous epileptic electrical activity eventually results in permanent facilitation of certain pathways of conduction."

The "kindling" phenomenon bears directly on these issues. Kindling is a term coined by Goddard and coworkers (12) to describe the progressive enhancement of electrical and clinical responses to short duration, initially subthreshold stimuli, which are applied at intervals of days or hours (13-19). Afterdischarges occur first, and sufficient repetition of the stimulus eventually results in a generalized convulsion of focal origin. Such kindled seizures have the advantage of being stereotyped, easily reproduced, and independent of tissue damage, gliosis, or metal ion deposits. General observations relevant to the kindling phenomenon follow [see (20-21) for reviews]. First, the enhanced responses, although diminished, persist over long periods of time (up to 12 months in some instances) without further stimulation. Second, wide variation in stimulus parameters does not significantly alter the time needed for kindling to occur, but a minimal interval between successive stimulations is critical. Third, "transfer" of this effect can be observed in that kindling in one amygdala facilitates subsequent kindling of contralateral amygdala and septal regions. Fourth, the appearance of motor-ictal concomitants can be correlated with an increase in amplitude of after-discharges particularly at the homotopic contralateral point. Of particular interest has been the finding that on occasion spontaneous interictal discharges may occur (19, 22). Most studies of the kindling phenomenon have utilized stimulation of the amydgala. Other areas of the brain are much less responsive but when subjected to repeated electrical stimulation over long periods may be kindled as well. These include hippocampus (23, 24), frontal lobe (25, 26,) and sensory thalamus (27). Normal primates are very resistant to kindling.

Although Goddard and coworkers (12) concluded that kindling "reflects a change in brain function, which is not merely threshold reduction but which involves relatively permanent trans-synaptic modifications in neural organization," there are only a few studies defining the actual cellular pathophysiology of the kindling phenomenon, and no structural or ultrastructural changes have yet been found. Kindling does appear to alter the general excitability level of brain tissue. Hippocampal slices from chemically-kindled guinea pigs generate epileptiform activity when exposed to elevated potassium levels in the perfusing medium (28). In contrast, control slices require both a high potassium concentration and addition of a convulsant drug. Further, kindling lowers the threshold for pentylenetetrazol-induced convulsions whether or not seizures developed during the kindling process (29). Several possibilities could explain the apparent increase in excitability even in the absence of detectable anatomic changes. These include increased firing of the afferent neurons, increased release of transmitter to a given stimulus, increased response of postsynaptic membrane to a given quantity of transmitter, decreased pre- or postsynaptic inhibition, and an increase in number of presynaptic release sites.

In attempting to understand the cellular basis of kindling, a number of pharmacological changes have been described in kindled animals, but the results of such studies have been difficult to relate to the kindling process itself. In addition, results from different laboratories have been variable and sometimes contradictory. Thus, there is suggestive evidence that catecholamines delay or suppress kindled seizure activity, since depletion of central catecholamines by reserpine, methyl-naphthyl-aziridine, and 6-hydroxydopamine facilitates the rate of amygdaloid kindling in rats and cats (30, 31). Catecholamine agonists have not been shown to affect amygdaloid seizure development (31, 32). Arnold and coworkers (30) reported that atropine blocks kindled seizures, but Corcoran and coworkers (33) were unable to confirm this effect. Frenk and coworkers (34) have postulated a role for opiate receptors in kindling since morphine enhanced the frequency of EEG spikes and postictal depression in their amygdaloid kindled rats. These effects were reversible with naloxone. Liebowitz and coworkers (23) showed a significant increase in potassium-induced release of gamma-aminobutyric acid (GABA) from hippocampal slices of rats which had generalized seizures induced by daily electrical stimulation of the entorhinal cortex. This change was selective in that it did not involve other hippocampal amino acids including glutamate. CA1 pyramidal neurons from rat hippocampus, when tested after a kindling stimulus, have been shown to be supersensitive to iontophoretic pulses of acetylcholine (35). There was no change in the sensitivity of neurons to glutamic acid or GABA. In contrast, Byrne and coworkers (36) have shown a decrease in muscarinic cholinergic receptors not only in the stimulated amygdala but in both ipsilateral and contralateral hippocampus. The decrease could not be related to development of either spikes or seizures.

Now, more than a decade after kindling was first described, it seems important to put the kindling phenomenon in some perspective as it relates to human epilepsy. In this regard several points deserve emphasis. First, it is not known if kindling can even occur in the human, and if it does occur, what the trigger parameters might be that correspond to the kindling stimulus in experimental animals. As with the mirror focus, evolutionary advancement is associated with progressively greater difficulty in kindling (12). Second, spontaneous seizures unrelated to a triggering stimulus are rare even in fully kindled animals (19) and have not been observed in primates except those with strong convulsive tendencies [*Papio papio*] (37). Finally, spontaneous interictal discharges are not universally seen and are most often observed in relation to the kindling process itself rather than at long intervals after kindling is complete (22, 38). While it is clear from experimental studies that interictal discharges can temporally disrupt neuronal function and influence seizure susceptibility, their long-term or permanent effects on epileptogenesis are not established. One of the most active EEGs in terms of frequency of focal interictal spiking is recorded in children with benign focal epilepsy of childhood (sylvian seizures). Yet it is characteristic of these children to be normal between attacks, for their seizures to be easily controlled, and for both the clinical and EEG manifestations to disappear in adolescence. Indeed, in any patient with epilepsy, there is only a rough correlation at best between the amount of interictal epileptiform activity on the EEG at any point in time and the frequency of clinical attacks. Further, cognitive deficits generally (39) and the behavioral syndrome of temporal lobe epilepsy in particular (40) relate to the duration of illness but not to seizure frequency, suggesting that both the seizures and the interictal psychological disturbance (if any) are only indirectly related.

In summary, we are skeptical of the existence of the mirror focus as an independent persistent phenomenon and feel that even as a concept it has little application to human epilepsy. Kindling remains an intriguing phenomenon. It is our present view, however, that it is a useful experimental model of central nervous system plasticity but one that currently has no direct relevance to the diagnosis and management of the patient with epilepsy.

CLASSIFICATION OF SEIZURES

The purpose of classifying seizures is to compress their many manifestations into a workable and logical scheme that is useful for easy and accurate communication and is compatible with effective diagnosis, treatment, and clinical investigation (41). The International Classification (42) and its currently proposed modifications (43) are the culmination of many years work toward those goals. It had become clear during the development of the classification that most recurrent seizures consistently begin in a localized area of the brain, and these were then called partial seizures. The main feature of the classification was the distinction between seizures which are generalized from the outset and those which originate locally. A subdivision of partial seizures was made into simple or complex depending upon whether or not consciousness is disturbed.

That seizures are often a sequence of symptoms which accompany abnormal electrical discharging in the brain as it spreads from one area to another is a concept that has now made its way into the classification. For example, where local excessive discharging ordinarily responsible for a simple partial seizure spreads into other areas of the brain sufficiently to cause a disturbance in consciousness, the attack has then evolved into a complex partial seizure. The newest version of the classification embodying this concept is given here in outline. A fuller account is published in *Epilepsia* (43).

PROGNOSIS OF SEIZURES

The application of population studies and other epidemiological methods to the problems of epilepsy is providing important new information of both practical and theoretical interest. In a longitudinal study of prognosis based in Rochester, Minnesota, Annegers and coworkers (44) studied the probability of patients with epilepsy becoming seizure-free. Patients with febrile seizures,

Table 1. Classification of Clinical Seizures

I. Partial Seizures (Focal and Local)
   A. Simple partial seizures
       1. With motor signs
       2. With somatosensory or special-sensory symptoms
       3. With autonomic symptoms or signs
       4. With psychic symptoms
   B. Complex partial seizures
       1. Simple partial onset followed by impairment of consciousness
       2. With impairment of consciousness at onset
   C. Partial seizures evolving to generalized tonic-clonic seizures (GTC)
       1. Simple partial seizures (A) evolving to GTC
       2. Complex partial (B) evolving to GTC
       3. Simple partial seizures evolving to complex partial seizures
          evolving to GTC
II. Generalized seizures
   A. Absence seizures ("Petit mal")
   B. Atypical absence
   C. Myoclonic seizures
   D. Tonic seizures
   E. Tonic-clonic seizures ("Grand mal")
   F. Atonic seizures

single seizures, and convulsions associated with acute illnesses were excluded. Among 457 patients followed for more than 5 years, it was estimated that 65% would be seizure-free for at least 5 consecutive years within 10 years of diagnosis. This estimate increased to 76% at 20 years. Relapses in the seizure-free group after this period occurred in 4%-6%. About 50% of patients surveyed were estimated to have been without seizures and off all medication for at least 5 years. The remission rate was higher for patients with primary (idiopathic) as opposed to secondary (symptomatic) epilepsy. Remission rate was also higher for patients with generalized tonic-clonic convulsions [GTC] (85% at 20 years) or absence seizures (80%) than for patients with complex partial seizures (65% at 20 years). If, however, a patient did not achieve remission within 5 years of the diagnosis being made, the chance of becoming seizure-free within the next 10 years was only 33%.

Partial confirmation of these data comes from a prospective study of 431 Japanese children followed for at least 5 years (45). Seizures were controlled for 3 years or more in 76% of the group as a whole. This favorable outcome was influenced in part by the prevalence of absent seizures and benign focal epilepsy of childhood, both conditions known to have a high incidence of age-related spontaneous remissions. In other subgroups the prognosis for becoming seizure-free was considerably worse. Seizures remitted in 58% of children with psychomotor attacks and in only 40% of cases diagnosed as Lennox-Gastaut syndrome. There was a general correlation between degree and type of EEG abnormality and the chance of becoming seizure-free. Patterns associated with good outcome included generalized 3/sec spike-wave bursts or atypical spike-wave paroxysms, and focal central-midtemporal spikes ("rolandic" or "sylvian" spikes). Diffuse slow-spike and wave discharges or focal spikes other than central-midtemporal were associated with a mixed prognosis.

Lindsay and coworkers (46) have followed the long-term social outcome of 100 children with temporal lobe epilepsy originally described in 1966 (47). The follow-up period ranged from 13 to 29 years with ages at follow-up between 19 to 39. Sixty-five percent were able to support themselves socially and economically. Only half, however, were seizure-free and off anticonvulsant medication. Thirty percent were disabled and dependent on family or institutional support. Five had died in childhood. Factors that were predictive of disability in later life included an IQ below 90, onset of seizures before age 2 1/2 years, frequent generalized convulsions, and severe behavior problems including rage attacks and hyperactivity.

Knowledge of remission rates for epilepsy is of obvious importance in orienting patients and their families for future planning, in making rational decisions about discontinuing antiepileptic drugs, and in assessing the efficacy of therapy. The remission rates found recently by Annegers and coworkers (44) are substantially higher than earlier reports would indicate (48). This emphasizes the difference between looking at entire populations at risk and specialty clinic populations which tend to select out more intractable, atypical, and complicated cases.

THE SINGLE SEIZURE

The patient who presents to the clinician after having a single seizure without obvious precipitating factors and who is otherwise healthy represents a special problem. If anticonvulsant drugs are prescribed, the patient is usually committed to 1 or more years of taking a drug which may or may not be necessary. While decisions about use of antiepileptic medication should be made guided by estimates of the likelihood of seizure recurrence and probable frequency, this information has until recently been unavailable. Now, the results of a study by Hauser and coworkers (49) provide new information that can directly affect management of the patient seen after a single seizure.

They studied 244 patients who presented with a single convulsive seizure. Patients whose seizures occurred in the context of an acute neurological or medical illness were not included. The risk of developing further seizures was greatest in the first year following the initial seizure. Recurrences occurred in 16% of all patients during the first 12 months, in 21% by 24 months, and in 27% by 36

months. No recurrences were observed beyond this time. Analysis of multiple variables showed that two factors were predictive of a higher recurrence rate—the EEG and past neurological illness. An EEG demonstrating generalized spike-wave discharges raised seizure recurrence to 50% at 24 months. A comprehensive EEG study was not possible, but other discriminating variables such as subtypes of generalized spike-wave patterns, location of focal spike discharges, and the circumstances under which the EEG is obtained—that is, sleep-deprivation, prolonged stage 2 sleep recording, and use of nasopharyngeal electrodes—should eventually be examined. The history of past neurological illness, including severe head injury, stroke, or intracranial infection, increased seizure recurrence to 27% at 12 months and 34% at 20 months. Seizure type, age, sex, findings on neurological examination, and family history did not seem to affect recurrence rate.

Physicians seeing patients after a single convulsive episode should seriously consider whether probability of seizure recurrence justifies use of antiepileptic drugs whose potential toxicity may not be inconsequential. This is particularly true for the patient whose EEG is normal and whose history does not provide a probable etiology for the seizure. In such an individual, the risk of further seizures within the next 12 months is about 10% and withholding medication until recurrence might be considered. Medication should be initiated promptly in patients with significantly abnormal EEGs or in those persons in whom the seizures are likely to be symptomatic of brain lesions.

FEBRILE SEIZURES

Febrile seizures are a common pediatric problem occurring in about 4% of children under 5 years of age, and the question of whether to initiate long-term anticonvulsant therapy after one or more febrile seizures has been controversial. Recent well-designed and well-conducted epidemiological studies by Nelson and Ellenberg at National Institutes of Health [NIH] (50-53) and by Annegers and coworkers (54) at the Mayo Clinic have provided a needed clear profile of the natural history of febrile seizures. Much of what follows is derived from these workers' data.

Febrile seizures may be diagnosed in a child less than 6 years of age who has a temperature greater than 38°C and in whom no acute neurological illness (e.g., meningitis, post-immunization syndrome, metabolic disorder) can be identified. The peak incidence occurs between 12 and 18 months of age. A second febrile convulsion will occur in 30% of children, and 10% will have 3 or more episodes. The risk of recurrence is greatest, about 50%, if the first seizure occurs before the age of 12 months. Three-quarters of recurrences take place within a year following the first convulsion.

Typical febrile seizures are usually brief, isolated generalized tonic or clonic convulsions. Atypical febrile seizures are those which last longer than 15 minutes, have prominent focal features, or recur in a prolonged cluster of attacks. If the first convulsion is a typical simple febrile seizure, only 1.4% of children will subsequently develop atypical febrile seizures.

The risk of epilepsy (i.e., recurrent afebrile seizures) is about 6% if all children with febrile seizures are considered. This figure can be subdivided into low risk and high risk groups. The risk of developing afebrile seizures has a high correlation with: (1) preexisting neurological or developmental abnormalities; (2) atypical febrile seizures; and (3) a family history of epilepsy. If none of these risk factors is present, the chance of developing epilepsy is only 1.3% or about twice the incidence in the general population. Children with both factors 1 and 2 have a 20-fold increased risk of developing chronic afebrile seizures with an actual incidence of later epilepsy of 13%. Death, persistent motor deficit, or impaired intellectual development are rare after febrile seizures. Simple febrile seizures do not appear to affect subsequent intellectual development.

The Proceedings of a Consensus Development Conference on Febrile Seizures sponsored by the NIH on May 19-21, 1980, will appear as a monograph. The salient conclusions have already been published in *Pediatrics* (55) and were: (1) Febrile seizures

are sufficiently benign that their recurrence does not justify chronic prophylaxis. (2) There is no information at the present time that anticonvulsant therapy reduces the risk of subsequent epilepsy. (3) A rational therapeutic approach takes into account the excellent long-term prognosis of the disorder in the vast majority of children. (4) Treatment should be considered in selected children if any of the risk factors for later epilepsy are present; if a child has had multiple febrile seizures; or if the initial febrile seizure occurs within the first year of life.

Phenobarbital prescribed continuously in daily doses to maintain a minimum serum concentration of 15 μg/ml is effective in reducing the risk of febrile seizure recurrence (56-58). Phenobarbital given intermittently at the time of fever is ineffective, but diazepam given acutely by rectum may provide protection (59, 60). Phenytoin is not an effective agent in preventing recurrences (61).

The role of the EEG in evaluating children with febrile seizures remains uncertain. It did not appear to predict development of later epilepsy in the Consensus Development Meeting, but this requires further study. We obtain EEGs to help identify children with epilepsy whose first seizure is merely triggered by or coincidental with a febrile illness. We consider focal or multifocal epileptiform discharges, or severely abnormal interictal background patterns as significant abnormalities that affect decisions about treatment. Timing of the EEG examination in relation to the seizure is important since nonspecific mild to moderate abnormalities may be seen as long as 7-10 days postictally.

DISCONTINUATION OF ANTIEPILEPTIC DRUGS

Discontinuing anticonvulsant drugs in patients who have been free of seizures even for years has been hazardous because of a paucity of reliable data on the risk factors involved. Emerson and coworkers (62) have assessed the risk factors and incidence of relapse in 68 children with epilepsy in whom anticonvulsant drugs were discontinued. All had been seizure-free on medication for at least 4 years and ranged in age from 6 to 22 years at the time of drug withdrawal. Statistical methods were used to control the different lengths of follow-up and to calculate the cumulative probability of patients remaining seizure-free over time. The overall probability of remaining seizure-free after 4 drug-free years was 69%. Most relapses (78%) occurred within the first year of drug withdrawal. Multivariate analysis was used to determine those factors most predictive of seizure recurrence. The two variables most strongly correlated with outcome were the number of generalized seizures that had occurred before control and the severity of the EEG abnormality (Fig. 1). Although mental retardation increased the risk of relapse by a factor of three, other abnormalities on neurological examination were not associated with increased risk of recurrence. Whether or not a presumed cause for the seizures was found was also not significant.

A number of important questions await future study. First, how important is the 4-year seizure-free interval before starting drug withdrawal? Would 2 or 3 years suffice? Second, is further refinement in predictive criteria possible so that antiepileptic drugs may be stopped sooner in selected cases? For example, a larger group of patients might show significant relationships of seizure type or the ease of achieving seizure control to relapse rate. Third, the predictive value of the EEG data needs further delineation as there are great differences among the various patterns of epileptiform activity, and certain epileptiform discharges may be inherited as traits distinct from overt seizures (63). Finally, does early discontinuation of anticonvulsants favorably affect cognitive function? This consideration is of special concern because of reports suggesting that duration of anticonvulsant therapy adversely

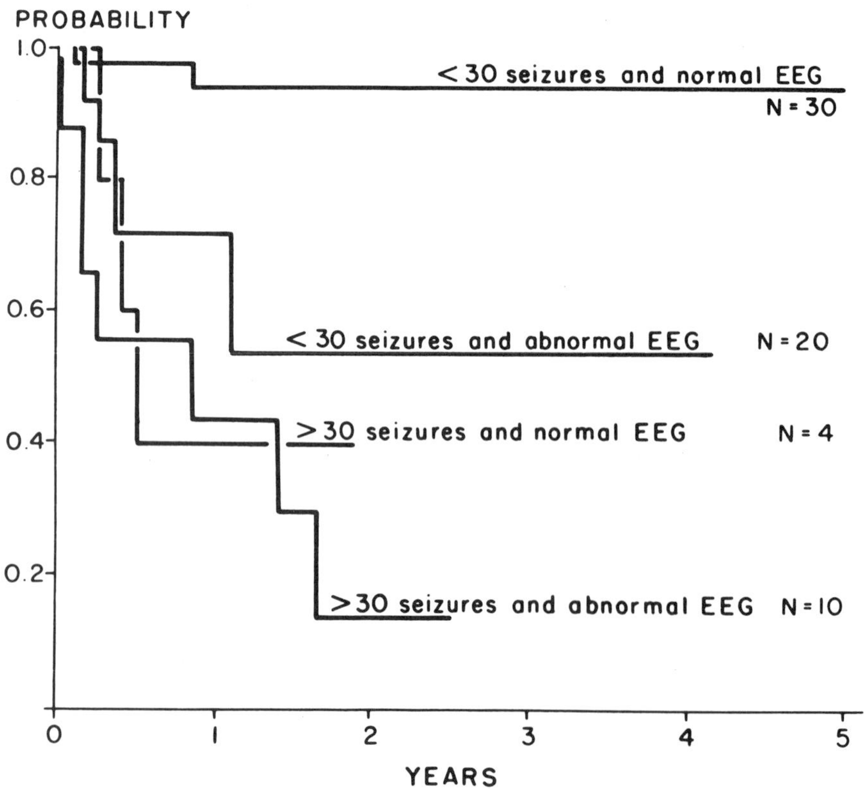

Figure 1. The cumulative probability of relapse plotted as a function of elapsed time following discontinuation of anticonvulsant drugs. The effect of seizure frequency and EEG findings on relapse rate are shown in four different combinations. (Reprinted with permission from Emerson RG, et al: Stopping medication in children with epilepsy. *N Engl J Med* 304:1125-1129, 1981.)

affects reading skills and memory concentration tasks (64-66).

In our practice, we attempt to discontinue drugs in children with simple absence attacks or benign focal epilepsy of childhood after a seizure-free interval of 12-18 months. In children with fully controlled primary GTC or simple partial seizures, we attempt drug withdrawal after 2 years if the neurological examination is normal, if there is no family history of seizures, and if the EEG is normal. In other epileptic children we prefer to wait at least 4 years or further into the indefinite future.

INFANTILE SPASMS

Massive myoclonus of infancy is associated with a wide variety of etiologies and in most instances is accompanied by mental and often by neurological retardation [see (67) for review]. The continuous interictal EEG is called hypsarrhythmia. During the brief myoclonic phase of each spasm, muscle and electrode artifacts tend to obscure a brief burst of bilaterally synchronous EEG spike and polyspike activity. In the subsequent tonic phase, a transient attenuation of EEG activity is referred to as an electrodecremental response. When massive myoclonus, neurological or developmental abnormalities, and a hypsarrhythmic EEG pattern occur together, the term "infantile spasm syndrome" is used. In one study from Japan, 85% of children with infantile spasms had varying degrees of developmental retardation at follow-up (68). Another study with generally similar findings clearly showed that cryptogenic cases fared much better both in seizure control and in neurological development than those having a known etiology (69).

Standard anticonvulsants, including phenobarbital, phenytoin, and carbamazepine, appear to have little lasting effect on either seizures or the infant's ultimate development. In a study of 19 patients, valproic acid decreased the frequency of attacks in about 50% of patients (70). In a more recent but preliminary study, valproic acid decreased seizure frequency in children who had been refractory to a 4-week trial of adrenocorticotropic hormone [ACTH] (P. Dyken, personal communication). While valproic acid reduced the number of spasms in most patients, none became completely seizure-free. Valproic acid must be used with caution in this age group as a significant number of cases of severe hepatic dysfunction and death have been reported in infants and young children.

The most widely used agent for treatment remains ACTH which recently has been shown to be more effective than steroids (71, 72). Singer and coworkers (73) in a retrospective study reported that doses of 40 units ACTH or greater per day begun within 1 month of seizure onset and used for extended periods produced a spasm-free condition in 87% of patients within 6 months. In a smaller controlled study Hrachovy and coworkers (71) indicated that using doses above 20 units of ACTH daily did not increase beneficial effects on neurological development. They emphasized the direct relationship between ACTH dosage and serious side effects, particularly hypertension. The frequency of side effects from ACTH therapy is usually underestimated. Serious hypertension, osteoporosis, electrolyte imbalance, and intercurrent infections occur in 37% of treated children and must be carefully watched for (74). The question of optimal dosage of ACTH and duration of treatment is still open, but we tend to use 4-5 units/kg/day. The mechanism of ACTHs action at a cellular or molecular level remains unknown.

POST-TRAUMATIC SEIZURES

There has been little uniformity among practicing physicians regarding the use of prophylactic antiepileptic drugs in patients with head trauma (75). Phenytoin or phenobarbital given in standard dosage schedules but without controlled plasma levels does not appear to affect the frequency of post-traumatic seizures (76). Young and coworkers (77) introduced a protocol specifically designed for head-injury patients, whereby a loading dose of phenytoin is given intravenously immediately after the trauma and therapeutic serum levels are rigidly maintained by serial measurements. The number of seizures observed during the first year was substantially below the expected incidence, a decrease the authors attribute to an effect of preventing the development of epileptogenic foci.

Part of the problem in developing guidelines for use of anticonvulsant drugs in patients with head injuries and in evaluating the effectiveness of prophylactic and therapeutic regimens has been due to a lack of information about risk factors predisposing to seizures in large civilian populations. Annegers and coworkers (78) studied 2747 residents of Olmsted County, Minnesota, who sustained head injuries between 1935 and 1974. Individuals with previous episodes of head trauma and prior epilepsy were excluded. Head injuries were categorized by severity. Seizures were designated as "early" (occurring as a direct effect of the injury) or "late" (occurring after recovery from acute effects of the trauma). The risk of developing post-traumatic epilepsy was related solely to the severity of the head injury. With severe trauma (brain contusion, intracranial hematoma, or unconsciousness or amnesia for at least 24 hours), the risk of late seizures was 7.1% at 1 year and 11.6% at 5 years. For mild trauma (no skull fracture but either unconsciousness or amnesia lasting less than 30 minutes), the risk of late seizures was only 0.1% at 1 year and 0.6% at 5 years, figures not significantly different than for the population at large. Early seizures were predictive of late seizures in adults with moderate or severe head trauma but not in cases of mild injury or in children with trauma of any severity.

In general, these data are in agreement with those of Jennett (79, 80) except as to the relationship between early seizures and the development of subsequent epilepsy. Jennett finds that early seizures increase the risk of late epilepsy regardless of the severity of head injury or age of the patient.

At the present time, it seems reasonable to consider prophylactic anticonvulsant medication in patients with severe head injury provided that compliance is assured. We prefer not to use prophylactic treatment in patients with mild or moderate injuries. No definite recommendation can be made about long-term drug treatment in children with early seizures whose trauma is assessed as being mild to moderate in degree. It is our current practice to treat prophylactically all children who have had early seizures but to discontinue medication after 1 year if no further seizures have occurred.

TERATOGENIC EFFECTS OF ANTIEPILEPTIC DRUGS

It is clear from a number of studies that there is a two- to threefold increase in the incidence of congenital malformations in infants born to epileptic mothers taking anticonvulsant drugs (81-86). Specific factors contributing to this risk have been disputed, but genetic considerations, drug exposure in utero, and frequency of seizures during pregnancy have all been implicated.

Shapiro and coworkers (87) found that the incidence of birth defects correlated with maternal epilepsy and not maternal anticonvulsant use. Friss and coworkers (88), who found that facial clefts are twice as prevalent among Danish epileptics than in the population at large, also suggested that parental factors related to the epilepsy rather than drug exposure per se may be operative. However, Annegers and coworkers (82) who also noted a maternal effect found it to be strongly related to drug use since mothers with active epilepsy but not taking medication did not bear as many babies with defects as those on medication.

The presence of seizures during pregnancy may be an additional element contributing to the risk of malformations, but this, too, remains controversial. Annegers and co-workers (82) did not find a significant difference in incidence of birth defects between children born to mothers not on anticonvulsants with epilepsy in remission and those born to mothers not on anticonvulsants who had seizures during pregnancy. This was also the conclusion of Lowe (89) and of Janz (85). On the other hand, Starreveld-Zimmerman and coworkers (86) found that women taking antiepileptic drugs had a greater chance of having a defective baby if they had GTC seizures during pregnancy than if they were seizure-free.

Several new experimental studies demonstrate direct teratogenic effects of antiepileptic drugs. Finnel (90) studied phenytoin-related teratogenesis in a mouse mutant (quaking) with genetic generalized seizures. The litters of heterozygous and homozygous females were used to discriminate between the effects of the quaking gene on birth defects from those of phenytoin alone. Both the homozygous females with daily seizures and the heterozygous females without seizures produced normal offspring. In contrast, both groups when given phenytoin produced offspring of low birth weight with a variety of malformations, the number and severity of which were dose-related. The defects were not related to fetal genotype. Maternal plasma concentrations of phenytoin were within the human therapeutic range. This study elegantly confirms the earlier report of Paulson and coworkers (91) showing a dose-related increase in phenytoin-induced cleft palates in mice.

Potential neuronal toxicity of chronic phenobarbital treatment has been studied in tissue cultures made from fetal mouse spinal cord (92). Exposure to phenobarbital for 2 to 6 weeks results in a dose-dependent decline in levels of choline acetyltransferase and in reduced numbers of spinal cord neurons. These effects appear to relate specifically to phenobarbital since they were not seen with the analog barbituric acid or with valproic acid.

A large collaborative study in Japan on fetal toxicity of anticonvulsant drugs has been completed (93). Fourteen percent of women receiving antiepileptic drugs had spontaneous abortions or stillbirths in contrast to four percent of the nonmedicated mothers. The incidence of malformations was 11.5% in the treated group but only 2.3% in epileptic women not taking medication. The risk of birth defects was somewhat higher (12.7%) in women on anticonvulsants who continued to have seizures during pregnancy. When the data were analyzed in terms of individual antiepileptic agents, trimethadione, phenobarbital, primidone, and acetazolamide were implicated most often. Teratogenic effects were not significantly increased after phenytoin, carbamazepine, or valproic acid. However, the number of patients in each drug group sample was small which may bias these findings. In addition, the majority of patients received two or more drugs, and analysis of

this variable showed that risk of malformation correlated positively with combination therapy. Feldman and coworkers (94) have also provided strong evidence that trimethadione has a significant teratogenic effect. Seven of eight infants exposed in utero to trimethadione alone had congenital anomalies. Given alone or in combination, trimethadione resulted in abortions or malformations in 87% of 53 pregnancies.

Specific fetal syndromes have been ascribed to both phenytoin (95) and trimethadione (94). It remains uncertain, however, whether these syndromes are truly drug-specific or whether they result from multiple and complex interrelating factors, only one of which is cellular toxicity from medication. The fetal hydantoin syndrome has been accepted as a definite entity by the American Teratology Society and is included in the Birth Defects Compendium (96). The syndrome is characterized by: (1) dysmorphic facies, including most commonly a broad, depressed nasal bridge, epicanthic folds, hypertelorism, ptosis, and ridging of the metopic suture; (2) cleft lip or palate: (3) deformities of the fingers including hypoplasia of the nails and distal phalanges; (4) cardiac anomalies; (5) growth retardation; and (6) microcephaly with mental retardation. In the mutant mouse model (90), this syndrome is reproduced in its entirety.

The fetal trimethadione syndrome was described by Zackai and coworkers (97) and further delineated by Feldman and coworkers (94). Major features include developmental delay, malformed or low-set ears, cleft lip and palate, mental subnormality, speech impairment, skeletal malformations, and congenital heart disease.

Use of Antiepileptic Drugs in Pregnancy

From information presently available on teratogenesis, it is possible to conclude the following. First, use of anticonvulsant drugs by epileptic women during pregnancy results in a two- to threefold increase in birth defects that is in large part due to teratogenic effects of the antiepileptic agents themselves. Second, individual drugs probably vary considerably in teratogenicity, and while current evidence is strongest for trimetha-dione, phenytoin and phenobarbital, all must be suspect. Third, the degree of risk is increased by use of two or more drugs, the presence of major seizures, and as yet incompletely-defined genetic factors.

The above considerations permit a reasonable approach toward pregnancy in women with epilepsy:

1. All women of child-bearing age should be informed of potential teratogenic effects of an antiepileptic drug at the time it is first prescribed.

2. Possible risks should be minimized before the patient becomes pregnant. The advisability of birth-control measures should be seriously considered by a woman with poorly-controlled major convulsive seizures who is taking multiple anticonvulsants.

3. When medication is required during pregnancy, attempts should be made to maintain satisfactory seizure control using a single agent at the lowest effective plasma concentration.

4. To avoid the slight but definite risk of having a deformed infant, the possibility of discontinuing medication altogether, at least for the first half of pregnancy, can be cautiously considered in patients with nonconvulsive generalized seizures or infrequent partial seizures that do not generalize. Some informed patients prefer occasional seizures of these types to the slight but definite risk of giving birth to a malformed baby.

5. Trimethadione should be eliminated from the medication regimen, and phenytoin and phenobarbital should be avoided when feasible. We also avoid valproic acid because of limited experience with this drug to date. The choice of "least risk" anticonvulsant is not clear cut but carbamazepine is the least implicated at the present time.

6. In the epileptic woman who has an unplanned pregnancy while on anticon-vulsant drugs, we agree with So and Penry (98) that medication should not be abruptly discontinued since the overall incidence of birth defects even while increased is still low, and the teratogenic insult may have already occurred.

7. We advise giving supplemental vitamin K throughout the last trimester to women receiving antiepileptic drugs to prevent vitamin K-dependent coagulation deficiency in the new-born.

SURGICAL THERAPY: SELECTION OF PATIENTS

In spite of the introduction of several completely new diagnostic methods and modification of existing techniques, the success rate of surgical treatment for intractable seizures of focal origin, although very good, remains at between 60% and 80% (99). The search for improved criteria to identify a larger number of patients who can benefit by resection of epileptogenic foci is a difficult one. This is, in part, because the extent of cortical tissue capable of epilepto-genesis in human focal epilepsy is not well defined. It appears to be composed of many small, potentially epileptogenic aggregates of cells in columnar arrangement which are spread over a wide area (100, 101). In addition, it is unusual to find a purely unilateral focal discharge in patients with epilepsy originating from the temporal lobe, the most common area extirpated. There is usually a degree of apparently independent firing from either hemisphere. The single most highly reliable localizing criterion is a discreet accessible structural lesion identified by radiological examinations, but this is found in only a minority of cases that come to surgery.

Engel and coworkers (102) analyzed 14 functional tests that can be used in presurgical evaluation. They found that the combined tests, which included the site of spontaneous interictal and ictal EEG spiking, evidence of decreased metabolic rate given by PET scanning, local relative decrease in thiopen-tal-induced fast activity, and intracarotid amobarbital testing for language and memory were reliable if consistent. However, when discrepancies occurred among the various tests, depth recording studies were considered decisive. In their study of 7 patients evaluated by the functional tests listed above, con-flicting information was found in several cases, and depth recording appeared to resolve the differences. In 1 patient, more

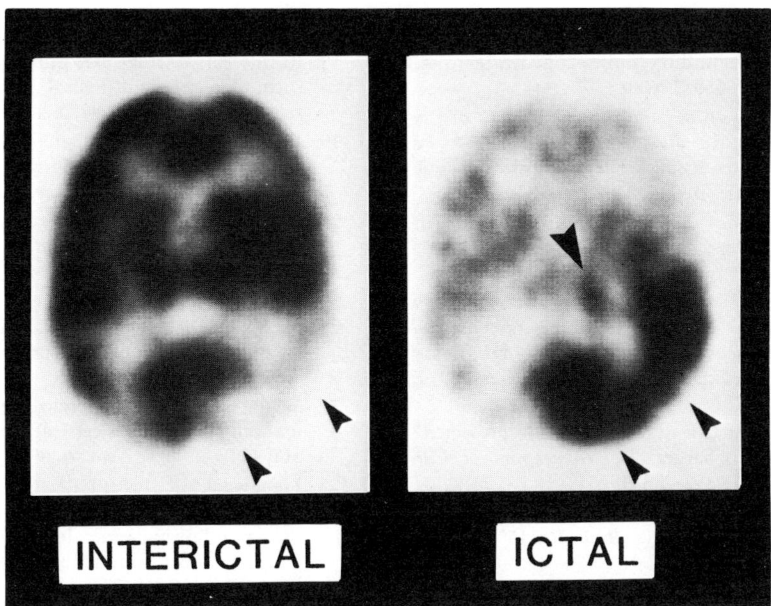

Figure 2. Position emission tomography (PET) scans are shown in a patient with complex partial seizures beginning with visual auras. Interictally, a zone of hypometabolic activity is seen in the right occipital area. During a seizure, the same region shows hypermetabolic activity. (Reprinted with permission from Phelps ME, et al: Topographic mapping of human cerebral metabolism: visual stimulation and deprivation. *Neurology* 31:517-529, 1981.)

seizures originated electrically from the side opposite to that eventually chosen for operation. Final decision in this case was made from the correlation of depth activity with the clinical pattern most typical of the patient's habitual seizures. In 4 of the 7 patients, the frequency of spontaneous interictal discharges from the depth recordings were of no value or misleading in lateralization.

The usefulness of PET scanning in focal seizures is demonstrated by Phelps and coworkers (103). In a patient whose complex partial seizures began with visual auras, a localized area of decreased metabolic activity was present in the right occipital lobe interictally. This was converted to a hypermetabolic zone during a clinical seizure (Fig. 2). The PET scan thus would appear to have considerable promise in the selection

and treatment of surgical candidates particularly since it may reliably demonstrate pathological alterations in local metabolic function even in the absence of gross anatomic changes. The computerized tomography (CT) scan itself identifies abnormalities in between 30% and 50% of patients with seizures (104, 105).

The combination of functional tests including PET scanning with CT and depth recording techniques have added new dimensions to the selection of patients who can benefit from surgical treatment. Nevertheless, definite criteria for identifying surgical candidates for the treatment of partial epilepsy cannot be made at this time. Indications for use of the various available techniques and the evaluation of their results depend on problems presented by the individual patient.

REFERENCES

1. Morrell F: Secondary epileptogenic lesions. *Epilepsia* 1:536-560, 1960

2. Morrell F: Physiology and histochemistry of the mirror focus. In *Basic Mechanisms of the Epilepsies*. Edited by Jasper HH, Ward AA, Pope A. Boston, Little, Brown. 1969, pp 357-370

3. Wilder BJ, Morrell F: Cellular behavior in secondary epileptic lesions. *Neurology* 17:1193-1204, 1967

4. Wilder, BJ: Projection phenomena and secondary epileptogenesis—mirror foci. In *Experimental Models of Epilepsy*. Edited by Purpura DP, Penry JK, Tower D, et al. New York, Raven Press, 1972, pp 85-111

5. Ajmone-Marsan C: Unitary analysis of "projected" epileptiform discharges. *Electroencephalogr Clin Neurophysiol* 15:197-208, 1963

6. Wyler AR: Single unit analysis of "mirror foci" in chronic epileptic monkeys. *Brain Res* 150:201-204, 1978

7. Lowrie MB, Ettlinger G: The development of independent secondary ("mirror") discharges in the monkey: failure to replicate earlier findings. *Epilepsia* 21:25-30, 1980

8. Harris, AB, Lockard JS: Absence of seizures or mirror foci in experimental epilepsy after excision of alumina and astrogliotic scar. *Epilepsia* 22:107-122, 1981

9. Wilder, BJ, King RL, Schmidt RP: Comparative study of secondary epileptogenesis. *Epilepsia* 9:275-289, 1968

10. Gupta PC, Dhrampaul, Pathak SN, Singh B: Secondary epileptogenic EEG focus in temporal lobe epilepsy. *Epilepsia* 14:423-426, 1973

11. Penfield W: Epileptogenic lesions. *Acta Neurol Psychiat Belg* 56:75-88, 1956

12. Goddard GV, McIntyre DC, Leech CK: A permanent change in brain function resulting from daily electrical stimulation. *Exp Neurol* 25:295-330, 1969

13. McIntyre DC, Goddard GV: Transfer, interference and spontaneous recovery of convulsions kindled from the rat amygdala. *Electroencephalogr Clin Neurophysiol* 35:533-543, 1973

14. Racine RJ: Modification of seizure activity by electrical stimulation. I. After-discharge threshold. *Electroencephalogr Clin Neurophysiol* 32:269-279, 1972

15. Racine, RJ: Modification of seizure activity by electrical stimulation. II. Motor seizure. *Electroencephalogr Clin Neurophysiol* 32:281-294, 1972

16. Racine RJ: Modification of seizure activity by electrical stimulation. III. Mechanisms. *Electroencephalogr Clin Neuophysiol* 32:295-299, 1972

17. Racine RJ, Burnham WM, Gartner JG: First trial motor seizures triggered by amygdaloid stimulation in the rat. *Electroencephalogr Clin Neurophysiol* 35:487-494, 1973

18. Racine RJ, Gartner JG, Burnham WM: Epileptiform activity and neural plasticity in limbic structures. *Brain Res* 47:262-268, 1972

19. Wada JA, Sato M, Corcoran ME: Persistent seizure susceptibility and recurrent spontaneous seizures in kindled cats. *Epilepsia* 15:465-478, 1974

20. Goldensohn ES: Epileptogenesis: recent neurobiological advances. In *Modern Perspectives in Epilepsy*. Edited by Wada JA. Montreal, Eden Press, 1978, pp 172-184

21. McNamara JO, Byrne MC, Dashieff RM, et al: The kindling model of epilepsy: a review. *Prog Neurobiol* 15:139-159, 1980

22. Wada JA, Sato M: Generalized convulsive seizures induced by daily electrical stimulation of the amygdala in cats. *Neurology* 24:565-574, 1974

23. Liebowitz NR, Pedley TA, Cutler RWP: Release of γ-aminobutyric acid from hippocampal slices of the rat following generalized seizures induced by daily electrical stimulation of entorhinal cortex. *Brain Res* 138:369-373, 1978

24. Sato M, Nakashima T: Kindling: secondary epileptogenesis, sleep and catecholamines. *Can J Neurol Sci* 2:439-446, 1975

25. Wada JA, Osawa T, Mizoguchi T: Recurrent spontaneous seizure state induced by prefrontal kindling in Senegales baboons (*Papio papio*). *Can J Neurol Sci* 2:477-492, 1975

26. Wake, A, Wada JA: Frontal cortical kindling in cats. *Can J Neurol Sci* 2:493-499, 1975

27. Cain DP: Kindling in sensory systems: thalamus. *Exp Neurol* 66:319-329, 1979

28. Oliver AP, Hoffer BJ, Wyatt RJ: Kindling induces long-lasting alterations in response of hippocampal neurons to elevated potassium levels in vitro. *Science* 208:1264-1265, 1980

29. Cain DP: Effects of kindling or brain stimulation on pentylenetetrazol-induced convulsion susceptibility. *Epilepsia* 21:243-249, 1980

30. Arnold P, Racine RJ, Wise R: Effect of atropine, reserpine, 6-OHDA and handling on seizure development in the rat. *Exp Neurol* 45:355-363, 1974

31. Wada JA: Pharmacological prophylaxis in the kindling model of epilepsy. *Arch Neurol* 34:389-395, 1977

32. Kamei C, Masuda Y, Oka M, et al: The effects of antidepressant drugs on amygdaloid after-discharges in rats. *Jpn J Pharmacol* 25:359-365, 1975

33. Corcoran ME, Wada JA, Wake A, et al: Failure of atropine to retard amygdaloid kindling. *Exp Neurol* 51:271-275, 1976

34. Frenk H, Engel J Jr, Ackermann RF, et al: Endogenous opioids may mediate post-ictal behavioral depression in amygdaloid-kindled rats. *Brain Res* 167:435-440, 1979

35. Burchfiel JL, Duchowny MS, Duffy FH: Neuronal supersensitivity to acetylcholine induced by kindling in the rat hippocampus. *Science* 204:1096-1098, 1979

36. Byrne MC, Gottlieb R, McNamara JO: Amygdala kindling induces muscarinic cholinergic receptor declines in a highly specific distribution within the limbic system. *Exp Neurol* 69:85-98, 1980

37. Wada JA, Osawa T: Spontaneous recurrent seizure state induced by daily electric amygdaloid stimulation in Senegalese baboons (*Papio papio*). *Neurology* 26:273-286, 1976

38. Fitz JG, McNamara JO: Spontaneous interictal spiking in the awake kindled rat. *Electroencephalog Clin Neurophysiol* 47:592-596, 1979

39. O'Leary DS, Seidenberg M, Berent S, et al: Effects of age of onset of tonic-clonic seizures on neuropsychological performance in childhood. *Epilepsia* 22:197-204, 1981

40. Bear DM, Fedio P: Quantitative analysis of interictal behavior in temporal lobe epilepsy. *Arch Neurol* 34:454-467, 1977

41. Goldensohn ES: The classification of epileptic seizures. In *The Nervous System*, vol 2, *The Clinical Neurosciences*. Edited by Tower DB. New York, Raven Press, 1975, pp 261-265

42. Gastaut H: Clinical and electroencephalographical classification of epileptic seizures. *Epilepsia* 11:102-113, 1970

43. Commission on Classification and Terminology of the International League against Epilepsy: Proposal for revised clinical and electroencephalographic classification of epileptic seizures. *Epilepsia* 22:489-501, 1981

44. Annegers JF, Hauser WF, Elveback LR: Remission of seizures and relapse in patients with epilepsy. *Epilepsia* 20:729-737, 1979

45. Ohtahara S, Yamatogi Y, Ohtsuka Y, et al: Prognosis in childhood epilepsy: a prospective follow-up study. *Folia Psychiatr Neurol Jpn* 31:301-313, 1977

46. Lindsay J, Ounsted C, Richards P: Long-term outcome in children with temporal lobe seizures. I. Social outcome and childhood factors. *Dev Med Child Neurol* 21:285-298, 1979

47. Ounsted C, Lindsay J, Norman RM: Biological factors in temporal lobe epilepsy. In *Clinics in Developmental Medicine,* no 22, Philadelphia, Lippincott, 1966

48. Rodin EA: Medical and social prognosis in epilepsy. *Epilepsia* 13:121-131, 1972

49. Hauser WA, Anderson E, Loewenson R, et al: Seizure recurrence following a first unprovoked seizure. *N Engl J Med.* In press, 1982

50. Nelson KB, Ellenberg JH: Predictors of epilepsy in children who have experienced febrile seizures. *N Engl J Med* 295:1029-1033, 1976

51. Nelson KB, Ellenberg JH: Prognosis in children with febrile seizures. *Pediatrics* 61:720-727, 1978

52. Ellenberg JH, Nelson KB: Febrile seizures and later intellectual performance. *Arch Neurol* 35:17-21, 1978

53. Ellenberg JH, Nelson KB: Sample selection and the natural history of disease. Studies of febrile seizures. *JAMA* 243:1337-1340, 1980

54. Annegers JF, Hauser WA, Elveback LR, et al: The risk of epilepsy following febrile convulsions. *Neurology* 29:297-303, 1979

55. Consensus Statement on Febrile Seizures: Long-term management of children with fever-associated seizures. *Pediatrics* 66:1009-1012, 1980

56. Faero O, Kastrup K, Nielsen E, et al: Successful prophylaxis of febrile convulsions with phenobarbital. *Epilepsia* 13:279-285, 1972

57. Wolf SM: The effectiveness of phenobarbital in the prevention of recurrent febrile convulsions in children with and without a history of pre-, peri- and post-natal abnormalities. *Acta Paediatr Scand* 66:585-587, 1977

58. Wolf S, Carr A, Davis DC, et al: The value of phenobarbital in the child who has had a single febrile seizure: a controlled prospective study. *Pediatrics* 59:378-385, 1977

59. Knudsen FU: Plasma diazepam in infants after rectal administration in solution and by suppository. *Acta Paediatr Scand* 66:563-567, 1977

60. Knudsen FU, Vestermark S: Prophylactic diazepam or phenobarbitone in febrile convulsions: a prospective controlled study. *Arch Dis Child* 53:660-663, 1978

61. Melchior J, Buchthal F, Lennox-Buchthal M: The ineffectiveness of diphenylhydantoin in preventing febrile convulsions in the age of greatest risk, under three years. *Epilepsia* 12:55-62, 1971

62. Emerson RG, D'Souza BJ, Vining EP, et al: Stopping medication in children with epilepsy. *N Engl J Med* 304:1125-1129, 1981

63. Pedley TA: Interictal epileptiform discharges: discriminating characteristics and clinical correlations. *Am J EEG Technol* 20:101-119, 1980

64. Camfield CS, Chaplin S, Doyle AB: Side effects of phenobarbital in toddlers: behavioral and cognitive effects. *J Pediatr* 95:361-365, 1979

65. MacLeod CM, Debaban AS, Hunt E: Memory impairment in epileptic patients: selective effects of phenobarbital concentration. *Science* 202:1102-1104, 1978

66. Stores G, Hart J: Reading skills of children with generalized or focal epilepsy attending ordinary school. *Dev Med Child Neurol* 18:705-716, 1976

67. Lacy JR, Penry JK: *Infantile spasms.* New York, Raven Press, 1976

68. Kurokawa T, Goya N, Fukuyama Y, et al: West syndrome and Lennox-Gastaut syndrome: a survey of natural history. *Pediatrics* 65:81-88, 1980

69. Matsumoto A, Watanabe K, Negoro T, et al: Long-term prognosis after infantile spasms: a statistical study of prognostic factors in 200 cases. *Dev Med Child Neurol* 23:51-55, 1981

70. Simon D, Penry JK: Sodium di-*N*-dipropylacetic acid (DPA) in the treatment of epilepsy. *Epilepsia* 16:549-573, 1975

71. Hrachovy RA, Frost JD, Kellaway P, et al: A controlled study of ACTH therapy in infantile spasms. *Epilepsia* 21:631-635, 1980

72. Hrachovy RA, Frost JD Jr, Kellaway P, et al: A controlled study of prednisone therapy in infantile spasms. *Epilepsia* 20:403-407, 1979

73. Singer WD, Rabe EF, Haller JS: The effect of ACTH therapy upon infantile spasms. *J Pediatr* 96:485-489, 1980

74. Riikonen R, Donner M: ACTH therapy in infantile spasms: side effects. *Arch Dis Child* 55:664-672, 1980

75. Rapport RL II, Penry JK: A survey of attitudes toward the pharmacological prophylaxis of post-traumatic epilepsy. *J Neurosurg* 38:159-166, 1973

76. Penry JK, White BG, Brackett CE: A controlled prospective study of the pharmacologic prophylaxis of post-traumatic epilepsy (abstract). *Neurology* 29:600, 1979

77. Young B, Rapp R, Brooks WH, et al: Post-traumatic epilepsy prophylaxis. *Epilepsia* 20:671-681, 1979

78. Annegers JF, Grabow JD, Groover RV, et al: Seizures after head trauma: a population study. *Neurology* 30:683-689, 1980

79. Jennett B: Post-traumatic epilepsy. In *Advances in Neurology*, vol 22. *Complications of Nervous System Trauma*. Edited by Thompson RA, Green JR. New York, Raven Press, 1979, pp 137-147

80. Jennett B, Teasdale G: *Management of Head Injuries*. Philadelphia, FA Davis, 1981, pp 281-288

81. Annegers JF, Elveback LR, Hauser WA, et al: Do anticonvulsants have a teratogenic effect? *Arch Neurol* 31:364-373, 1974

82. Annegers JF, Hauser WA, Elveback LR, et al: Congenital malformations and seizure disorders in the offspring of parents with epilepsy. *Int J Epidemiol* 7:241-247, 1978

83. Bodendorfer TW: Fetal effects of anticonvulsant drugs and seizures disorders. *Drug Intell Clin Pharm* 12:14-21, 1978

84. Hill, RM, Vermiand WM, Horning MG, et al: Infants exposed in utero to antiepileptic drugs. *Am J Dis Child* 127:645-653, 1974

85. Janz D: The teratogenic risk of antiepileptic drugs. *Epilepsia* 16:159-169, 1975

86. Starreveld-Zimmerman AAE, van der Kolk WJ, Elshove J, et al: Teratogenicity of antiepileptic drugs. *Clin Neurol Neurosurg* 77:81-95, 1975

87. Shapiro S, Slone D, Hartz SC, et al: Anticonvulsants and parental epilepsy in the development of birth defects. *Lancet* 1:272-275, 1976

88. Friis ML, Broeng-Nielsen B, Sindrup EH, et al: Facial clefts among epileptic patients. *Arch Neurol* 38:227-229, 1981

89. Lowe CR: Congenital malformations among infants born to epileptic women. *Lancet* 1:9-10, 1973

90. Finnel RH: Phenytoin-induced teratogenesis: a mouse model. *Science* 211:483-484, 1981

91. Paulson RB, Paulson GW, Jreissaty S: Phenytoin and carbamazepine in production of cleft palates in mice. *Arch Neurol* 36:832-836, 1979

92. Bergey GK, Swaiman KF, Schrier BK, et al: Adverse effects of phenobarbital on morphological and biochemical development of fetal mouse spinal cord neurons in culture. *Ann Neurol* 9:584-589, 1981

93. Nakane Y, Okuma T, Takahashi R, et al: Multi-institutional study on the teratogenicity and fetal toxicity of antiepileptic drugs: a report of a collaborative study group in Japan. *Epilepsia* 21:663-680, 1980

94. Feldman GL, Weaver DD, Lovrien E: The fetal trimethadione syndrome. Report of a family and further delineation of this syndrome. *Am J Dis Child* 131:1389-1392, 1977

95. Hanson JW, Smith DW: The fetal hydantoin syndrome. *J Pediatr* 87:285-290, 1975

96. *Birth Defects Compendium*, 2nd ed. Edited by Bergsma D. New York, National Foundation March of Dimes, 1979

97. Zackai EH, Mellman WJ, Neiderer B, et al: The fetal trimethadione syndrome. *J Pediatr* 87:280-284, 1975

98. So EL, Perry JK: Epilepsy in adults. *Ann Neurol* 9:3-16, 1981.

99. Spencer SS: Depth electroencephalography in selection of refractory epilepsy for surgery. *Ann Neurol* 9:207-214, 1981

100. Goldensohn ES, Zablow L, Salazar A: The penicillin focus. I. Distribution of potential at the cortical surface. *Electroencephalogr Clin Neurophysiol* 42:480-492, 1977

101. Lueders H, Bustamante LA, Zablow L, et al: The independence of closely spaced discrete experimental spike foci. *Neurology* 31:846-851, 1981

102. Engel J Jr, Rausch R, Lieb JP, et al: Correlation of criteria used for localizing epileptic foci in patients considered for surgical therapy of epilepsy. *Ann Neurol* 9:215-224, 1981

103. Phelps ME, Mazziotta JC, Kuhl DE, et al: Tomographic mapping of human cerebral metabolism: visual stimulation and deprivation. *Neurology* 31:517-529, 1981

104. Bogdanoff BM, Stafford CR, Green L, et al: Computerized transaxial tomography in the evaluation of patients with focal epilepsy. *Neurology* 25:1013-1017, 1975

105. Gastaut H, Gastaut JL: Computerized axial tomography in epilepsy. In *Epilepsy, The Eighth International Symposium*. Edited by Penry, JK. New York, Raven Press, 1977, pp 5-15

11
NEUROLOGICAL DISORDERS OF THE NEONATE

Janette Goddard, Daniel G. Glaze, and Marvin A. Fishman

This chapter will review the two most common neurological disorders affecting premature and full-term neonates: intraventricular hemorrhage (IVH) and seizures. Although recent developments have been stressed, where appropriate, sufficient background material and references to earlier studies have been provided to give the reader more thorough information. In addition to the relevant clinical advances, experimental research leading to better understanding of the problems has been reviewed. This is particularly pertinent in relation to the pathogenesis of IVH in prematures. Multiple clinical and biochemical disturbances occur simultaneously in the premature infant. Only in the experimental model can these factors be studied individually or in various combinations in an effort to determine which are relevant and contribute to the production of hemorrhages. The adverse effects of seizures on the morphological and biochemical development of the immature and developing brain can be studied only in the experimental model, so this material has also been, reviewed. In addition, recent investigations have raised questions regarding the effects of antiepileptic drugs on the developing nervous system. Therefore, these studies have been briefly reviewed to provide the reader with an appropriate balance of information regarding experimental epilepsy. However, the clinical relevance of the effects of seizures and their treatment in the experimental model to human disease remains to be determined.

AN UPDATE OF NEONATAL IVH

Incidence and Associated Clinical Factors

Neonatal IVH and its sequelae are problems predominantly of the premature infant but have also now been recognized in the term neonate (1-5). Fedrick and Butler in 1970 documented the occurrence of IVH at 1.1 per 1000 live births, but they found an incidence of 176 per 1000 in babies of less than 28 weeks gestation (6). The incidence has varied from 10% to 40% in neonates studied at autopsy (7-9). Recent prospective studies utilizing computerized tomographic scanning (CT) or ultrasound examination to detect hemorrhages during life show incidences of 43% to 90% in premature infants during the first hours to days after birth (10-12). These studies have been done in infants of less than 1500 g birth weight or less than 34-35 weeks of gestation.

Of interest, however, both in autopsy studies and from reports of clinical evaluations, are the number of infants at term found to have IVH (1-5). Donat and coworkers (1), in a series of babies autopsied in the first 2 months after birth, identified the choroid plexus as the source of IVH in 100% of the full-term infants as opposed to premature infants in whom germinal layer hemorrhage was the probable source of the IVH in 87% of the cases. This study suggests that the origin of hemorrhage differs in the term baby compared to the premature.

In a recent survey by Armstrong and co-workers (13), the choroid plexus and the germinal matrix layer (GML) were sources of hemorrhage in both premature and term infants, although there was a trend toward more choroid plexus hemorrhages in older gestational-aged infants. Of interest also in the studies of Armstrong was the correlation of intraparenchymal hemorrhages predominantly with white matter infarction; in fact, direct primary extension of blood from the ventricles into surrounding white matter was not seen in the 43 cases of IVH.

IVH has been associated clinically with prematurity, the presence of respiratory distress syndrome, and factors such as hypoxemia, hypercarbia, mechanical ventilation, high peak inflation pressures, and pneumothorax (13). Other related factors have included patent ductus arteriosus, sodium bicarbonate administration, early volume expansion, hypotension, and intrauterine growth retardation (13).

The possible role of therapeutic interventions in the pathogenesis of hemorrhage has been raised (14-17). Although the role of sodium and sodium bicarbonate administration has been controversial (15-17), in the prospective study of Dykes and coworkers (14) early sodium bicarbonate administration, sodium administration in doses greater than 8 mEq/kg/day, acidosis, and birth weight less than 1200 g were associated with IVH. Guggenheim and coworkers (18) found that infants of gestational age less than 31 weeks had a hemorrhage occurrence rate of 67% and that male gender, assisted ventilation during the first day of life, and blood transfusion during the first day were significant risk factors for germinal matrix hemorrhage.

Clark and coworkers (19) stated that outborn birth is the most significant factor related to IVH (19). They also recognized that outborn babies received more sodium bicarbonate and more intravenous fluid therapy and sustained prolonged hyperoxemia more frequently. Vaginal breech delivery has been correlated with IVH by DeLemos and coworkers (20).

These factors may vary for a given institution and population. What seems clear is that the insults in the perinatal period may be multiple, and that therapies must be instituted with iatrogenic consequences as well as benefits in mind.

Why has the discussion of IVH reached such a peak? Neonatologists, neurologists, and pediatricians are now faced with a growing population of survivors of IVH. While those with isolated subependymal hemorrhages, without other lesions such as periventricular leukomalacia, may do quite well, IVH and its associated lesions are responsible for handicapping many infants (21). In most follow-up studies to date, the mortality from IVH and associated lesions has been as high as 50%, and the incidence of handicapping lesions in the survivors has been as high as 60% (21-23). These infants often exhibit motor deficits, visual deficits, learning disabilities, mental retardation, seizures, and most commonly, posthemorrhagic hydrocephalus (21).

Experimental Models: Concepts of Etiopathogenesis

A search for pathogenetic mechanisms to account for these hemorrhages began long ago in autopsy studies of stillborn and perinatally deceased infants (8). Recently, the histopathology of this lesion has been correlated with physiological studies in animal models (24, 25). Experimental models have aided our concepts of the etiopathogeneses of IVH and may aid in the testing of pharmacological agents, which may prove to be useful for intervention in these babies.

Two animals, the fetal lamb and the newborn beagle puppy, have shown isolated germinal matrix, tela choroidea, choroid plexus, and IVH similar to those found in humans under experimental conditions. (24-26). Both of these animals have substantial germinal matrices. That of the newborn term puppy resembles the immature human GML of approximately 30-32 weeks gestation. It is very vascular and most prominent in the first 72 hours of life before dissipating by 7 days of age in most cases (25). During the first 3 days of life, hemorrhages have been produced in this model. The hemorrhages are similar in site of origin and extent to those found macroscopically and microscopically in human brains at autopsy (25, 26).

The physiological changes associated with hemorrhages in the fetal sheep have included increases in arterial or venous pressures together with asphyxia and large increases in arterial pressure without asphyxia (24). In the newborn beagle pup, hemorrhages have occurred after the animals have been rendered hypercarbic along with a modest elevation in systemic blood pressure, after blood pressure has been increased rapidly by a mean of 30 mm Hg with phenylephrine HCl, and after volume reperfusion following acute (5 minutes duration) hemorrhagic hypotension, which reduces systemic arterial pressure to one-half control values (25-27). During the reperfusion of blood volume in the last series of experiments, blood pressure increased significantly over initial normovolemic values. Hemorrhages have occurred in up to 75% of these animals after phenylephrine-induced hypertension and after volume reperfusion. In saline perfused animals (15% of blood volume) jugular venous pressures have increased significantly, and two-thirds of the animals have shown microscopic subependymal hemorrhages without IVH. Pups rendered hypotensive for only 5 minutes and sacrificed immediately have not had any significant hemorrhages (27). The effects of longer periods of hypotension on the production of hemorrhages have not yet been studied. Therefore, hypotension has not been excluded as being important in the pathogenesis of bleeding.

Cerebral blood flow (CBF) studies indicate that blood flow to the brain, especially the brain stem, thalamus, and basal ganglia, is maintained during the acute hemorrhagic hypotension and, in fact, may exceed the normovolemic, normotensive flows of these regions. After 10-20 minutes of hypotension, blood flows to cortical structures fall, and brain-stem flow is maintained longest. Flows to all regions of the brain are increased during reperfusion of volume and during phenyl-

ephrine-induced hypertension. These flows, which have been quantitated by the radioactive microsphere method, may be greater than 300% of initial flow values in the steady state (28-30). These findings suggest that the brain is protected under conditions in which the immature animal has undergone peripheral vasoconstriction. However, rapid pharmacologically induced central increases in flow with peripheral vasoconstriction, and volume expansion in a vascular bed already dilated, combined with immature vessels in a poor supporting matrix, may cause hemorrhage. Hemorrhage and its associated lesions, such as ischemic infarction, may then be worsened by factors such as the poor clotting ability of the newborn or the release of endogenous substances such as thromboxanes and prostaglandins, which, in addition to other agents, have been thought to play a role in posthemorrhagic vasospastic states.

Earlier studies of autopsy specimens had implicated elevated venous pressures, possibly secondary to venous thromboses and associated infarctions as prominent in the pathogenesis of these lesions (31, 32). Cole and coworkers (33) felt that venous stasis would lead to transudation and hemorrhage and could be accounted for in premature infants by congestive heart failure and hypoxia. Hambleton and Wigglesworth (34) were the first to suggest that the capillary bed of the germinal matrix was the predominant source of these hemorrhages in the preterm infant. Although Goddard and coworkers have shown that increased arterial and venous pressures and CBF may play important roles in the genesis of hemorrhages, they have not proved that the capillary-venule junction is the source of the hemorrhage. Asphyxia, acidosis or other insults may set off a chain of reactions which lead to altered cerebrovascular hemodynamics that contribute to the production of hemorrhages.

Indeed, most premature infants are asphyxiated at birth and after birth. If, as Dawes, Modanlou and others (35, 36) have observed, the very first response to asphyxia is an elevation of blood pressure, and if, as Lou (37) speculates from his CBF studies in fetal sheep and in neonates, blood flow is relatively pressure passive (especially after asphyxia) in the newborn brain, then these factors may precipitate hemorrhage directly through increased pressure and flow in a poorly supported GML vessel bed. If a premature infant is in shock from hemorrhage and is quickly infused with blood, albumin, or saline, then these same vascular beds may be overwhelmed and overdistended by volume in the face of systemic but not cerebral vasoconstriction.

Attempts to eliminate IVH by prevention of rapid elevations in blood pressures may lead to decreased cerebral perfusion in the vascular border zones and centrum semiovale if the systemic hypotension is sustained. The resulting periventricular leukomalacia in these infants may cause motor deficits. Blood flow may be severely compromised by modest increases in intracranial pressure (ICP) secondary to hemorrhage or ischemic infarction, especially if blood flow is already at a borderline level [i.e., 20-30 ml/min/100 g] (29, 38). Although infants with open sutures only rarely herniate, increases in IPC of only a few mm Hg may severely compromise brain perfusion. All of these factors make resuscitation and handling of the newborn premature very delicate matters; approaches must include continuous monitoring of arterial pressures, P_{O_2}, P_{CO_2}, and intracranial pressures in noninvasive ways. Thus, the appropriate clinical management of these problems is very complicated and requires careful balancing of many factors.

New Methods of Clinical Evaluation and Timing of Hemorrhages

The CT scan has been most useful in the prospective and clinical evaluations of IVH in the newborn population at risk. The studies of Papile and Burstein not only showed the incidence of IVH in infants of birth weights lower than 1500 g to be 43% but also showed that asymptomatic infants could have significant hemorrhages (10, 40). These asymptomatic infants may be at risk for the development of sequelae, especially for posthemorrhagic hydrocephalus. Thus, routine scanning of infants at risk may be of great value.

The transport and care of ill premature newborn infants are not simple tasks. These infants easily become hypothermic, lose intravenous feeding lines in transit, may have apneic attacks, and often are being maintained on ventilators. The use of ultrasound scanning at the bedside has thus begun to replace the CT examination because it obviates the difficulties of transporting patients. Also, although ultrasound may have side effects not yet determined, it does not subject the immature infant and his brain to ionizing radiation (41). Bejar and coworkers (12), utilizing this technique, have reported an incidence of IVH or periventricular hemorrhage in 90% of infants less than 34 weeks gestation who were examined in the first day of postnatal life, often within the first few hours after birth. This early and almost universal onset of IVH has not been confirmed in other studies. Armstrong and coworkers (13) found that 25% of the infants in their autopsy series dying before 24 hours of age had IVH. Bejar and coworkers (12) also noted rapid changes in ventricular size after the hemorrhages or after ventriculo-peritoneal shunting or repeated lumbar punctures for hydrocephalus. In these authors' experience, at least one IVH (hematocrit 0.5%) was echodense by real time ultrasound and isodense with brain by CT scan. Thus, ultrasound is sensitive to small amounts of blood. Silverboard and coworkers (41) showed a correlation of 77% between ultrasound and CT scan. Some of the hemorrhages, which could not be detected on ultrasound and were proven by CT scan, became evident on subsequent ultrasound scans 2-3 days later. Thus, they point out that while clots may be more striking on ultrasound scan, fresh blood may appear sonolucent (41).

Several techniques have been utilized to assess CBF including transfontanelle Doppler ultrasound, which estimates blood flow in the anterior cerebral arteries. Bada and coworkers (42) have used this extensively and have calculated an anterior cerebral artery pulsatility index. This index varies inversely with flow and directly with vascular resistance in these vessels, that is, vasodilatation (decreased vascular resistance) is correlated with increased blood flow and a lower pulsatility index. Bada and coworkers (42) have shown that pulsatility indices are low prior to onset of symptoms of IVH; following IVH, the pulsatility index increases.

Another method which measures an apparent total CBF is venous occlusion plethysmography (43). The expansion of the compliant skull is measured by a strain gauge during bilateral jugular occlusions for several seconds. This change in skull diameter with arterial pulsations against a temporarily occluded venous outflow can be translated into flow (43). Studies by Milligan using this method have indicated a pressure-passive response of the cerebrovasculature to pressure changes induced by blood transfusion or exchange blood transfusion (44). Of the infants studied, 80% suffered fatal IVH within 12 hours of observed increases in blood flow (44). This may be a useful technique in predicting IVH, but there may be hazard to bilateral jugular occlusion in these infants, even if the procedure is carried out for only a few seconds.

No other currently available methods for blood flow measurement in infants are noninvasive and nonradioactive. The 133 Xenon inhalation technique has been used to measure hemispheric blood flows in newborn infants (45, 46). However, in addition to the complication of total-body-radiation absorption and significant extra cranial contamination, this procedure is expensive and requires a team with much expertise. Inevitably, the least expensive, safest, and most portable method will help the neonatologist, the neurologist, and the pediatrician to evaluate these infants.

Pharmacological Intervention: One Study*

IVH has been shown to occur with symptoms most frequently on the second day of life, and as the latest ultrasound studies indicate, these hemorrhages may be present in asymptomatic babies as early as 1 hour after birth (11). The birth process, the transition period, shock and asphyxial insults, and resuscitation and

evolution of RDS may all contribute to IVH (20). Can anything be done to prevent these hemorrhages, and, if so, when should prophylaxis be instituted? Donn and coworkers (47) have embarked upon a randomized controlled study of the effects of phenobarbital in preventing IVH. To date, 60 infants ($<$ 1500 g and $<$ 6 hours of age) have been enrolled in the study—30 have been in the treatment group, given phenobarbital intravenously, 10 mg/kg, upon admission and 12 hours later, followed by 2.5 mg/kg every 12 hours for 7 days. Thirty have been in the control group. Out of the treatment group, 4 have had IVH (13.3%), while 14 of the control group have had hemorrhages (46.7%). No differences were found between the groups when compared for birth weights, gestational ages, Apgar scores, or other risk factors. The difference in the incidences of hemorrhages in these two groups is significant to $P < 0.01$ (47). Phenobarbital in similar dosages has been used in neonates with seizures and appears to be safe. Data regarding the effect of the drug on blood flow and metabolism in many regions of the premature brain may be helpful in determining the mechanisms by which it seems to prevent IVH. Further studies confirming this original report should be completed before recommending phenobarbital as routine therapy. The thought of possible prophylactic pharmacological intervention is exciting, since the basic problem—the elimination of prematurity—is not likely to soon be solved.

Difficulties: Prevention and Alleviation of Posthemorrhagic Hydrocephalus

Posthemorrhagic hydrocephalus is the most common immediate sequela of IVH (10, 40, 48-50). Progressive ventricular enlargement may be apparent on CT scans or ultrasound scans weeks before an appreciable increase in head circumference (50). Attempts to prevent the development of hydrocephalus have been undertaken. Serial lumbar punctures beginning at the time of diagnosis of IVH have been performed by Mantovani and coworkers (48).

---

*Since the preparation of this chapter Hope and coworkers have published a letter to the editor in *Lancet* reporting their failure to demonstrate a reduction in the incidence of germinal layer or intraventricular hemorrhage after treatment of babies with phenobarbital at the doses suggested by Donn et al. *Lancet* (Feb. 20, 1982) pp. 442-445.

The expectation has been that a decrease in blood and protein in the basilar cisterns would hasten recovery and help re-establish normal cerebrospinal fluid (CSF) flow (48). This has not been proved to be efficacious. A different approach, that of alleviating increased intracranial pressure and reducing ventricular size by serial lumbar punctures after the presence of ventricular dilatation has already been established, has been tried by Papile and coworkers (49). The main goal has been to reduce ventricular size and to obviate the need for ventriculoperitoneal shunting, which has major complications when performed in small infants. They reported success in alleviating ventricular enlargement in 11 out of 12 cases (49).

Others have used osmotic agents—especially glycerol—to reduce hydrocephalus. Taylor and coworkers (51) report that glycerol has been of benefit to infants with slowly progressive hydrocephalus that persists beyond the first month of life.

Conclusion

This update and summary of some of the current laboratory research, clinical investigations, and treatment of IVH reflect a surge of interest in this condition, which, with its associated lesions, is the major cause of neurological morbidity and mortality in babies in newborn intensive care units. Understanding of its etiologies and pathogeneses will lead not only to possible therapeutic interventions but also to a better understanding of the immature cerebrovascular system—its structure, regulation, and responses to physiological changes.

NEONATAL SEIZURES

Introduction

Neonatal seizures are the most distinctive signs of many neurological diseases affecting the neonate (52). The underlying disease processes responsible for the seizures may produce irreversible damage to the nervous system and cause significant morbidity and mortality if not promptly recognized and treated. Neonatal seizures which persist may interfere with cardiopulmonary function and produce metabolic injury to the brain (52-57).

Seizures in the newborn period differ from seizures in later childhood in their characteristics, causes, management, and prognoses. These differences have been explained on the basis of the morphological and physiological organization of the immature cortex of the neonate (52, 54-58). The full complement of neurons have not completed cytoplasmic and membranous differentiation. The completion of these processes and the proper orientation, alignment, and layering of the cortical neurons are necessary for the cortical organization to propagate and sustain generalized seizures. Lacking this degree of cortical organization, neonates tend to have fragmentary and focal appearing seizures. The difficulty of focal discharges in exciting adjacent areas of the brain and thus the rarity of generalized seizures in neonates may be further explained by observations of Purpura and coworkers (58-60). In newborn kittens, evoked potentials from neocortex have predominant inhibitory activities, and there is a delay in the maturation of excitatory synaptic activities. In contrast, the hippocampus and other limbic structures have been observed to have advanced maturational features with excitatory characteristics (60). This and the connection of these structures to diencephalon and brain stem may underlie such frequent manifestations of neonatal seizures as oral-buccal, sucking, chewing, blinking, and pedaling movements, as well as respiratory changes and apnea. These aspects of neurophysiological development and neuroanatomical development complement each other in inhibiting the propagation of synchronous, generalized cortical seizures in newborn infants and in producing the unusual manifestations of neonatal seizures.

Clinical Aspects

Retrospective and prospective studies, including the recent report of the National Institutes of Health (NIH) Collaborative Perinatal Project of neonatal seizures have been reviewed, and their data form the basis of several tables included in this discussion

(61-83). Similar to Volpe's earlier review, these tables have been organized into two groups, pre-1970 and post-1970 studies and the Collaborative Study. Table 1 summarizes the incidence of neonatal seizures, which varies from 0.2% to 1.4%. This variation most likely reflects patient selection, inclusion or omission of preterm infants, and the prevalence of different etiologies. In three recent studies, the incidence ranged from 0.15% to 0.5% (81-83). The low incidence of 0.15% in a Swedish study during 1970-1976 contrasts with an earlier report which found an incidence of 0.37% for years 1960-1962 (82). In part, this decrease may be attributed to better perinatal care but also may reflect a lower incidence of primary hypocalcemia which followed the introduction of improved modified cow's milk formula. The most recent United States' study also reports a lower incidence than in the past but does not provide a breakdown by etiological factors (83). Similarly, the lower incidence, 0.42% reported by the recent Oxford study, is likely due to a combination of a lower incidence of primary hypocalcemia (14% of all neonatal seizures in this study versus 53% in an earlier English study) and variation in maternal health status (81).

Table 1. Incidence of Neonatal Seizures

Study	*Incidence*
Burke, 1954 (61)	0.2%
Craig, 1960 (62)	0.8%
Carbonell, et al., 1969 (70)	1.4%
Keen, 1969 (72)	0.86%
Hopkins, 1972 (74)	0.38%
Brown, et al. 1972 (75)	1.4%
Keen and Lee, 1973 (76)	1.22%
Knauss and Marshall, 1977 [intensive care unit (ICU) study] (79)	0.74%
Dennis, 1978 (81)	0.42%
Eriksson and Zetterstrom, 1979 (82)	0.15%
Holden, et al., 1980 [NIH Collaborative Perinatal Project] (83)	0.50%

In the past, seizures were observed less frequently in premature infants than in full-term infants. Monod and associates rarely recorded electrographic seizures in infants of less than 32 weeks conceptional age (84). In their series infants under 36 weeks conceptional age accounted for only 10% of recorded seizures. However, recent studies have reported a significant incidence of seizures in premature infants (79, 85). The neonatal seizure population of the Collaborative Study was characterized by an excess of infants less than 2500 g as compared to the whole Collaborative Study population (83). Two other recent studies each reported that 20% of the neonatal seizures occurred in premature infants (81, 82). Thus, the incidence of seizures in prematures is less than full-term infants but may be increasing because of increased survival of premature infants and heightened awareness and improved recognition of seizures in premature infants.

The characteristics of seizures in neonates differ considerably from those of older children. The recognition of a neonatal seizure may be difficult. True tonic-clonic seizures are rare, and neonatal seizures tend to be focal, migratory, or fragmentary, often quite anarchic, polymorphic, and poorly organized. Premature infants have even less organized seizures. Five broad categories of clinical seizures have been described by Volpe. (1) Subtle seizures may consist of any one or combination of jerking horizontal deviation of eyes, repetitive blinking or fluttering of the eyelids, drooling, sucking, tonic posturing of the extremities, short apneic spells, or changes in the respiratory pattern. They are often associated with perinatal hypoxia, neonatal meningitis, and other severe central nervous system (CNS) insults and may be seen in term and preterm infants. This was the most common seizure type observed. (2) Multifocal clonic seizures consist of clonic movements of one or more extremities that rapidly migrate to another part of the body in a nonordered fashion at irregular intervals. These seizures are particularly characteristic of the full-term infant, and in one series 75% of infants with these seizures weighed over 2500 g. This seizure pattern is often associated with metabolic aberrations such as hypocalcemia or hypoglycemia (86). (3) Focal clonic seizures are relatively uncommon and characterized by well localized clonic jerking. These may be seen following focal trauma, cerebral contusion, and often in conjunction with other seizure phenomena. (4) Tonic seizures when generalized appear like decerebrate posturing with body stiffening and arching, and may be accompanied by respiratory pattern changes or eye signs. Volpe observed that these seizures are characteristic of the premature infant and that 70% of infants with tonic seizures weighed less than 2500 g (1). In another series, tonic seizures were equally prevalent among infants of all birth weights (79). (5) Myoclonic seizures consist of rapid synchronous single or multiple flexion jerks of extremities. In all series, myoclonic seizures were infrequently observed.

The variability of neonatal seizures is reflected in electrographic patterns as well as clinical manifestations. Electrographic seizures in neonates are often characterized by the buildup and abrupt termination of sharp transients, spikes, rhythmic 6-10 hertz (Hz) activity, or a succession of different patterns including rhythmic 6-10 Hz activity, spikes, slow waves, and polymorphic bursts (85). The interictal record may show a normal background, disrupted sleep cycling, focal or multifocal spikes, heterochronism, or focal or generalized depression (85). Two studies have reported similar electrographic correlations with the various types of seizures (87, 88). Subtle seizures were associated with rhythmic delta and alpha patterns and accompanied by occasional spikes or sharp waves and burst-suppression patterns. Multifocal and focal clonic seizures were accompanied by repeated spikes or sharp waves and often had a rolandic location. During tonic seizures, rhythmic delta waves were most frequently seen, but rhythmic alpha waves and repeated sharp and slow waves were also observed. Clinical myoclonic seizures were associated with suppression-burst patterns or no paroxysmal discharges. The most frequent

initial sites of paroxysmal discharges were the central or occipital areas. Utilizing polygraphic recordings, Wantanabe and co-workers (88) observed that neonatal seizures most often occurred in active sleep when the state could be determined and that the sleep cycle was usually altered in cases in which seizures occurred mainly in quiet sleep. In half the infants, seizures had no preference for any particular sleep state. In newborn infants, the relation between clinical seizures and the behavioral state is different than in older children in whom seizures usually occur in nonrapid eye movement sleep. This difference may be related to the immaturity of the CNS of these infants (88). Heart rate has been noted to be increased in multifocal clonic, tonic, or apneic seizures, though tonic and apneic seizures have also been associated with bradycardia. No change in heart rate was associated with focal clonic, myclonic, or subtle seizures without apnea. Respiratory rate was often observed to be irregular with multifocal seizures and little affected with focal clonic or myoclonic seizures. Tonic seizures were usually accompanied by apnea or dyspnea (88).

There are many causes of neonatal seizures, but relatively few etiologies account for the majority of these seizures. Perinatal asphyxia, birth injury, hypocalcemia, and hypoglycemia account for 90% of these seizures with identifiable etiologies (55). Specific etiologies may be defined in as many as 75% of all neonatal seizures (64). Table 2 provides an extensive list of the various etiologies of neonatal seizures and Table 3 the frequencies of various etiologies. There have been several comprehensive reviews of these etiologies and only some brief comments will be made here (52-57).

The category of fundamental perinatal problems includes those cases of hypoxic-ischemic encephalopathy. This is a frequent cause of seizures in full-term and premature infants and is usually related to intrauterine hypoxia (52, 55). Volpe reported 60%-65% of patients had this as the cause of their seizures (52). In other recent series, Dennis reported a 44% incidence and Eriksson and Zetterstrom a 48% incidence (81, 82). In all series, seizures secondary to hypoxia most frequently

Table 2. Etiologies of Neonatal Seizures (52, 54, 55, 81)

I. The Fetus with a Problem

    A. Major cerebral or noncerebral structural anomalies
        1. Cerebral cortical dysgeneses
            a) Lissencephaly
            b) Pachygyria
            c) Polymicrogyria
        2. Systemic congenital anomalies
            a) Congenital heart disease
            b) Trisomies
    B. Neurodermatoses
        1. Incontinentia pigmenti
        2. Neurofibromatosis
        3. Sturge-Weber disease
        4. Tuberous sclerosis

II. Fundamental Perinatal Factors

    A. Perinatal asphyxia
    B. Perinatal trauma
        1. Subarachnoid hemorrhage
        2. Subdural hemorrhage
    C. Intraventricular hemorrhage
    D. Hyperviscosity
        1. Intrauterine asphyxia
        2. Placental hypertransfusion

III. Metabolic Factors

    A. Hypocalcemia
        1. Early (secondary)
            a) Perinatal asphyxia trauma (hemorrhage)
            b) Small-for-gestational age
            c) Infant of diabetic mother
            d) Postexchange transfusion
            e) DiGeorge syndrome
            f) Septicemia
            g) Maternal hyper- or hypoparathyroidism
        2. Late (primary)
            a) Diet—low calcium/phosphorous ratio
        3. Hypomagnesemia
            a) Associated with hypocalcemia
            b) Magnesium malabsorption syndrome
    B. Hypoglycemia
        1. Transient
            a) Small-for-gestational age
            b) Prematurity
            c) Hyperinsulinemia, infant of diabetic mother
            d) Perinatal asphyxia or trauma (hemorrhage)
            e) Meningitis
            f) Postexchange transfusion
        2. Persistent
            a) Galactosemia
            b) Fructosemia
            c) Leucine sensitivity
            d) Glycogen storage disease (glucose-6-phosphatase deficiency)

            e) Beckwith syndrome
            f) Pancreatic islet cell tumor
            g) Anterior pituitary hypoplasia
    C. Hyponatremia and hypernatremia
            a) Inappropriate fluid therapy
            b) Sodium bicarbonate therapy in prematures
            c) Inappropriate antidiuretic hormone
    D. Inborn errors of metabolism
        1. Aminoaciduria
            a) Phenylketonuria
            b) Maple sugar urine disease
            c) Hyperglycinemia
            d) Congenital lysinuria
         2. Urea cycle defects
            a) Carbamyl phosphate synthetase deficiency
            b) Ornithine carbamyl transferase deficiency
            c) Citrullinemia
            d) Argininosuccinic aciduria
            e) Transient hyperammonemia of preterm and associated with perinatal asphyxia
        3. Organic acidurias
            a) Propionic acidemia
            b) Methylmalonic acidemia
            c) Methylmalonyl-CoA mutase deficiency
         4. Pyridoxine
            a) Deficiency
            b) Dependency (autosomal recessive)
    E. Toxins
        1. Endogenous
            a) Bilirubin encephalopathy
         2. Exogeneous
            a) Mercury
            b) Hexachlorophene
            c) Injected penicillin or anesthetics (for labor)
    F. Maternal drug dependency
        1. Narcotics
        2. Barbiturates (short- versus long-acting)

IV. Infection

    A. Septicemia
    B. Meningitis
        1. Group B *β-Streptococcus*
        2. *E. coli*
    C. Meningoencephalitis
        1. Toxoplasmosis
        2. Herpes simplex
        3. Coxsackie B
        4. Rubella
        5. Cytomegalovirus

V. Familial

    A. Benign familial neonatal seizures

VI. Unknown

Table 3. Incidence of Neonatal Seizures by Etiologies

| | *Etiology (%)* | | | | | |
Study	Perinatal	Metabolic	Infection	CNS* Anomoly	Unknown	Premature
Pre-1970 Total number of patients—1305 (61–69, 71, 72)	21[†]/17[‡]	13[§]/2[∥]	5	4	24	5
Post-1970 Total number of patients—641 (73–76, 79–82)	24[†]/14[‡]	11[§]/6[∥]	6	4	26	10

*Central nervous system.
†Hypoxia.
‡Hemorrhage.
§Hypocalcemia.
∥Hypoglycemia.

occurred within the first 24 hours of life, and Volpe found the onset was within 12 hours of birth in 60% of these neonates (52). Subtle seizures, multifocal clonic seizures in term infants, and tonic seizures in prematures are common in infants with hypoxic injuries. Also included in this category is intracranial hemorrhage of which the most frequent form is IVH, a lesion found most frequently in premature infants. The predominant seizure type is the generalized tonic variety, which most often is part of a catastrophic deterioration in these infants (52). This etiology accounted for 87% of seizures in 1 study exclusively reviewing infants weighing less than 2500 g and was associated with a 95% mortality (71).

Hypocalcemia (primary and secondary) and hypoglycemia are the most frequent metabolic abnormalities associated with neonatal seizures. Previous studies reported a high incidence of primary hypocalcemic seizures (72-76); however, more recent reviews found a much lower incidence of seizures secondary to primary hypocalcemia, possibly reflecting improved infant formulas, better quality of maternal health care, and sampling differences (52, 81, 82). Hypomag-

nesia may accompany hypocalcemia (75, 89). Administration of calcium may further lower magnesium and aggrevate seizures, while an infusion of magnesium may correct both problems (89, 90). Hypocalemia and hypoglycemia are frequently associated with perinatal asphyxia, hemorrhage, and infection and are not the primary aberrations responsible for the seizures following these insults. However, these metabolic disturbances may contribute to and sustain the seizure activity. Glucose and calcium may not immediately abort the seizure activity but may be helpful in preventing greater brain injury associated with prolonged seizures (52, 79).

Included in the metabolic category are seizures associated with drug withdrawal, a cause of increasing importance. Seizures are an infrequent manifestation of narcotic withdrawal. In two large series the incidence was 3% and 6% of passively addicted infants (91, 92). Seizures are more likely to occur in neonates passively addicted to short-acting barbiturates while jitteriness is associated with withdrawal from longer-acting barbiturates (52). Withdrawal signs and jitteriness may occur in the first 24 hours of life and precede seizures which begin on days 2-3 (93). In infants passively addicted to narcotics the mean time of seizure onset is 10 days, with seizures occurring as late as 34 days (92). Seizures were more frequent in infants exposed to methadone (7.8%) than to heroin [1.2%] (92). The mechanism of withdrawal seizures is unknown. The structural or biochemical immaturity of the neonatal brain and the narcotic-induced disturbances in the synthesis and utilization of neurotransmitters have been proposed as having a role in the pathogenesis of withdrawal seizures (92).

Benign familial neonatal convulsions have been reported in 11 families (73, 94-100). The inheritance pattern is autosomal dominant. Family members usually have frequent seizures beginning on the third to tenth day of life. All studies have indicated a favorable outcome, though as many as 50% of the affected family members in one series had recurrent seizures but otherwise no remarkable neurological deficits (94). The seizures have been observed to be focal or multifocal clonic in character, and the interictal electroencephalogram (EEG) appeared normal (94, 95, 97, 98).

The onset of neonatal seizures is influenced by the underlying etiology. In general, three peaks occur. (1) During the first 48 hours of life, seizures are most likely to be secondary to asphyxia, trauma, secondary hypocalcemia, or hypoglycemia. (2) On days 4-7, primary hypocalcemia seizures occur. (3) On days 7-10, seizures secondary to infection or congenital anomalies are more likely to occur. The initial seizure occurred during the first 24 hours of life in 37.9% of the neonates with seizures enrolled in the Collaborative Perinatal Project and by the end of the first week of life in 86.3% of the cases (83). These data and data from pre- and post-1970 studies concerning day of onset of seizures are summarized in Table 4.

Table 4. Day of Initial Seizure

	Day (%)				
Study	*1*	*2*	*3*	*4–7*	*7–28*
Pre-1970 Total number of patients—414 (61, 63, 64, 72)	43	25	11	12	8
Post-1970* Total number of patients—401 (73, 75, 76)	19	16.5	12	27	25.5
Total	31	21	12	20	16
Collaborative Project (83)	37.9	24.9	14.4	9	13.7

*Represents early 1970 studies with high incidence hypocalcemic seizures.

Prognosis

The prognosis in neonatal seizures is determined by the underlying disease causing the convulsions. Overall outcome and outcome by etiology are reviewed in Tables 5 and 6. In general, primary hypocalcemia has an excellent prognosis, 80%-100% of infants are normal at follow-up, while with secondary hypocalcemia or hypoglycemia this figure drops to 50%. Infants with infection of the CNS have a 20%-50% chance of being normal at follow-up, while infants with seizures following hypoxia have only a 10%-20% chance of normal developmental and neurological outcome (52). In all series, infants who have seizures associated with anomalies of the CNS are reported to have little chance of nor-nal outcome.

Neonatal seizures carry an increased statistical risk of residual brain damage (motor deficits, mental retardation, or recurrent seizures) whatever the cause (53, 83). In patients studied prior to 1970 (Table 5),

mortality was 40%, and only 40% of infants were normal at follow-up. In recent reports, mortality has declined, and morbidity has risen. Dennis noted a 22% mortality rate, and only 40% of the entire group was found to be normal at 2½ year follow-up (81). Eriksson and Zetterstrom reported a 13% mortality rate (82). At 1 year, 53% of the infants had no signs of sequelae. In both of these studies, the authors observed that the highest mortality and morbidity were related to perinatal as-phyxia and anomalies of the CNS (81, 82). The Collaborative Perinatal Project (83) reported a 34.7% mortality in infants with seizures; of the survivors 11.6% had moderate or severe cerebral palsy, and 18.8% had a full scale IQ less than 70. Infants with seizures were 55-75 times more likely to have cerebral palsy than other infants enrolled in the Collaborative Study. Approximately 40% of the infants with seizures survived without major neurological difficulties. In this study there were significant correlations between presence of mental retardation and the types

Table 5. Outcome

	Status (%)				
Study	Normal	Deaths	Abnormal	Recurrent Seizures	Survivors without Deficits or Seizures
Pre-1970 Total number of patients— 1205 (61–69, 71)	46	30(1)*	4[†]/19[‡]	8	66
Post-1970 Total number of patients— 826 (73, 75–82)	52	18(3)	10/16	10	63
Collaborative Project Total number of patients— 277 (83)	46	23(12)	9/20	17	70.7

* Late death.
† Mild deficit (attentional deficit disorders, seizures alone).
‡ Severe (mental retardation, cerebral palsy).

Table 6. Prognosis by Etiology

| | | | | Etiology (%) | | | |
Outcome*	Hypoxia	CNS† Hemor- rhage	CNS Infection	CNS Anomalies	Hypo- calcemia	Hypo- glycemia	Unknown
Normal	43	33	53		91	42	63
Death	16.5	50	22	63	3‡	14	8
Mild residual	6			16			4
Severe residual	34	17	25	21	6‡	44	25

Note.—Data taken from references (61, 63, 67, 71, 73, 76, 79, 81, 82).
* Total number of patients–709.
† Central nervous system.
‡ All with secondary hypocalcemia.

of neonatal seizures (tonic and myoclonic), number of days of seizures persisted (4.5 versus 2.5 days), and seizures lasting longer than 30 minutes. Afebrile seizures occurred in 22% of the survivors. The data from the Collaborative Perinatal Project have also been reviewed by Nelson and associates who concluded that in the neonatal period, intracranial hemorrhage and neonatal seizures were the most potent predictors of severe neurological handicap (100, 101). In studies of neonatal asphyxia (defined as the requirement of more than 1 minute of positive pressure ventilation before sustained respiration occurred), MacDonald and associates (102, 103) observed that seizure postasphyxia was associated with a higher incidence of severe sequelae. The incidence of seizures was significantly less for infants who established respiration with 5 minutes (2 of 41, 5%) than for those who established respiration after 5 minutes [11 of 21, 52%] (102, 103). In addition, infants with seizures persisting for more than 48 hours had a higher incidence of severe sequelae than those who had seizures for less than 48 hours. This finding is similar to those of the Collaborative Project (83). Contrastingly, Finer and associates (104) did not find a similar correlation between outcome and the presence of seizures following perinatal asphyxia. However, infants with seizures in the first 24 hours of life were at greater risk for an abnormal outcome, with 48% of these infants being significantly handicapped compared to 24% of infants with seizures after 24 hours.

Finer and coworkers (104) found an association between the presence of a low voltage back group on the EEG and subsequent outcome, a relationship previously observed by Sarnat and Sarnat (105). The interictal EEG in some full-term infants has been reported to have prognostic significance (66, 73, 87, 106). In general, a normal interictal record has been observed to correlate with a favorable outcome, while a markedly abnormal record has been associated with major sequelae. Table 7 reviews association of EEG patterns with outcome. Certain specific abnormal patterns indicate a poor prognosis, and these include multifocal, inactive or paroxysmal burst-suppression tracings, low voltage records with theta rhythm, absence of lability, and isoelectric records (73, 106, 107). Borderline abnormal records have not been helpful in predicting outcome. In two recent studies the prognostic value of the EEG has been reviewed (107, 108). Lombroso (107) found that certain ictal and interictal EEG patterns during the newborn period had some validity in predicting neurological outcome but proved to be unreliable for at least 25% of term

Table 7. Electroencephalogram (EEG) Pattern in Various Clinical Outcomes

	EEG				
Outcome	*Normal*	*Focal*	*Multifocal*	*Periodic*	*Flat*
Normal (total number of patients—208)	62	17	21	. . .	. . .
Died (total number of patients—72)	29	1	56	8	6
Residual severe (total number of patients—93)	16	14	61	8	1
Residual mild (total number of patients—12)	50	. . .	50	. . .	. . .

Note.—Data taken from references (63, 64, 66, 73).

infants and were of doubtful assistance when applied to premature infants (107). Tharp and associates (108) reviewed the EEG recorded during the neonatal period in a long-term follow-up of a group of premature infants (gestational age under 36 weeks). They found that infants with normal serial EEGs were usually normal at follow-up or had only minor sequelae, but all infants who had at least one markedly abnormal EEG during the neonatal period suffered some type of neurological sequelae or died. The markedly abnormal patterns included isoelectric or paroxysmal backgrounds and electrographic seizures. These authors as well as others emphasized the inadequacy of recording a single EEG and stressed the importance of obtaining serial EEGs to increase their prognostic value (106-108). EEG recordings done in the first week of life were recommended since certain abnormal patterns may disappear by the second week of life.

The report of the Collaborative Perinatal Project and other studies concluded that the occurrence of neonatal seizures correlates with a higher incidence of neurological sequelae (83, 100-102). The outcome is mainly determined by the etiology of the seizures, but in infants who have similar clinical problems, those with seizures are at higher risk for neurological sequelae. The reported poor prognosis following neonatal seizures raises the question of whether the seizure itself causes further injury to the immature brain.

Experimental Models

Experimental animal models of seizures provide data that may be relevant to human epilepsy. In paralyzed ventilated rats a single seizure is associated with an increase in cortical glycolytic flux, pyruvate and lactate:pyruvate ratio, and a decline in high energy phosphates (109, 110). With repetitive seizures the above biochemical changes are accompanied by cerebral vasodilatation, an increase in CBF, CMR_{O_2}, and cerebral glucose consumption (111). When body temperature was kept at 37°C and arterial hypotension, arterial hypoxemia, and hypoglycemia was prevented, a fall in cortical glucose concentration to 30% of control occurred after 1 minute of seizure activity, followed by a subsequent rise to 50% after 1 hour of seizure activity and finally a fall to the 30% level of control after 2 hours [of seizure activity] (112). Similar results including a fall in high energy phosphate stores following prolonged seizures was observed by Duffy and coworkers (110).

In newborn rats, Wasterlain and associates (113) have investigated the effects of single and repetitive seizures on the developing brain. One electroconvulsive seizure per day for 10 days in rats between postnatal days 2 to 11 was associated with a significant reduction in brain weight, deoxyribonucleic acid (DNA) and ribonucleic acid (RNA). Seizures from days 9 to 18 reduced brain weight, protein, and RNA, and from days 19-28 no changes occurred in brain weight, cell number, or cell size (114). No gross or microscopic evidence of damage secondary to the electroconvulsive shock was noted. Similar significant reductions in brain weight and cell number were observed when nutritional factors were controlled (115). Flurothyl-induced status epilepticus in 4-day-old rats was also found to curtail brain weight and DNA (116). Immature rats with flurothyl-induced status epilepticus and rats with single repetitive electroconvulsive seizures both showed delayed developmental milestones and reduced seizure thresholds in comparison to controls without seizures, some of which received subthreshold electroconvulsive treatment (116-118). In rats with bicuculline or flurothyl-induced status epilepticus, pretreatment with glucose reduced mortality by 90% in rats under 1 week of age, 80% in 10-day-old rats, 50% in 15-20-day-old rats, and not at all in adult rats (119). Glucose-treated infant rats showed significantly less reduction in brain weight, DNA, RNA, protein, and cholesterol than in saline-treated litter mates. In the saline group, seizures caused a progressive fall in brain glucose level but no fall in blood glucose level; while in glucose treated rats, blood and brain glucose concentrations remained elevated throughout the convulsive period. These findings emphasize that during seizures the presence of a normal blood glucose concentration does not ensure adequate supplies of glucose to the brain. Cerebral adenosine triphosphate (ATP) and phosphocreatine levels remained intact in the 4-day-old rats in contrast to

a situation in adult rats, in which there is a decline in cerebral energy reserves during prolonged seizures. This suggests that lack of glucose during seizures may have impaired brain growth by depletion of its main carbon source, which is necessary for the synthesis of macromolecules, neurotransmitters, and growth-related hormones (119). Two mechanisms have been suggested to underly these effects: impaired glucose transport and inhibition of DNA synthesis (113, 118). The above experiments suggest that seizures too mild to damage the adult rat brain may irreversibly impair brain development when they occur during vulnerable periods (113, 118). Volpe (52) has criticized these studies on the basis that Golgi studies were not done, that it is unclear if the biochemical effects observed were irreversible, and that the period of 2 to 11 days is comparable to a period from 6 months of gestation to approximately 1 year postnatally. He does emphasize though, that the data raise important questions concerning the possibility of deleterious, long-term biochemical effects from recurrent seizures in the human infants (52).

The kindling model of experimental epilepsy warrants brief discussion. Kindling, as originally described by Goddard, refers to the development of an electroclinical seizure after repeated administration of an initially ineffective, low intensity brain stimulation (120). Repeated electrical stimulation of various limbic, extrapyramidal, thalamic, and cortical loci in various species, including rats, cats, and subhuman primates, gradually leads to the development of overt motor convulsions evoked by stimulation that had been initially ineffective (120-124). Wada and Sato demonstrated that cats once kindled retain their induced seizure susceptibility, as measured by the generalized seizure-triggering threshold and interictal spike discharge in the ipsilateral midbrain reticular formation, for more than 12 months without further brain stimulation (122). Wada and associates observed the development of spontaneous clinical (partial and generalized) seizures in kindled cats and in baboons (123, 125). These results suggest that repeated seizures induced by daily amygdaloid stimulation result in a widespread secondary functional alteration and reorganization of brain function and in a persistent state of epileptogenicity. The application of kindling phenomenon to human conditions is not proven, but the findings of kindling experiments may support the implication that seizures in themselves may be injurious to the developing brain by engendering a propensity to recurrent seizures.

Treatment

The treatment of neonatal seizures has been adequately reviewed elsewhere and will not be fully discussed here (52-58). Treatment depends upon defining the etiology of the seizures so that infectious, metabolic, and deficiency syndromes can be specifically treated. The infants' pulmonary and cardiovascular functions must be supported, and serum glucose levels should be maintained at increased levels in an attempt to provide greater amounts of substrate to the brain for energy metabolism.

The pharmacokinetics of phenobarbital and phenytoin in neonates are different from those in older infants and children. Lockman and coworkers (126) have demonstrated that seizure control in a newborn may not be achieved until phenobarbital blood levels are greater than 15 μg/ml. Such levels can be achieved with loading doses of 15-20 mg/kg intravenously or intramuscularly if the former route of administration cannot be accomplished and cardiovascular function is adequate to support peripheral perfusion (126, 127). Higher loading doses and blood levels may be necessary in some cases. Drug levels do not vary significantly for the first 24 hours following loading doses. Daily maintenance does of phenobarbital above 5 mg/kg may result in the accumulation of excessive amounts of the drug and thereby may produce toxicity (127). Therapeutic plasma levels of phenytoin may be achieved with doses of 15-20 mg/kg given intravenously (127). Oral and intramuscular administration are not advisable because of poor and erratic absorption from the gastrointestinal tract and poor absorption of phenytoin from the peripheral tissues (127). The loading doses of phenobarbital and phenytoin required to achieve adequate plasma levels have been found not to vary with birth weight or gestational age (126, 127). There is significant interpatient variability in the metabolism of anticonvulsants, and the half-life of the drugs, particularly phenytoin, may change in the first few weeks of life (128). Therefore, the frequent determination of plasma levels of the anticonvulsants is necessary to maintain blood levels in the appropriate ranges.

Several recent reports have raised questions concerning the effects of phenobarbital on the developing brain (129-132). The administration of phenobarbital to infant rats or fetal mice has been associated with retarded brain growth and a decrease in large neurons (129-131). In cell cultures of fetal rodent spinal cord, phenobarbital (30-120 μg/ml) treatment produced dose dependent decreases in choline acetyltransferase, which were reversible after withdrawal of the drug (132). There was also a reversible decrease in large spinal cord neuron cells. Phenytoin has also been reported to have adverse effects on cultured neurons (133, 134). In one experiment, a dose-related neurotoxic effect was reported (133). Cell cultures of dissociated chick embryo brain treated with various phenytoin concentrations (27.4 to 137 μg/ml) exhibited fewer cell aggregates and neurons and less prominent neuronal processes. In this experiment the effects of phenobarbital were similar to the controls. In an earlier experiment utilizing a cell-free protein synthesizing system derived from 7-day-old rat brain, dose-related inhibition of leucine incorporation into protein was observed (134). While antiepileptic drugs may adversely affect the developing nervous system in experimental animals, repeated seizures negatively influence brain growth and development. While these animal studies are not directly applicable to human infants, they do raise questions regarding the possible long-term effects of seizures and antiepileptic drugs on developing brain.

Conclusion

This brief overview of seizures in preterm and full-term neonates reflects the current interest and increased awareness of this problem by pediatricians, neonatologists, and neurologists. A better undestanding of the pathophysiology, clinical manifestations, EEG correlates, and natural history has evolved. Studies of experimental models have raised important concerns regarding the effects of seizures on the developing brain as well as the possible adverse effects of antiepileptic drugs on the immature nervous system. These issues have to be resolved in the future as well as the question of how long to treat neonates with seizures not caused by metabolic aberrations. Hopefully, these answers will be provided as a result of ongoing clinical and basic scientific research.

REFERENCES

1. Donat JF, Okazaki H, Kleinberg F, et al: Intraventricular hemorrhage in full-term and premature infants. *Mayo Clin Proc* 53:437-441, 1978

2. Mitchell W, O'Tuama L: Cerebral intraventricular hemorrhages in infants: a widening age spectrum. *Pediatrics* 65:35-40, 1980

3. Chaplin ER, Goldstein GW, Norman D: Neonatal seizures, intracerebral hematoma, and subarachnoid hemorrhage in full-term infants. *Pediatrics* 63:812-815, 1979

4. Cartwright GW, Culbertson K, Schreiner RL, et al: Changes in clinical presentation of term infants with intracranial hemorrhage. *Dev Med Child Neurol* 21:730-737, 1979

5. Palma PA, Miner ME, Morriss FH, et al: Intraventricular hemorrhage in the neonate born at term. *Am J Dis Child* 133:941-944, 1979

6. Fedrick J, Butler NR: Certain causes of neonatal death. II. Intraventricular hemorrhage. *Biol Neonate* 15:257-290, 1970

7. Craig WS: Intracranial hemorrhage in the newborn. *Arch Dis Child* 13:89-124, 1938

8. Gröntoft O: Intracerebral and meningeal haemorrhages in perinatally deceased infants. I. Intracerebral haemorrhages. A pathologico-anatomical and obstetric study. *Acta Obstet Gynecol Scand* 32:308-333, 1953

9. Leech RW, Kohnen P: Subependymal and intraventricular hemorrhage in the newborn. *Am J Pathol* 77:465-475, 1974

10. Ahmann PA, Lazzara A, Dykes FD, et al: Intraventricular hemorrhage in the high risk preterm infant: incidence and outcome. *Ann Neurol* 7:118-124, 1980

11. Papile LA, Burstein J, Burstein R, et al: Incidence and evolution of subependymal and intraventricular hemorrhage: a study of infants with birthweights less than 1500 grams. *J Pediatr* 92:529-534, 1978

12. Bejar R, Curbelo V, Coen RW, et al: Diagnosis and follow-up of intraventricular and intracerebral hemorrhages by ultrasound studies of infants' brain through the fontanelles and sutures. *Pediatrics* 66:661-673, 1980

13. Armstrong DL, Goddard J, Schwartz M, et al: Another look at the pathology of intraventricular hemorrhage. *Ross Conference on Perinatal Intracranial Hemorrhage, Dec. 11-13, 1980,* Washington, DC, pp 1-21

14. Dykes FD, Lazzara A, Ahmann PA, et al: Intraventricular hemorrhage: a prospective evaluation of etiopathogenesis. *Pediatrics* 66:42-49, 1980

15. Simmons MA, Adcock EW, Bard H, et al: Hypernatremia and intracranial hemorrhage in neonates. *N Engl J Med* 291:6-10, 1974

16. Papile LA, Burstein J, Burstein R, et al: Relationship of intravenous sodium bicarbonate infusions and cerebral intraventricular hemorrhage. *J Pediatr* 93:834-836, 1978

17. Corbet DJ, Adams JM, Kenny JP, et al: Controlled trial of bicarbonate therapy in high-risk premature newborn infants. *J Pediatr* 91:771, 1977

18. Guggenheim MA, Rumack C, Langendorfer S, et al: Risk factors in germinal matrix hemorrhage. *Ann Neurol* 8:225, 1980

19. Clark CE, Lane B, Clyman RI, et al: Risk factor analysis for intraventricular hemorrhage in infants of very low birth weight. *Ann Neurol* 8:227, 1980

20. DeLemos RA, Tomasovic JJ, Null DM: The role of post natal factors in the pathogenesis of subependymal and intraventricular hemorrhage in the premature infant. *Ross Conference on Perinatal Intracranial Hemorrhage Dec. 11-13, 1980,* Washington, DC, pp 63-86

21. Papile LA, Munsick G, Weaver N, et al: Cerebral intraventricular hemorrhage (CVH) in infants < 1500 grams: developmental follow-up at one year. *Pediatr Res* 13:528, 1979

22. Krishnamoorthy KS, Shannon DC, DeLong GR, et al: Neurologic sequelae in the survivors of neonatal intraventricular hemorrhage. *Pediatrics* 64:233-237, 1979

23. Williamson WD, Wilson GS, Desmond MM, et al: Early neurodevelopmental outcome of low birth weight infants surviving neonatal intraventricular hemorrhage. *Ross Conference on Perinatal Intracranial Hemorrhage Dec. 11-13, 1980,* Washington, DC, pp 736-751

24. Reynolds MG, Evans EAN, Reynolds EOR, et al: Intracranial haemorrhage in the preterm sheep fetus. *Early Hum Dev* 3/2:163-186, 1979

25. Goddard J, Lewis RM, Alcala H, et al: Intraventricular hemorrhage—an animal model *Biol Neonate* 37(1/2):39-52, 1980

26. Goddard J, Lewis RM, Armstrong DL, et al: Moderate, rapidly induced hypertension as a cause of intraventricular hemorrhage with newborn beagle model. *J Pediatr* 96:1057-1060, 1980

27. Goddard J, Lewis RM, Armstrong DL, et al: Intraventricular and subependymal cell plate hemorrhages following hypovolemic hypotension and volume expansion in the newborn beagle: relationship to hemodynamic changes. *Ann Neurol* 8:224, 1980

28. Goddard J, Lewis RM, Michael LH, et al: Preliminary studies of regional cerebral blood flow in hypovolemic and hypertensive newborn beagle pups. *Ann Neurol* 8:224-225, 1980

29. Goddard J: Unpublished observations

30. Goddard J, Armstrong DL, Michael LH: Regional cerebral blood flow (rCBF) in an experimental model of intraventricular hemorrhage. *J Neuropathol Exp Neurol* 40:344, 1981

31. Towbin A: Cerebral intraventricular hemorrhage and sub-ependymal matrix infarction in the fetus and premature newborn. *Am J Pathol* 52:121-139, 1968

32. Larroche JC: Hemorrhagies cerebrales intraventriculaires chez le premature. 1. Anatomic et physiopathologie. *Biol Neonate* 7:36-56, 1974

33. Cole VA, Durbin GM, Olaffson A, et al: Pathogenesis of intraventricular hemorrhage in newborn infants. *Arch Dis Child* 79:722-728, 1974

34. Hambleton G, Wigglesworth JS: Origin of intraventricular hemorrhage in the preterm infant. *Arch Dis Child* 51:651-659, 1976

35. Dawes GS: *Fetal and Neonatal Physiology.* Chicago, Yearbook Medical Publishers, 1968, p 149

36. Modanlou H, Yeh SY, Siassi B, et al: Direct monitoring of arterial blood pressure in depressed and normal newborn infants during the first hour of life. *J. Pediatr* 85:553-559, 1974

37. Lou HC, Lassen NA, Tweed WA, et al: Pressure passive cerebral blood flow and breakdown of the blood-brain barrier in experimental fetal asphyxia. *Acta Paediatr Scand* 68:57-63, 1979

38. Volpe JJ: *Neurology of the Newborn.* Philadelphia, WB Saunders, 1981. p 279

39. Lou HC, Lassen NA, Friis-Hansen B: Impaired autoregulation of cerebral blood flow in the distressed newborn infant. *J Pediatr* 94:118-121, 1979

40. Burstein J, Papile LA, Burstein R: Intraventricular hemorrhage and hydrocephalus in premature newborns: a prospective study with CT. *AJR* 132:631-635, 1979

41. Silverboard G, Horder MH, Ahmann PA, et al: Reliability of ultrasound in diagnosis of intracerebral hemorrhage and post hemorrhagic hydrocephalus: comparison with computed tomography. *Pediatrics* 66:507-514, 1980

42. Bada HS, Hajjar W, Chua C, et al: Noninvasive diagnosis of neonatal asphyxia and intraventricular hemorrhage by Doppler ultrasound. *J Pediatr* 95:775-779, 1979

43. Cooke RWI, Rolfe P, Howat P: A technique for the non-invasive estimation of cerebral blood flow in the newborn infant. *J Med Eng Technol* 263-266, 1977

44. Milligan DWA: Failure of autoregulation and intraventricular hemorrhage in preterm infants. *Lancet* 1:896-898, 1980

45. Ment LR, Lange R, Ehrenkranz R, et al: Cerebral blood flow determinations in preterm neonates. *Ann Neurol* 8:225, 1980

46. Younkin D, Reivich M, Delivoria-Papadopoulos M, et al: Regional cerebral blood flow in high risk neonates: technique and preliminary results. *Ann Neurol* 8:226, 1980

47. Donn SM, Goldstein GW, Roloff DW: Phenobarbital for the prevention of neonatal intracranial hemorrhage: a controlled trial. *Lancet* 2:215, 1981 1982

48. Mantovani JF, Pasternak JK, Mathew OP, et al: Failure of daily lumbar punctures to prevent the development of hydrocephalus following intraventricular hemorrhage. *J Pediatr* 97:278-281, 1980

49. Papile LA, Burstein J, Burstein R, et al: Posthemorrhagic hydrocephalus in low birth-weight infants: treatment by serial lumbar punctures. *J Pediatr* 97:273-277, 1980

50. Volpe JJ, Pasternak JF, Allan WC: Ventricular dilation preceding rapid head growth following neonatal intracranial hemorrhage. *Am J Dis Child* 131:1212-1215, 1977

51. Taylor DA, Hill A, Fishman MA, et al: Treatment of post hemorrhagic hydrocephalus with glycerol (abstract). *Ann Neurol* 10:297, 1981

52. Volpe JJ: Neonatal seizures. *Clin Perinatol* 4:43-63, 1977

53. Paine R: Characteristics of fits in the newborn period. *Clin Dev Med* 27:70-77, 1968

54. Freeman JM: Neonatal seizures—diagnosis and management. *J Pediatr* 77:701-708, 1970

55. Brown JK: Convulsions in the newborn period. *Dev Med Child Neurol* 15:823-846, 1973

56. Snodgrass GJ: Seizures in newborn infants. *Dev Med Child Neurol* 16:92-94, 1974

57. Solomon GE: Neonatal seizures. *Pediatr Ann* 34-50, 1975

58. Purpura DP: Relationship of seizure susceptibility to morphologic and physiologic properties of normal and abnormal immature cortex. In *Neurological and Electroencephalographic Correlative Studies in Infancy.* Edited by Kellaway P, Petersen I. New York, Grune and Stratton, 1964, pp 117-157

59. Purpura DP: Factors contributing to abnormal neuronal development in the cerebral cortex of the human infant. In *Brain Fetal and Infant.* Edited by Berenberg SR. The Hague, Martinus-Nijhoff, 1977, pp 54-78

60. Purpura DP: Stability and seizure susceptibility of immature brain. In *Basic Mechanisms of the Epilepsies.* Edited by Jasper HH, Ward AA, Pope A. Boston, Little, Brown, 1969, p 481

61. Burke JB: Prognostic significance of neonatal convulsions. *Arch Dis Child* 29:342-345, 1954

62. Craig WS: Convulsive movements occurring in the first 10 days of life. *Arch Dis Child* 35:336-344, 1960

63. Harris R, Tizard JPM: The EEG in neonatal convulsions. *J Pediatr* 57:501-520, 1960

64. Prichard JS: The character and significance of epileptic seizures in infancy. In *Neurological and Electroencephalographic Correlative Studies in Infancy.* Edited by Kellaway P, Petersen I. New York, Grune and Stratton, 1964, pp 273-286

65. Keith HM: Convulsions in children under three years of age. *Mayo Clin Proc* 39:895-907, 1964

66. Tibbles JAR, Prichard JS: The prognostic value of the EEG in neonatal convulsions. *Pediatrics* 35:778-786, 1965

67. Schulte FJ: Neonatal convulsions and their relations to epilepsy in early childhood. *Dev Med Child Neurol* 8:381-392, 1966

68. Degen R, Koschtial I: The late prognosis of convulsions in the newborn. *Nschr Kinderheilk* 116:133-139, 1968

69. Massa T, Niedermeyer E: Convulsive disorders during the first three months of life. *Epilepsia* 9:1-9, 1968

70. Carbonell JM, Carbonell EM, Carbonell EX, et al: Diagnostic assessment of neonatal convulsions. *Rev Esp Pediatr* 25:85-96, 1969

71. McInerny TK, Schubert WK: Prognosis of neonatal seizures. *Am J Dis Child* 117:261-264, 1969

72. Keen JH: Significance of hypocalcaemia in neonatal convulsions. *Arch Dis Child* 44:356-361, 1969

73. Rose AL, Lombroso CT: Neonatal seizures states. *Pediatrics* 45:404-425, 1970

74. Hopkins IS: Seizures in the first week of life. A study of etiological factors. *Med J Aust* 2:647-651, 1972

75. Brown, JK, Cockburn F, Forfar JO: Clinical and chemical correlates in convulsions of the newborn. *Lancet* 1:135-138, 1972

76. Keen JH, Lee D: Sequelae in neonatal convulsions. *Arch Dis Child* 48:542-546, 1973

77. Combes JC, Rufo M, Vallade MJ, et al: Neonatal seizures. Etiology and prognosis. *Pediatrie* 30:477-492, 1975

78. Bawdon JJ, Bouillie J, Gleizes H: Clinical, etiologic and prognostic aspects of neonatal convulsions. *Rev Pediatr* 11:457-462, 1975

79. Knauss TA, Marshall RE: Seizures in a neonatal intensive care unit. *Dev Med Child Neurol* 19:719-728, 1977

80. Seay A, Bray PF: Significance of seizures in infants weighing less than 2500 grams. *Arch Neurol* 34:381-382, 1977

81. Dennis J: Neonatal convulsions: etiology, late neonatal status and long-term outcome. *Dev Med Child Neurol* 20:143-158, 1978

82. Ericksson M, Zetterstrom R: Neonatal convulsions. *Acta Paediatr Scand* 68:807-811, 1979

83. Holden KR, Freeman JM, Mellits ED: Outcomes of infants with neonatal seizures. In *Advances in Epileptology,* vol 10, *Epilepsy International Symposium.* Edited by Wada JA, Penry JK. New York, Raven Press, 1980, pp 155-158

84. Monod N, Dreyfus-Brisac C, Sfaello Z: Depistage et prognostic de l'etat de mal neonatal (d'apres l'etude electroclinique de 150 cas). *Arch Fr Pediatr* 26:1085-1102, 1969

85. Werner S, Stockard J, Bickford R: *Atlas of Neonatal Electroencephalography.* New York, Raven Press, 1977, pp 106-149

86. Marshall R, Sheehan M, Escobedo M, et al: Seizures in a neonatal intensive care unit: a prospective study. *Pediatr Res* 10:450, 1976

87. Dreyfus-Brisac C, Monod N: Electroclinical studies of status epileptus and convulsions in the newborn. In *Neurological and Electroencephalographic Correlative Studies in Infancy.* Edited by Kellaway P, Petersen I. New York, Grune and Stratten, 1964, pp 250-271

88. Watanabe K, Hara K, Miyazaki S, et al: Electroclinical studies of seizures in the newborn. *Folia Psychiatr Neurol Jap* 31:383-392, 1977

89. Cockburn F, Brown JK, Belton NR, et al: Neonatal convulsions associated with primary disturbance of calcium, phosphorus, and magnesium metabolism. *Arch Dis Child* 48:99-108, 1973

90. Clark PCN, Carre IJ: Hypocalcemia, hypomagnesemic convulsions. *J Pediatr* 70:806-809, 1967

91. Zelsin C: Infant of the addicted mother. *N Eng J Med* 288:1393-1395, 1973

92. Herzlinger RA, Kandall SR, Vaughan HG: Neonatal seizures associated with narcotic withdrawal. *J Pediatr* 91:638-641, 1977

93. Bleyer WA, Marshall NE: Barbiturate withdrawal syndrome in a passively addicted infant. *JAMA* 221:186-186, 1972

94. Bjerre I, Corelius E: Benign familial neonatal convulsions. *Acta Paediatr Scand* 57:557-561, 1968

95. Carton D: Benign familial neonatal convulsions. *Neuropediatrie* 9:167-171, 1978

96. Quattlebaum TG: Benign familial convulsions in the neonatal period and early infancy. *J Pediatr* 94:257-259, 1979

97. Pettri RE, Fenichel GM: Benign familial neonatal seizures. *Arch Neurol* 37:47-48, 1980

98. Tibbles JAR: Dominant benign neonatal seizures. *Dev Med Child Neurol* 22:664-667, 1980

99. Gross S, Schubert W, Silka M: Benign convulsions in infancy. *J Pediatr* 96:952, 1980

100. Nelson KB, Bromen SH: Perinatal risk factors in children with serious motor and mental handicaps. *Ann Neurol* 2:371-377, 1977

101. Nelson KB, Ellenberg J: Neonatal signs as predictors of cerebral palsy. *Pediatrics* 64:225-232, 1979

102. MacDonald H, Mulligan J, Allen A, et al: Neonatal asphyxia. I. Relationship of obstetric and neonatal complications to neonatal mortality in 38,405 consecutive deliveries. *J Pediatr* 96:898-902, 1980

103. Mulligan J, Painter M, O'Donoghue P, et al: Neonatal asphyxia. II. Neonatal mortality and long term sequelae. *J Pediatr* 96:903-907, 1980

104. Finer NN, Robertson CM, Richards RT, et al: Hypoxic-ischemic encephalopathy in term neonates: perinatal factors and outcome. *J Pediatr* 98:112-117, 1981

105. Sarnat H, Sarnat MS: Neonatal encephalopathy following fetal distress. *Arch Neurol* 33:696-705, 1976

106. Monod N, Pajot N, Guidasa S: The neonatal EEG: statistical studies and prognostic value in full-term and pre-term babies. *Electroencephalogr Clin Neurophysiol* 32:529-544, 1972

107. Lombroso CT: Quantified electrographic scales on 10 pre-term healthy newborns followed up to 40-43 weeks of conceptional age by serial polygraphic recordings. *Electroencephalogr Clin Neurophysiol* 46:460-474, 1979

108. Tharp BR, Cukier F, Monod N: The prognostic value of the electroencephalogram in premature infants. *Electroencephalogr Clin Neurophysiol* 51:219-236, 1981

109. Plum F, Wasterlain C: Developmental retardation in rat brain after perinatal seizures. In *Brain Fetal and Infant*. Edited by Berenberg, S. The Hague, Martinus-Nijhott, 1977, pp 274-294

110. Duffy TE, Howse DC, Plum F: Cerebral energy metabolism during experimental status epilepticus. *J Neurochem* 24:925-934, 1975

111. Meldrun BS, Nilsson B: Cerebral blood flow and metabolic rate early and late in prolonged epileptic seizures induced in rats by bicuculline. *Brain* 99:523-542, 1976

112. Chapman AG, Meldrum BS, Siesjo BK: Cerebral metabolic changes during prolonged epileptic seizures in rats. *J Neurochem* 28:1025-1035, 1977

113. Wasterlain CG: Neonatal seizures and brain growth. *Neuropadiatrie* 9:213-228, 1978

114. Wasterlain CG, Plum F: Vulnerability of developing rat brain to electroconvulsive seizures. *Arch Neurol* 29:38-45, 1973

115. Wasterlain CG: Developmental effects of seizures: role of malnutrition. *Pediatrics* 51:197-200, 1976

116. Wasterlain CG: Effects of neonatal status epilepticus on rat brain development. *Neurology* 26:975-986, 1976

117. Wasterlain CG, Plum F: Retardation of behavioral landmarks after neonatal seizures in rats. *Trans Am Neurol Assoc* 98:320-321, 1973

118. Wasterlain CG, Duffy TE: Pathophysiologic basis for the selective vulnerability of the immature rat brain to seizures. In *Brain Fetal and Infant*. Edited by Berenberg S. The Hague, Martinus-Nijhott, 1977, pp 274-294

119. Wasterlain CG, Duffy TE: Status epilepticus in immature rats. *Arch Neurol* 33:821-827, 1976

120. Goddard GV, McIntyre DC, Leech CK: A permanent change in brain function resulting from daily electrical stimulation. *Exp Neurol* 25:295-330, 1969

121. Racine RJ: Modification of seizure activity by electrical stimulation: I. After-discharge threshold. *Electroencephalogr Clin Neurophysiol* 32:269-279, 1972

122. Wada JA, Sato M: Generalized convulsive seizures induced by daily electrical stimulation of the amygdala in cats. *Neurology* 24:565-574, 1974

123. Wada JA, Osawa T: Spontaneous recurrent seizure state induced by daily electric amygdaloid stimulation in Senegalese baboons (*Capio papio*) *Neurology* 26:273-286, 1976

124. Wada JA, Mizoguchi T, Osawa T: Secondarily generalized convulsive seizures induced by daily amygdaloid stimulation in rhesus monkeys. *Neurology* 28:1026-1036, 1978

125. Wada JA, Sato M, Corcoran ME: Persistent seizure susceptibility and recurrent spontaneous seizures in kindled cats. *Epilepsia* 15:465-478, 1974

126. Lockman LA, Kriel R, Zaske E, et al: Phenobarbital dosage for control of neonatal seizures. *Neurology* 29:1445-1449, 1979

127. Painter MS, Pippenger C, MacDonald H, et al: Phenobarbital and diphenylhydantoin levels in neonates with seizures. *J Pediatr* 92:315-319, 1978

128. Loughnam PM, Greenwald A, Purton WW, et al: Pharmacokinetic observations of phenytoin disposition in the newborn and young infant. *Arch Dis Child* 52:302-309, 1977

129. Schain RJ, Watanabe K: Origin of brain growth retardation in young rats treated with phenobarbital. *Exp Neurol* 50:806-809, 1976

130. Diaz J, Schain RJ, Barky BJ: Phenobarbital-induced brain growth retardation in artificially reared rat pups. *Biol Neonate* 32:77-82, 1977

131. Yanai J, Rosselli-Austin L, Tohakoff B: Neuronal deficits in mice following prenatal exposure to phenobarbital. *Exp Neurol* 64:237-244, 1979

132. Bergey GK, Swaiman KF, Schrier BK, et al: Adverse effects of phenobarbital on morphological and biochemical development of fetal mouse spinal cord neurons in culture. *Ann Neurol* 9:584-589, 1981

133. Culver B: Effects of anticonvulsant drugs on chick embryonic neurons and glia in cell culture. *Dev Neurosci* 2:74-85, 1979

134. Swaiman KF, Stright PL: The effects of anticonvulsants on in vitro protein synthesis in immature brain. *Brain Res* 58:515-518, 1973

Index

Note: Page numbers in *italics* denote illustrations; those followed by (t) denote tables.